# Handbook of Evidence-Based Psychodynamic Psychotherapy

For other titles published in this series, go to
www.springer.com/series/7634

Raymond A. Levy • J. Stuart Ablon
Editors

# Handbook of Evidence-Based Psychodynamic Psychotherapy

## Bridging the Gap Between Science and Practice

Foreword by Glen O. Gabbard

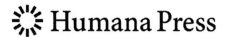 Humana Press

*Editors*
Raymond A. Levy
Clinical Director
Psychotherapy Research Program
Massachusetts General Hospital
Boston, MA 02114
RLEVY2@PARTNERS.ORG

J. Stuart Ablon
Director
Psychotherapy Research Program
Massachusetts General Hospital
Boston, MA 02114
sablon@cprinstitute.org

*Series Editor*
Jerrold F. Rosenbaum
Chief of Psychiatry
Massachusetts General Hospital
Stanley Cobb Professor of Psychiatry
Harvard Medical School
Boston, MA 02114

ISBN: 978-1-934115-11-4          e-ISBN: 978-1-59745-444-5
DOI: 10.1007/978-1-59745-444-5

Library of Congress Control Number: 2008933513

*Cover images provided by Raymond A. Levy, Psy.D.*

Printed on acid-free paper

9  8  7  6  5  4  3  2  1

springer.com

*We would like to dedicate this book to remembering the life and legacy of one of the world's greatest psychodynamic treatment researchers – the late Dr. Enrico Jones. It gives us great satisfaction to know how proud he would be of the contribution this volume makes to the evidence base for psychodynamic psychotherapy.*

*To my family – Nonny, Ben and Hannah – my love for you and from you has sustained me.*

*To my friends, patients, and teachers who have inspired me.*

*Raymond Levy*

*To Christina who always stands by me.*
*To Jack, Carter and Paige who make me proud to be their father.*

*John S. Ablon*

# Foreword

There can be little doubt that psychoanalysis and the psychodynamic therapies that arise from it are currently in a beleaguered state. The average educated reader today is likely to be confronted with a series of statements in the popular press that are variations on the following themes: Freud is dead; psychoanalysis is more religion than science; psychodynamic psychotherapy has no research to support its efficacy; cognitive-behavior therapy has surpassed psychoanalytic therapy as the most accepted form of psychotherapeutic treatment; psychodynamic psychotherapy is too long and too expensive; and the fundamental psychoanalytic concepts are too vague to be rigorously studied. The common wisdom among psychoanalysts these days is that if a patient asks you if you are "a Freudian," the correct answer is "no."

One could argue, of course, that psychoanalytic theory and practice have always been subversive. Indeed, psychoanalytic thinking thrives in exile from the cultural mainstream. In *fin de siecle* Vienna, the social structure was scandalized by ideas such as infantile sexuality, parental seduction of children, and the notion that we are consciously confused and unconsciously controlled. More than 100 years later, Freud is regularly killed off in the pages of *Time*, *Newsweek*, and *The New York Review of Books*, only to be resurrected. Hence a successive series of declarations that he is once again dead are required to keep him in his grave.

Perhaps the most persuasive evidence of the core truths inherent in psychoanalytic thinking can be found in this need to repeatedly proclaim their irrelevance and the fundamental flaws in the theory. The emotional frenzy stirred by psychoanalytic ideas may best be illustrated by the recent comment of an academic I know who confessed, "Even if it were scientifically proven, I still wouldn't believe it. I can assure you that I never wanted to have sex with my mother."

In any case, the contempt for psychodynamic psychotherapy and psychoanalytic thought has been intensified in recent years by the rise of evidence-based medicine and the empirically supported therapy movement. According to these trends in science and clinical practice, a treatment approach can be proven only by the findings of randomized controlled trials

(RCT). The methodology and research design of the RCT derive from medication studies in which an active agent is shown to be more effective in the improvement of symptoms than a placebo. Even though placebo has actually been shown to be a pretty good treatment for many psychiatric symptoms, this approach to research has helped us learn which medications may be better than others.

When worship at the altar of the randomized controlled trial is transferred to psychotherapy research, we are confronted with a host of problems. The most striking difficulty is that pills and psychotherapists are different. Pills are smaller than psychotherapists; pills are not living, breathing organisms like psychotherapists; pills do not have personalities like psychotherapists; and perhaps most important, a pill and a patient do not have a complex human relationship in the way that a psychotherapist and a patient do. Another point is of particular importance – a specific technique applied mechanistically is unlikely to be effective in any sort of psychotherapy. The quality of the therapeutic relationship appears to be far more important in terms of outcome than any specific technique of psychotherapy.

The methodology of the RCT has other problems when applied to psychotherapy research as well. Is the type of person who is highly motivated to seek out long-term psychoanalytic psychotherapy to gain a thoroughgoing understanding of herself really interested in being randomized to an alternative treatment or a waiting list condition? In addition, manualization of psychotherapy, while essential for rigorous research, introduces a highly artificial technique that does not reflect what practitioners actually do in therapy. Moreover, a focus on specific psychiatric disorders and their symptoms is misleading in that many patients require an exploration of fundamental characterological themes that make them vulnerable to psychiatric illnesses, as well as the inevitable existential problems of being human, such as the inescapability of ambivalence and conflict in relationships, the necessity of mourning losses with each developmental phase, and the randomness of tragedy in our lives and its consequences.

In spite of this catalogue of difficulties in the systematic study of psychodynamic psychotherapy, an intrepid group of psychodynamic researchers has doggedly pursued scientific method in a series of psychodynamic studies. As this splendid new volume demonstrates, this courageous assortment of investigators has succeeded against all odds to demonstrate the efficacy of psychodynamic psychotherapy and even some of the crucial processes that underlie change or therapeutic action in such treatments.

To be sure, not all of the resistance to the acceptance of psychodynamic research has come from external sources. Psychoanalysts and psychodynamic researchers were far too complacent and smug for decades while cognitive therapists turned out one study after another. Even now, many psychoanalysts feel that the complexity of psychoanalytic work cannot possibly be demonstrated by the relatively superficial and simple-minded approaches of researchers, who must have measurable variables that lend themselves to quantitative analysis.

Still more would argue that psychoanalytic treatments belong more to hermeneutics than to science, and therefore research is irrelevant. This dichotomizing is unfortunate since there is certainly room for both disciplines within psychoanalytic theory and practice.

In any case, when we read in the popular press that psychodynamic psychotherapy has no support from empirical research, this statement is simply no longer true. A skeptic can be referred to the research that is encyclopedically described in the pages of this book. More research is certainly needed, but as a field, psychodynamic psychotherapy is well on its way to establishing respectability in the scientific community.

The investigations described in this volume go beyond the demonstration of efficacy. Process factors in psychotherapy are also discussed. Clinicians need to know which interventions are most likely to lead to positive outcomes. Those that facilitate the forging of a therapeutic alliance and those that increase patient awareness of affect states appear to be particularly useful. In addition, the notion that psychoanalytic concepts are too ill-defined and subjective to lend themselves to research is also refuted in this book. Even a highly subjective construct, such as countertransference, can be systematically measured and quantified in a way that is generalizable from one treatment to another. Finally, the interface of neurobiology and psychodynamic ideas are soon to be far more than a pipe dream of Freud's. The new techniques of neuroimaging and the understanding of brain structures allow us to begin to conceive of a marriage between mind and brain that informs technique as well as the understanding of how neurobiology informs psychology.

In summary, psychodynamic psychotherapy has come a long way since its inception, and it can hold its head high rather than bury it in ignominious shame. What psychoanalysts and psychodynamic psychotherapists do has a rationale based in science. Even though therapeutic action may ultimately be mysterious in a given case, we now have an empirical basis for choosing our interventions and monitoring the progress of patients. We should not expect to be welcomed with open arms by the scientific community, but we really wouldn't want that anyway. That has never been our role. We are fortunate to have this volume and the comprehensive perspective it provides on the current state of the art in psychodynamic psychotherapy research. It not only provides a useful reference for those who want to know what has already been studied, it also paves the way for the future. We are all in the authors' debt.

Brown Foundation Chair of Psychoanalysis and       Glen O. Gabbard, MD
Professor of Psychiatry, Baylor College of Medicine
Houston, Texas

# Preface

The papers presented together in this volume, entitled *Handbook of Evidence-Based Psychodynamic Psychotherapy: Bridging the Gap Between Science and Practice*, make a convincing case for the importance of empirical research for the future of psychodynamics for two primary reasons. The first reason concerns the current marginalization of psychodynamic work within the mental health field which we see partially as a result of a lack of empirical grounding relative to other therapeutic modalities. Sound empirical research has the potential to affirm the important role that psychodynamic theory and treatment have in modern psychiatry and psychology. The second reason that research is crucial to the future of psychodynamic work concerns the role that systematic empirical investigations can have in developing and refining effective approaches to a variety of clinical problems. Empirical research functions as a check on our subjectivity and theoretical alliances in our on-going attempts to determine the approaches most helpful in working with our patients clinically. When familiar theories guiding our approaches do not seem to yield promising clinical results, it is our hope that clinicians will add systematic empirical research to their means of improving treatment. It is in this spirit of inquiry and on-going dialogue between clinicians and researchers that we present the following research papers. We are enthusiastic about offering work from experienced clinician–researchers who, in many cases, have been publishing their findings for decades. We believe that the uniform immediate interest in contributing reflects the feeling that such a volume is overdue. We are pleased to be adding to the evidence that psychodynamic psychotherapy is an effective treatment for many common psychological problems.

Raymond A. Levy, PsyD
J. Stuart Ablon, PhD

# Acknowledgments

We are fortunate to have many people and groups to thank for their contributions to this volume. First of all, we are grateful to Dr. Jerry Rosenbaum, Chief of Psychiatry at Massachusetts General Hospital, the Series Editor who offered us the opportunity to assemble a volume on Psychodynamic Psychotherapy Research. He has been supportive of our research group s efforts over the past decade and has encouraged us to persevere by including a broader perspective of inquiry.

We are also grateful to the larger Department of Psychiatry at MGH for its excellence and innovative and creative research initiatives which have inspired us to continue our own research efforts and expand our thinking. Often it seems that there is hardly an area of study within psychiatry, psychology, and psychotherapy research that is not addressed at MGH by one individual or research group or another. The Department is relentless in its pursuit of creative clinical, assessment, and research initiatives. We have borrowed from this ethos.

Our own research group, the Psychotherapy Research Program, is a source of inspiration to us. The seven faculty, visiting psychiatry residents and four research assistants have coalesced into a cohesive working group that pursues multiple areas of inquiry including psychotherapy process research and process correlates of outcome, the use of physiological measures in psychotherapy research, empathic doctor–patient interviewing, assessment of the impact of the psychoanalytic couch in creating psychoanalytic process, the study of the placebo effect and neuroimaging assessment of changes in the brain pre- and post-short-term, manualized psychotherapy treatment for depression. The members of the program function in a collaborative manner that has lead to productive work. We have benefited from the advice and consultation of members of the Psychotherapy Research Program.

Clearly, we owe our strongest debt to the clinician researchers who have contributed chapters to this volume. Most have been in the forefront of psychodynamic psychotherapy research for years and, in some cases, decades. Their work has often been undervalued by the larger mental health community. They are the true leaders of our attempts to provide the evidence base for psychodynamic psychotherapy toward the goal of refining and improving the treatment while preserving these valued ideas and clinical interventions to serve our patients as needed. Every contributor immediately agreed to write for the book when asked and cooperated with us in any dialog about the nature of their chapter. The experience has been an exciting one for us in large part due to the inspired and eager attitude of the contributors.

And finally, we would like to thank our Research Assistant, Julie Ackerman, who worked tirelessly and without strict attention to time boundaries, to help organize and execute the endless demands, small and large, of publishing such a volume. Additionally, her passionate interest in the subject matter and her ambition to take her place as a future psychotherapy researcher were inspiring along the way. Our professional requests of her went far beyond the usual organizational demands given to a Research Assistant.

Clinical Director                                          Raymond A. Levy, PsyD
Psychotherapy Research Program
Massachusetts General Hospital
Boston, MA 02114


Director                                                      J. Stuart Ablon, PhD
Psychotherapy Research Program
Massachusetts General Hospital
Boston, MA 02114

# Contents

# Contributors

J. Stuart Ablon, PhD
Department of Psychiatry, Massachusetts General Hospital, Suite 402, 313 Washington Street, Boston, MA 02458, USA,
e-mail: sablon@cpsinstitute.org

Anne Alonso, PhD
Center for Psychoanalytic Studies and Department of Psychiatry, Massachusetts General Hospital, Boston, MA, USA.

Matthew R. Baity, PhD
Department of Psychiatry, Massachusetts General Hospital, Boston, MA, USA,
e-mail: asher1208@hotmail.com

Stephen M. Beck PhD
The Institute of Community and Family Psychiatry, Sir Mortimer B. Davis Jewish General Hospital, 4333 Chemin de la Côte Ste-Catherine, Montréal, Québec H3T 1E4, Canada, and McGill University, Montreal, Québec, Canada,
e-mail: smbeck@sympatico.ca

Ephi J. Betan, PhD
Clinical Pshycology Program at Argosy University, Suite 1100, 990 Hammond Dr., Atlanta, GA, USA, e-mail: ebetan@argosy.edu

Sidney J. Blatt, PhD
Department of Psychiatry, Yale University School of Medicine, Suite 901, 300 George Street, New Haven, CT 06511, USA,
e-mail: Sidney.blatt@yale.edu

Frederic N. Busch, MD
New York Presbyterian Hospital/Weill Cornell, 10 East 78th Street Apt. 5A, New York, NY 10021, USA,
e-mail: FNB80@aol.com

Prometheas Constantinides, MD
The Institute of Community and Family Psychiatry, Sir Mortimer B. Davis
Jewish General Hospital, 4333 Chemin de la Côte Ste-Catherine, Montréal,
Québec H3T 1E4, Canada, and McGill University, Montreal, Québec, Canada;
Louis-H Lafontaine, 7401, Rue Hochelaga, Montréal, Québec H1N 3M5,
Canada, e-mail: prometheas@videotron.ca

Jared A. Defife, MA
Massachusetts Mental Health Center, Jamaica Plain, MA, USA,
e-mail: jareddefife@yahoo.com

Marc J. Diener, PsyD
The Addiction Institute of New York, St. Luke's- Roosevelt Hospital Center,
1000 Tenth Avenue, New York, NY 10019, USA, e-mail: mdiesner@chpnet.org;
American School of Professional Psychology, Argosy University/Washington
DC, Suite 600, 1550 Wilson Blvd., Arlington, VA 22209, USA,
e-mail: melekhdiener2@aol.com

J. Elizabeth Foley, PhD
The Institute of Community and Family Psychiatry, Sir Mortimer B. Davis
Jewish General Hospital, 4333 Chemin de la Côte Ste-Catherine, Montréal,
Québec H3T 1E4, Canada, and McGill University, Montreal, Québec,
Canada, e-mail: elizabeth foley@mcgill.ca

Glen O. Gabbard, MD
Brown Foundation Chair of Psychoanalysis and Professor of Psychiatry,
Baylor College of Medicine, Training and Supervising Analyst, Houston-
Galveston Psychoanalytic Institute, Houston, TX, USA,
e-mail: ggabbard@bcm.edu

Andrew J. Gerber, MD, PhD
New York State Psychiatric Institute, Columbia University, College of Physician
and Surgeons, 1051 Riverside Drive, New York, NY 10032, USA,
e-mail: asher1208@hotmail.com

Lance Hawley, PhD
Department of Psychology, McGill University, Quebec, Canada,
e-mail: lance hawley@camh.net

Mark J. Hilsenroth, PhD
Derner Institute of Advanced Psychological Studies, Adelphi University,
Garden City, NY, USA, e-mail: hilsenro@adelphi.edu

Tai Katzenstein, PhD
Department of Psychiatry, Massachusetts General Hospital, 15 Parkman Street,
WAC 812, Boston, MA 02114-3117, USA,
e-mail: tkatzenstein@partners.org

John M. Kelley, PhD
Department of Psychiatry, Massachusetts General Hospital, Boston, MA,
USA; Departments of Psychology and Statistics, Endicott College, 376 Hale
Street, Beverly, MA 01915, USA,
e-mail: JKelley@Endicott.Edu.

Ira Lable, MD
Department of Psychiatry, Massachusetts General Hospital, WACC 805,
15 Parkman St., Boston, MA 02114, USA,
e-mail: ira_lable@hms.harvard.edu

Falk Leichsenring, DSc
Department of Psychosomatics and Psychotherapy, University of Giessen,
35392 Giessen, Germany,
e-mail: Falk.Leichsenring@psycho.med.uni-giessen.de

Kenneth N. Levy, PhD
Department of Psychology, Pennsylvania State University, 521 Moore Bldg,
University Park, PA 16802, USA, e-mail: klevy@psu.edu

Raymond A. Levy, PsyD
Department of Psychiatry, Massachusetts General Hospital, Parkman Street,
WACC-805, Boston, MA 02114, USA,
e-mail: RLEVY2@PARTNERS.ORG

Molly Magill, PhD
Boston College Graduate School of Social Work, 193 Hampshire St.,
Cambridge, MA 02139, USA, e-mail: magillmo@bc.edu

Carl D. Marci, MD
Department of Psychiatry, Massachusetts General Hospital, 15 Parkman Street,
WAC 812, Boston, MA 02114-3117, USA,
e-mail: cmarci@partners.org

Leigh McCullough PhD
Harvard Medical School, and Modum Bad Research Institute, 3370 Vikersaud,
Norway, e-mail: leigh@hms.harvard.edu

Barbara Milrod, MD
Department of Psychiatry, Weill Cornell Medical College, 525 East 68th Street,
New york, NY 10065, e-mail: bmilrod@med.cornell.edu

J. Christopher Muran, PhD
Division of Psychology, Beth Israel Medical Center, New York, NY, USA,
e-mail:jcmuran@chpnet.org

J. Christopher Perry, MPH, MD
The Institute of Community and Family Psychiatry, Sir Mortimer B.
Davis Jewish General Hospital, 4333 Chemin de la Côte Ste-Catherine,
Montréal, Québec H3T 1E4 Canada, and McGill University, Montreal,
Québec, Canada; The Erikson Institute for Training and Research at the
Austen Riggs Center, Stockbridge, MA 01262-0962, USA,
e-mail: jchristopher.perry@mcgill.ca

Bella Proskurov
New School for Social Research, New York, NY, USA,
e-mail: bellaprv@yahoo.com

Helen Riess, MD
Department of Psychiatry, Massachusetts General Hospital, Boston, MA,
USA, e-mail: hriess@partners.org

Joshua L. Roffman, MD
Psychiatric Neuroscience Program, MGH-East, Bldg 149, 13th Street, 2nd Floor,
Charlestown, Boston, MA 02129, USA,
e-mail: jroffman@partners.org

Jeremy D. Safran, PhD
Department of Psychology, New School University, 65 Fifth Avenue, New York,
NY 10003, USA, e-mail: Safranj@newschool.edu

Rolf Sandell, MD
Department of Clinical Psychology, Linkoping University, Fredrikshovsgatan
3A, SE-11523 Stockholm, Sweden, e-mail: rolf.sandell@liu.se

Lori N. Scott, MS
Department of Psychology, Pennsylvania State University, University Park,
PA, USA, e-mail: lscott@psu.edu

Caleb J. Siefert, PhD
Department of Psychiatry, Massachusetts General Hospital, 15 Parkman Street,
WAC 812, Boston, MA 02114-3117, USA, e-mail: csiefert@partners.org

Heather Thompson-Brenner, PhD
Department of Psychology, Boston University, 648 Beacon Street, Boston,
MA 02215, USA, e-mail: ht141@hotmail.com

Rachel H. Wasserman, MS
Department of Psychology, Pennsylvania State University, University Park,
PA, USA, e-mail: rwasserm@psu.edu

Jolie Weingeroff, MA
Department of Psychology, Boston University, Boston, MA, USA,
e-mail: jollew@bu.edu

Anthony P. Weiss, MD, MSc
Department of Psychiatry, Massachusetts General Hospital, One Bowdoin
Square, Room 734, Boston, MA 02114, USA, e-mail: aweiss@partners.org

Drew Westen, PhD
Departments of Psychology and Psychiatry and Behavioral Sciences, Emory
University, Atlanta, GA, USA, e-mail: dwesten@emory.edu

Frank E. Yeomans, PhD
Joan and Sanford I. Weill Medical College, Cornell University, NY, USA,
e-mail: Fyeomans@nyc.rr.com

David C. Zuroff, PhD
Department of Psychology, McGill University, Quebec, Canada,
 e-mail: zuroff@ego.psych.mcgill.ca

# Introduction

This introduction is organized into two parts: one focusing on empirical research testing the efficacy and effectiveness of psychodynamic psychotherapy and the other focusing on how research can improve outcomes by advancing theory, technique, and process.

## Effectiveness of Psychodynamic Psychotherapy: What we Know and New Directions

Although the general benefits of psychotherapy have clearly been established beyond a shadow of a doubt by meta-analyses [1], psychodynamic treatment remains scientifically speaking, the poor cousin to other treatments such as cognitive and behavioral therapies and pharmacologic regimens for which efficacy has been well-established through empirical methods. Thus, the perception remains that psychodynamic psychotherapy for many disorders is ineffective or inferior. In recent years, perhaps as a reaction to this perception, the field of psychodynamic psychotherapy has begun to look more seriously toward process and outcome research and attribute increased value to it, but this change has not been entirely for voluntary reasons. It has come about partially because the field has lost status and been marginalized within psychiatry and psychology by these other approaches to treatment that have shown efficacy through a plethora of research studies. Regardless of the motivation behind it, the recent movement from within psychodynamic circles toward integrating research into clinical training programs has emphasized the scholarly need to gather data about the validity of psychodynamic theory and treatment through accepted scientific research initiatives. Significant changes need to be made to professional organizations to enable this shift to happen. Some have proposed a science-based conception of psychoanalysis, which equally values clinical expertise and research expertise. It is imperative to modify our professional organizations to foster the development of researchers who can generate data elucidating empirically based tenets that will inform psychoanalytic theory and practice.

Even when there is great motivation and willingness to put the outcomes of psychodynamic treatments to the test empirically, researchers are then faced with a lack of consensus as to the acceptable methodological approaches for a treatment to meet criteria as an empirically supported treatment (EST). Currently, the gold standard for research methodology is the randomized controlled trial (RCT), which is intended to provide proof of the efficacy of a given treatment. The central features of a RCT are (1) the random assignment of subjects to the different treatment conditions in an attempt to ensure that existing differences among subjects are equally distributed and (2) the use of controlled treatments with manuals and adherence checks to ensure treatment fidelity. The goal of randomization and monitoring of treatment fidelity then is to attribute the observable effects of a treatment condition exclusively to the applied therapy. The RCT design has been adopted as the sole standard for an experimental treatment to be considered an EST. According to Fonagy et al. [2], "research that is considered empirically supported tends to have three characteristics: (1) studies address a single disorder (usually Axis I) with diagnostic assessments to ensure homogeneity of samples, (2) treatments are manualized and are of brief and fixed duration to ensure the integrity of the 'experimental manipulation,' and (3) outcome assessments focus on the symptom(s) that represent the declared priority of the study (and often the intervention). The underlying aim is the maximization of internal validity by random assignment, controlling confounding variables, and standardizing procedures."

Westen et al. [3] have expertly and aggressively challenged the notion that psychotherapy treatments studied through RCTs are scientifically unassailable and worthy of being the sole gatekeeper for admission to the private world of the empirically supported (see Westen et al. [3] for full discussion). For the purpose of this discussion, probably the primary objection to the position of the sole legitimacy of the RCT is that RCTs tend to test treatments in the artificial environment of the researcher's laboratory, which has the effect of limiting interventions to overly simplistic manualized responses that are not transferable to treatment in the community. RCTs also tend to evaluate treatments for specific disorders, which have not been found to exist in isolation very often in epidemiological studies [4]. These considerations limit the generalizability of findings from the laboratory to the community, where most treatment occurs [5]. Additionally, the question of the degree to which laboratory treatments actually conform to the stated brand name treatments has also been raised through research findings [6–8].

Westen et al., the 2005 APA Division 12 Task Force [9], and others [2, 5, 10–12] have called for the inclusion of effectiveness research, including naturalistic studies, to help determine which treatments achieve status as an empirically supported treatment. Effectiveness studies are carried out under usual conditions of clinical practice and include patients most often carrying their expected co-morbid diagnostic complexity through the research protocol. The duration of the treatment is often determined by the clinical requirements and, most importantly, therapists treat patients with the same methods and techniques they usually would, that is, adherence to treatment manuals is not aspired to or measured. Process measures can be utilized in effectiveness studies to determine what occurred in the treatments and therefore what interventions were the active ingredients in the treatment of the complex disorders often seen in treatment in the community rather than laboratory settings. The primary criticism of naturalistic research has to do with the diminished possibility of controlling factors influencing outcome separate from the experimental condition, in this case the psychotherapy treatment. It appears that the pendulum has begun to swing away from the extreme of embracing only efficacy studies. For example, the National Institute of Mental Health has called for more naturalistic research in testing treatment hypotheses [13].

This movement to grant official acceptance of specific research-based treatments is well developed, with the American Psychiatric Association adhering to the methodological gold standard of RCTs to officially support specific brand name treatments. The American Psychiatric Association has a three-tiered system in which a treatment is labeled as Level 1, recommended with substantial clinical confidence; Level 2, recommended with moderate clinical confidence; or Level 3, may be recommended on the basis of individual circumstances. The placement of treatments at different levels is determined by the presence of outcome data from RCTs that demonstrates the efficacy of manualized treatments for specific disorders.

The American Psychological Association, after much controversy, has included data collected from naturalistic studies as well as from randomly controlled trials, in establishing criteria for treatments to gain status as empirically supported. However, this has not always been the case. The initial 1995 Task Force on Promotion and Dissemination of Psychological Procedures Report [14, 15] established 18 empirically validated treatments, originally established to combat the perception that most psychotherapy treatments were inferior to psychopharmacologic treatment, and included data only from randomly controlled trials of diagnostic-specific groups treated with a manualized treatment. While this Division 12 Task Force Report did indeed make certain psychological treatments more visible to the general public and to members of the mental health field, it excluded, until 2005, data from sources other than RCTs and thus excluded psychodynamic treatments for which no RCTs existed at that time. As a result of the initial criticism of the 1995 report, however, data from naturalistic research (including process studies) was included in the 2005 revision of criteria by the Task Force [9]. The Task Force adapted a definition of evidence-based practice from Sackett et al.'s well-known Institute of Medicine Report [16] and concluded that "Evidence-based practice is the integration of best research evidence with clinical expertise and patient values" (p. 147). With the publication of this report, the scope of acceptable data used to determine status as an EST was significantly expanded, thereby making room for psychodynamic treatments. Clinical judgments, patient values, and the larger clinical context are integrated as well. Although the definition of acceptable data has been expanded for the American Psychological Association, this expansion is far from broadly accepted in the larger mental health field at this time.

In this volume, readers will see state-of-the-art examples of RCTs as well as naturalistic studies of psychodynamic treatment. A chapter by Busch and Milrod presents the results of an RCT demonstrating the efficacy of a short-term (24 sessions) manualized psychodynamic treatment with patients diagnosed with panic disorder. This study represents a wonderful example of how psychodynamic treatment can indeed be studied using a rigorously designed RCT. In another chapter, Levy and Wasserman report findings from efficacy studies of three different treatments for borderline personality disorder, including another psychodynamic treatment: transference focused psychotherapy. Thompson-Brenner, Weingeroff, and Westen then provide a review of psychodynamic treatments of eating disorders that includes data from both efficacy and naturalistic studies. The case for the utility of psychodynamic approaches in the treatment of patients with eating disorders is made convincingly and then demonstrated with a clinical example that describes both the researchers' case conceptualization and treatment approach. Finally, using meta-analysis, Leichsenring offers an exhaustive review of all studies of short-term psychodynamic psychotherapy (STPP), demonstrating that STPP is an efficacious treatment in specific disorders although the same evidence base is yet to be built for long-term psychodynamic psychotherapy or psychoanalysis. As Fonagy and Roth state, when it comes to the evidence base for long-term psychodynamic psychotherapy, "...here the evidence base becomes rather patchy" [2]. On a more positive note however, Fonagy continues, "In no area is the evidence compelling, but in most areas where systematic investigation has been carried out, outcomes are comparable to those obtained by other therapeutic methods." Clearly, psychodynamic psychotherapy is in need of a commitment from within to conduct rigorous empirical research to investigate clinical process and outcomes of long-term psychodynamic treatment.

## Can Empirical Research Inform and Improve Clinical Outcomes?

"What have we learned from psychotherapy research that we use in clinical practice?" is often the first question raised when conversation among a group of clinicians turns to research. This volume, written exclusively by clinician researchers, is an attempt to address this issue with the belief that clinical practice and research are mutually dependent and should co-exist in training, clinical and academic circles. Many others have attempted to "bridge the gap" between clinicians and researchers in the world of psychodynamic psychotherapy (see, e.g., [17–19]), and it seems the success of these efforts has been gradual and incremental but slow. There are clearly several oft-noted obstacles to further integration of clinical and research efforts. Often research findings seem so far removed from the front line of clinical work that clinicians pay little attention, leaving the value to remain purely within academic, non-treatment circles. And clinicians, for their part, often feel that their own clinical work allows them to test their theories and approaches, and the complexity of the clinical situation does not translate into measurable phenomena. We see this volume as evidence that clinical research into psychodynamic theories and approaches can, at its best, support a spirit of inquiry by helping clinicians' evaluate their own complex theories in light of observable phenomena while maintaining clinical complexity and meaning. Toward this end, all chapters that discuss research findings also offer a clinical example that demonstrates the importance of the research for clinical work. A spirit of inquiry has been a hallmark of psychodynamic psychotherapy since its inception, expressed through individual supervisions, case conferences for individual cases and theoretical development. This volume provides some of the most powerful examples of empirical research as an equally important avenue of exploration.

We are at the stage in development within psychodynamic theory and therapy in which we have accepted that no one theory captures all the important insights for treatment with all patients by all therapists. This realization leaves the door open for a crucial potential role for research. Jimenez [20] explains that "research might indicate which forms of intervention are most appropriate in terms of producing therapeutic change, given the characteristics of the patient and the relationship established with the analyst/therapist." He further points out that we no longer try to fit all patients to a standard technique. Rather, "modified techniques allow for a flexible set of indications whereby the treatment is adapted to the characteristics of each patient" [21]. Some clinicians would argue that this has always been the case, but certainly supporters of particular theoretical models have not heralded this approach. One clear value of research in this context can be to help determine effective therapeutic techniques and processes in various disorders and therapeutic dyads. To accomplish these goals, the focus needs to shift from outcome studies (that tell us if a patient improves as a result of treatment) to process studies (which aim to determine how a patient changes as a result of treatment). According to Jimenez, "Process research holds the promise of matching therapist and patient based on patient needs and therapist techniques" [20].

With the emerging evidence base stating the case for the effectiveness of psychodynamic treatment, many researchers have turned their attention to better understanding therapeutic action. Several chapters in this volume reflect this emphasis on process research. Siefert, Defife, and Baity begin by presenting 10 process measures in depth that they value as significant for researchers' consideration when initiating process research. Then several chapters demonstrate the use of some of these specific process measures. The findings reported by Katzenstein, Ablon, and Levy emerge from a process and outcome study on the naturalistic treatment of panic disorder and reveal specific active ingredients that correlate with positive outcome that are empirically identified through the use of the Psychotherapy Process Q-set (PQS). The study complements Milrod's RCT for panic disorder nicely and indicates the salience of an emotion-focused approach to psychotherapy with a population of patients with panic disorder. The authors also discuss empirical findings concerning the presence of and correlation with positive outcome of three brand name treatment processes with this population. In their chapter, Diener and Hilsenroth emphasize process variables in reviewing both the theory and research findings of affect-focused treatments for anxiety. Additionally, they offer clinical examples of affect-focused interventions that are applicable in a broad range of clinical cases. McCullough and Magill also focus on process variables in designing short-term dynamic therapy that also emphasizes a patient's affect as the focus of treatment. Through the use of a detailed case example presented with narration, the authors describe their empirical findings that support their particular approach to working with a patient's previously defended or split off affect. This approach aims to minimize a patient's resistance to experiencing their emotions, their "affect phobia" as McCullough labels it. The narration of the therapeutic approach allows the reader to be part of their thinking and treatment techniques in detail from the inside out. The chapter offers an interesting approach to treatment of a broad spectrum of disorders from the perspective of a clinician – researcher who was originally trained in a behavioral approach to treatment before moving toward a more interactive, affect-based model of conceptualizing and working that grew from a focus on treatment process. Finally, in their chapter, Blatt, Zuroff, and Hawley call upon researchers to de-emphasize their preferred brand name treatments when developing research initiatives in favor of a focus on discovering specific process variables that correlate with positive outcome in psychotherapy treatments. They call on clinician researchers to "...identify the central features of the treatments we provide and the dimensions that contribute to constructive and sustained therapeutic change." Their chapter describes research into understanding factors contributing to sustained therapeutic gain in outpatient treatments of depression, a clear emphasis on determining salient process variables in treatments that transcend brand names.

Two additional chapters introduce and demonstrate the use of a new empirical measure to assess complex clinical phenomena and arrive at clinically useful conclusions that can contribute to guiding a treatment. Betan and Westen present a countertransference measure that details eight factors or groupings of dozens of clinician responses to working with personality disordered patients, a patient diagnosed with narcissistic personality disorder in the case example provided. As the authors explain, their findings suggest that "countertransference reactions occur in coherent and predictable patterns in the treatment of personality pathology." The presence of such a measure implies that clinicians will be better prepared to maintain a therapeutic alliance and sustain their own engagement with the patient if they are able to welcome and identify their emotional reactions to their patients. The chapter reveals the specific constellation of counter transference reactions that a psychotherapist treating such a patient is likely to have. Similarly, Safran, Muran, and Proskurov introduce a Rupture Resolution Questionnaire that details the specific process variables contained in the repair of a therapeutic alliance rupture. This group has focused their clinical and research initiatives on the alliance over time and reminds us that research has repetitively shown that "specific techniques account for only 5–15% of outcome variance." They remind us that all interventions are relational acts, that is, they occur in the context of a specific dyadic relationship. The therapeutic alliance remains the most robust predictor of therapeutic outcome, and the authors offer four-stages of interactions between patient and therapist, empirically validated, to repair ruptures. Again, Safran's research is aimed squarely at helping clinicians in their frontline psychotherapy with patients. An excellent clinical example is offered to demonstrate the power of their method.

In addition to process research, another clear wave of the future centers on neuroscience research. In the coming years, neuroscience methods will continue to be integrated with more traditional process and outcome studies in helping to develop different therapeutic options for different therapeutic treatment dyads. In their chapter, Roffman and Gerber declare that psychotherapy and neuroscience have reached an historic crossroad. In their remarkable review of neuroscience findings that are relevant to psychotherapy, they elucidate the current emerging data from brain imaging studies that they see contributing to the improvement of psychotherapy technique. In a second chapter relevant to psychotherapy and neuroscience research, Marci and Reiss review the history of physiologic monitoring during psychodynamic psychotherapy and present recent findings that complement neuroimaging results and support recent advances in interpersonal neurobiology and social neuroscience. The presentation of a clinical case in which physiological monitoring is utilized informs us about the relevance of such technique for improving psychotherapy outcome.

Finally, this volume includes a section of writing not often found in research-oriented books. We have included a section of letters from five members of the mental health community on a variety of subjects. Anne Alonso, from the perspective of a well-respected clinician and teacher of psychodynamic ideas and approaches to treatment, writes about her heartfelt history of concerns about the limitations of research for the clinical enterprise. Her letter is made more poignant by the fact that, with her passing, it is her final written contribution, among many, to the field. Her insights, dedication, and devotion to psychodynamic work will sorely be missed. She ends her letter with a more optimistic view of the possibility of integrating research into clinical curricula. Ira Lable, a psychoanalyst and clinician for decades, gives us a moving glimpse of his thought processes and personal experience in embracing research as a means of promoting learning within the field of psychoanalysis. His path embraces his research study on the effect of the presence and absence of the couch on analytic process. John Kelley, a statistician and researcher, offers an in-depth warning about the use and misuse of research findings from a statistical perspective. He clarifies and emphasizes what research findings do and don't tell us and expresses concern about how researchers and institutions have utilized findings in the past. Rolf

Sandell, a psychoanalyst – researcher, in a creative letter to a fictional colleague, places before us a new direction for research initiatives. He asks us to consider the meaning of individual subjects whose data is outside the main thrust of findings. What can we learn from trying to discover the variables responsible for their position as research outliers? Anthony Weiss, in an approach he calls bibliometrics, traces the path from journal publication to general availability of information and research findings to other mental health practitioners for use in improvement of treatment. His findings are interesting and powerful for those of us who research and practice psychodynamic treatment. He concludes through data analysis that researchers and we psychodynamic clinicians exist inside a bubble, in a state of "splendid isolation," as Fonagy has described [2], our work visible almost exclusively to ourselves. This conclusion should stand as a call to action for clinicians and researchers alike and one which we hope this volume helps address.

## References

1. Smith M.L., Glass G.V., Miller T.I. (1980). *The benefits of psychotherapy*. Baltimore, MD: John Hopkins University Press.
2. Fonagy P., Roth A., Higgitt A. (2005). Psychodynamic psychotherapies: Evidence-based practice and clinical wisdom. *Bulletin of the Menninger Clinic 69 (1)*: 1–58.
3. Westen D., Morrison K., Thompson-Brenner H. (2004). The empirical status of empirically supported psychotherapies: Assumptions, findings, and reporting in controlled clinical trials. *Psychological Bulletin 130 (4)*: 631–663.
4. Kessler R.C., McGonagle K.A., Zhao S., Nelson C.B., Hughes M., Eshleman S., Wittchen H.U., Kendler K.S. (1994). Lifetime and 12-month prevalence of DSM-III-R psychiatric disorders in the United States. *Archives of General Psychiatry 51*: 8–19.
5. Leichsenring F. (2004). Randomized controlled versus naturalistic studies: A new research agenda. *Bulletin of the Menninger Clinic 68 (2)*: 137–151.
6. Ablon J.S., Jones E.E. (1998). How expert clinicians' prototypes of an ideal treatment correlate with outcome in psychodynamic and cognitive-behavioral therapy. *Psychotherapy Research 8*: 71–83.
7. Ablon J.S., Jones E.E. (2002). Validity of controlled clinical trials of psychotherapy: Findings from the NIMH Treatment of Depression Collaborative Research Program. *American Journal of Psychiatry 159*: 775–783.
8. Ablon J.S., Levy R.A., Katzenstein T. (2006). Beyond brand names of psychotherapy: identifying empirically supported change processes. *Psychotherapy: Theory, Research, Practice, Training 43 (2)*: 216–231.
9. Levant R.F., et al. (2006). Evidence-based practice in psychology. *American Psychologist 61 (4)*: 271–285.
10. Seligman M.E.P. (1995). The effectiveness of psychotherapy. The Consumer Reports study. *American Psychologist 50*: 965–974.
11. Beutler L.E. (1998). Identifying empirically supported treatments: What if we didn't? *Journal of Consulting and Clinical Psychology 66*: 113–20.
12. Roth A.D., Parry G. (1997). The implications of psychotherapy research for clinical practice and service development: Lessons and limitations. *Journal of Mental Health 6*: 367–380.
13. Krupnick J.L., Sotsk S.M., Simmens S., Moyer J., Ein I., Watkins J., Pilkonis P. (1996). The role of the therapeutic alliance in psychotherapy and pharmacotherapy outcome:

Findings in the National Institute of Mental Health Treatment of Depression Collaborative Research Program. *Journal of Consulting and Clinical Psychology 64*: 532–539.

14. Chambless D.L., Hollon S. (1998). Defining empirically supported therapies. *Journal of Consulting and Clinical Psychology 66*: 7–18.

15. Chambless D.L., Sanderson W.C., Shoham V., Johnson S.B., Pope K.S., Crits-Christoph P., et al. (1996). An update on clinically validated therapies. *Clinical Psychologist 49*: 5–18.

16. Sackett D.L., Strauss S.E., Richardson W.S., Rosenberg W., Hayes R.B. (2000). *Evidence-based medicine: How to practice and teach EBM* (2nd Edition). New York: Churchill Livingstone.

17. Orlinsky D.E. (1994). Research-based knowledge as the emergent foundation for clinical practice in psychotherapy. In: Talley PF, Strupp HH, Butler SF, editors. *Psychotherapy research and practice: Bridging the gap*, pp. 99–23. New York: Basic Books.

18. Safron J.D., Muran J.C. (1994). Toward a working alliance between research and practice. In: Talley PF, Strupp HH, Butler SF, editors. *Psychotherapy research and practice: Bridging the gap*, pp. 206–26. New York: Basic Books.

19. Miller N.E., Luborsky L., Barber J.P., Docherty J.P. (1993). *Psychodynamic treatment research: A handbook for clinical practice*. New York: Basic Books, 577pp.

20. Jiménez J.P. (2007). Can research influence clinical practice? *International Journal of Psychoanalysis 88*: 661–79.

21. Thoma H., Kachele H. (1987). *Psychoanalytic practice*, Vol. 1: *Principles*, Wilson M, Roseveare D, translators. New York: Springer, 421pp.

# Part I
# Efficacy and Effectiveness Studies
# for Specific Disorders

# Chapter 1
# Psychodynamic Psychotherapy: A Review of Efficacy and Effectiveness Studies

Falk Leichsenring

## Introduction

Having seen a patient and having carried out diagnostic assessment on both a phenomenological and a psychodynamic level, psychodynamically oriented clinicians have to decide what kind of treatment they recommend to a patient. For this reason, it is useful for them to know which treatment approach has been shown to be effective in the treatment of the respective disorder. In this chapter, a review of the efficacy and effectiveness of psychodynamic psychotherapy is given. First, randomized controlled trials (RCTs) of psychodynamic psychotherapy in specific mental disorders are reviewed. After that, effectiveness studies of long-term dynamic therapy are presented. Studies of psychodynamic psychotherapy published between 1960 and 2006 were identified by a computerized search using MEDLINE, PsycINFO, and Current Contents. In addition, textbooks and journal articles were used.

## Evidence-Based Medicine and Empirically Supported Treatments

Several proposals have been made to evaluate the available evidence of both medical and psychotherapeutic treatments [1–5]. All of these proposals regard RCTs as the "gold standard" to demonstrate that a treatment is effective. RCTs (efficacy studies) are conducted under controlled experimental conditions; thus, they allow one to control for variables systematically influencing the outcome apart from the treatment. For this reason, RCTs are especially appropriate to ensure the internal validity of a study [6]. However, the exclusive position of RCTs in psychotherapy research has recently been questioned [7–14]. Following the methodology of pharmacological research, which is based on the RCT approach, is questionable with regard to psychotherapy research. In

F. Leichsenring
Department of Psychosomatics and Psychotherapy, University of Giessen, 35392, Giessen, Germany
e-mail: Falk.Laichsenring@psycho.med.uni-giessen.de

R.A. Levy, J.S. Ablon (eds.), *Handbook of Evidence-Based Psychodynamic Psychotherapy*, DOI: 10.1007/978-1-59745-444-5_1, © Humana Press 2009

psychotherapy research the defining features of RCTs such as randomization, use of treatment manuals, focus on specific mental disorder and frequently excluding patients with a poor prognosis raise the question as to whether RCTs are sufficiently representative of clinical practice [7–14]. Furthermore, the methodology of RCT with its use of treatment manuals and randomized control conditions is hardly applicable to long-term psychotherapy lasting several years [12, 15]. Contrary to RCTs, naturalistic studies (effectiveness studies) are conducted under the conditions of clinical practice. Thus, their results are highly representative for clinical practice with regard to patients, therapists, and treatments (external validity) [16]. Effectiveness studies cannot control for outside variables affecting the outcome to the same extent as RCTs (internal validity). However, the internal validity of effectiveness studies can be improved by quasi-experimental designs using other methods than randomization to rule out alternative explanations of the results [6, 9]. According to several studies, there is evidence that effectiveness studies do not overestimate effect sizes compared to RCTs [16–18].

According to these considerations, efficacy and effectiveness studies address different questions of research: RCTs examine the efficacy of a treatment under controlled (laboratory) conditions, whereas effectiveness studies address the effectiveness under clinical practice conditions [9]. As a consequence, the results of an efficacy study cannot be directly transferred to clinical practice and vice versa [9]. Thus, the relationship between RCTs and effectiveness studies is not a rivalrous one, but rather a complementary one. Some authors have emphasized that evidence RCT methodology is not the one and only approach to prove that a treatment works. From this perspective, a distinction is required between empirically supported therapies (ESTs) and RCT methodology [9, 13].

## Evidence for Psychodynamic Psychotherapy in Specific Mental Disorders

One aim of this review is to identify for which mental disorders RCTs of both short-term psychodynamic psychotherapy (STPP) and long-term psychodynamic psychotherapy (LTPP) are available. Here, the criteria proposed by the Task Force on Promotion and Dissemination of Psychological Procedure of the American Psychological Association [19], modified by Chambless and Hollon [20], to define efficacious treatments were applied. Thus, one aim of this review is to examine the evidence for psychodynamic psychotherapy under the requirements of the criteria proposed by Chambless and Hollon [20]. Previous reviews were given, for example, by Fonagy et al. [21] and by Leichsenring [22]. As the methodology of RCT is hardly applicable to long-term psychotherapy lasting several years, naturalistic (effectiveness) studies of LTPP are reviewed in a specific section of this chapter.

## Method

### *Definition of Psychodynamic Psychotherapy*

Psychodynamic psychotherapy operates on an interpretive–supportive continuum. The use of more interpretive or supportive interventions depends on the patient's needs [23–25]. Gabbard [23] has suggested regarding therapies of more than 24 sessions or lasting longer than 6 months as long-term. In this review, the definition of STPP or LTPP given by Gabbard [23] is applied. With regard to STPP, different models have been developed, which were reviewed by Messer and Warren [26]. Gabbard's definition of LTPP is the working model of this chapter [23, p. 2]: "...a therapy that involves careful attention to the therapist–patient interaction, with thoughtfully timed interpretation of transference and resistance embedded in a sophisticated appreciation of the therapist's contribution to the two-person field."

## Disorder-Specific Manuals of Psychodynamic Therapy as Helpful Guides for Clinicians

Apart from their use in RCTs discussed above, treatment manuals are very useful for therapists in clinical practice. They describe both the interventions specific to the respective approach and its indications. Thus, they facilitate treatment implementation in clinical practice. Meanwhile, manual-guided models of psychodynamic psychotherapy for a variety of specific psychiatric disorders are available for depression [27–29], chronic depression [30], anxiety disorders [31–33], posttraumatic stress disorder (PTSD) [34, 35], pathological grief [36], bulimia nervosa [37], somatoform disorders [27, 38, 39], borderline personality disorder [40, 41], avoidant and obsessive-compulsive personality disorder [42], or substance-related disorders [43, 44]. Owing to lack of space, these manuals cannot be discussed here in detail. Clinical recommendations for the treatment of specific mental disorders are given, for example, by Gabbard [45].

## Results

Thirty-one RCTs providing evidence for psychodynamic psychotherapy have been included in this review. These studies are presented in Table 1.1.

*Therapy duration*: In the RCTs of psychodynamic psychotherapy, between 7 and 46 sessions were conducted (Table 1.1). The duration of STPP ranged from 7 to 24 sessions. According to the definition given above, 19 studies (61%) examined STPP and 12 studies (39%) examined LTPP. The efficacy studies of

**Table 1.1** Randomized controlled studies of psychodynamic psychotherapy (PP) in specific psychiatric disorders

| Study | Disorder | $N$ (PP) | Comparison group | Concept of PP | Treatment duration |
|---|---|---|---|---|---|
| Thompson et al. (1987) | Depression | 24 | BT: $N = 25$, CBT: $N = 27$, waiting list: $N = 19$ | Horowitz and Kaltreider | 16–20 sessions |
| Shapiro et al. (1994) | Depression | 58 | CBT: $N = 59$ | Shapiro and Firth | 8 vs. 16 sessions |
| Gallagher-Thompson and Steffen (1994) | Depression | 30 | CBT: $N = 36$ | Mann; Rose, and DelMaestro | 16–20 sessions |
| Barkham et al. (1996) | Depression | 18 | CBT: $N = 18$ | Shapiro and Firth | 8 vs. 16 sessions |
| Maina et al. (2005) | Dysthymic disorder | 10 | Supportive therapy: $N = 10$, waiting list: $N = 10$ | Malan | 15–30, $M = 19.6$ |
| Milrod et al. (2007) | Panic disorder | 26 | CBT (applied relaxation), $N = 23$ | Milrod et al. | 24 sessions |
| Knijnik et al. (2004) | Social phobia | 15 | Credible placebo control group: $N = 15$ | Knijnik et al. | 12 sessions |
| Crits-Christoph et al. (2005) | Generalized anxiety disorder (GAD) | 15 | Supportive therapy: $N = 16$ | Luborsky; Crits-Christoph et al. | 16 sessions |
| Leichsenring, Winkelbach, and Leibing (2006) | GAD | 25 | 25 | Luborsky; Crits-Christoph et al. | 30 |
| Bögels et al. (2003, 2004) | Social phobia | 22 | CBT: $N = 27$ | Malan | 36 |
| Brom et al. (1989) | PTSD | 29 | Desensitization: $N = 31$, hypnotherapy: $N = 29$ | Horowitz | 18.8 sessions |
| Dare et al. (2001) | Anorexia nervosa | 21 | Cognitive-analytic therapy (Ryle): $N = 22$, family therapy: $N = 22$, routine treatment: $N = 19$ | Malan; Dare | $M = 24.9$ sessions |

**Table 1.1** (continued)

| Study | Disorder | N (PP) | Comparison group | Concept of PP | Treatment duration |
|---|---|---|---|---|---|
| Gowers et al. (1993) | Anorexia nervosa | 20 | Treatment as usual: N = 20 | Crisp | 12 sessions |
| Fairburn et al. (1986) | Bulimia nervosa | 11 | CBT: N = 11 | Rosen; Stunkard; Bruch | 19 sessions |
| Garner et al. (1993) | Bulimia nervosa | 25 | CBT: N = 25 | Luborsky | 19 sessions |
| Bachar et al. (1999) | Anorexia nervosa, bulimia nervosa | 17 | Cognitive therapy: N = 17, nutritional counseling: N = 10 | Barth; Goodsitt; Geist | 46 sessions |
| Svartberg et al. (2004) | Cluster C Personality Disorders | 25 | CBT: N = 25 | Malan; McCullough; Vaillant | 40 sessions |
| Muran et al. (2005) | Cluster C personality disorders | 22 | Brief relational therapy: N = 33, CBT: N = 29 | Pollack et al. | 30 sessions |
| Munroe-Blum and Marziali (1995) | Borderline personality disorder | 31 | Interpersonal group therapy: N = 25 | Kernberg | 17 sessions |
| Bateman and Fonagy (1999, 2001) | Borderline personality disorder | 19 | Treatment as usual: N = 19 | Bateman and Fonagy | 18 months |
| Clarkin et al. (2007, in press) | Borderline personality disorder | 30 | Dialectical behavioral therapy: N = 30, supportive therapy: N = 30 | Clarkin et al. | 12 months |
| Giesen-Bloo et al. (2006) | Borderline personality disorder | 42 | CBT: N = 44 | Clarkin et al. | 3 years with sessions twice a week |
| Emmelkamp et al. (2006) | Avoidant personality disorder | 23 | CBT: N = 21, waiting list: N = 18 | Malan; Luborsky; Luborsky and Mark; Pinsker et al. | 20 sessions |

Table 1.1 (continued)

| Study | Disorder | N (PP) | Comparison group | Concept of PP | Treatment duration |
|---|---|---|---|---|---|
| Woody et al. (1983, 1990) | Opiate dependence | 31 | Drug counseling (DC): $N = 35$, CBT + DC: $N = 34$ | Luborsky + drug counseling | 12 sessions |
| Woody et al. (1995) | Opiate dependence | 57 | Drug counseling: $N = 27$ | Luborsky + drug counseling | 26 sessions |
| Sandahl et al. (1998) | Alcohol dependence | 25 | CBT: $N = 24$ | Foulkes | 15 sessions ($M = 8.9$) |
| Crits-Christoph et al. (1999, 2001) | Cocaine dependence | 124 | CBT + group drug counseling (DC): $N = 97$, individual DC: $N = 92$, individual DC + group DC: $N = 96$ | Mark and Luborsky + group DC | Up to 36 individual and 24 group sessions, 4 months |
| Guthrie et al. (1991) | Irritable bowel | 50 | Supportive listening: $N = 46$ | Hobson; Shapiro and Firth | 8 sessions |
| Creed et al. (2003) | Irritable bowel | 59 | Paroxetine: $N = 43$, treatment as usual: $N = 86$ | Hobson; Shapiro and Firth | 8 sessions |
| Hamilton et al. (2000) | Functional dyspepsia | 37 | Supportive therapy: $N = 36$ | Shapiro and Firth | 7 sessions |
| Monsen and Monsen (2000) | Somatoform pain disorder | 20 | Treatment as usual/no therapy: $N = 20$ | Monsen and Monsen | 33 sessions |
| Psychodynamic psychotherapy plus medication | | | | | |
| Burnand et al. (2002) | Major depression | STPP + Clomipramine $N = 35$ | Clomipramine alone: $N = 39$ | Androli; Safran | 10 weeks |
| De Jonghe et al. (2001) | Major depressive disorder | $N = 106$, STPP + medication | STPP combined with antidepressant medication: $N = 85$ | Werman; Strupp and Binder; Rockland; de Jonghe et al. | Up to 16 sessions |

**Table 1.1** (continued)

| Study | Disorder | N (PP) | Comparison group | Concept of PP | Treatment duration |
|---|---|---|---|---|---|
| McCallum and Piper (1990) | Prolonged or delayed grief | STPP + medication, N = 45 (?) | Waiting list combined with medication: N = 35 (?) | Piper et al. | 12 weeks |
| Piper et al. (2001) | Complicated grief | STPP + medication, N = 53 | Supportive group therapy combined with medication: N = 54 | Piper, McCallum, and Joyce; McCallum, Piper, and Joyce | $M = 10.7$, $M = 10.6$ |
| Wiborg and Dahl | Panic disorder | STPP + clomipramine, N = 20 | Clomipramine: N = 20 | Davanloo; Malan, Strupp, and Binder; Wiborg | 9 months |

LTPP examined time-limited psychodynamic psychotherapy as contrasted to open-ended LTPP (Table 1.1) (for this differentiation, see Luborsky [46]).

*Models of psychodynamic psychotherapy*: In the studies identified, different forms of psychodynamic psychotherapy were applied (Table 1.1). The models developed by Luborsky [27, 34, 46], Shapiro and Firth [27], and Horowitz [34] were used most frequently.

## Evidence for the Efficacy of Psychodynamic Psychotherapy in Specific Mental Disorders

The studies of psychodynamic psychotherapy included in this review will be presented for the different mental disorders. However, from a psychodynamic perspective, the results of a therapy in a specific psychiatric disorder (e.g., depression, agoraphobia) are influenced by the underlying psychodynamic features (e.g., conflicts, defenses, personality organization), which may vary considerably within one category of psychiatric disorder [47]. These psychodynamic factors may affect treatment outcome and may have a greater impact on outcome than the phenomenological *Diagnostic and Statistical Manual of Mental Disorders* (DSM) categories [36].

## Major Depression

Cognitive-behavioral therapists get the patients to be more active and work through depressive cognitions. Psychodynamic therapists focus on the conflicts or ego functions associated with the depressive symptoms. At present, four RCTs are available that provide evidence for the efficacy of STPP compared to cognitive-behavioral therapy (CBT) in depression [29, 48–50]. Different models of STPP were applied (Table 1.1). In these studies, STPP and CBT proved to be equally effective with regard to depressive symptoms, general psychiatric symptoms and social functioning [51]. A more detailed discussion of these results has been presented in another paper [52]. In the above-mentioned meta-analysis, STPP achieved large pre–post effect sizes in depressive symptoms, general psychiatric symptoms and social functioning [51]. The results proved to be stable in follow-up studies [53, 54]. These results are consistent with the findings of the meta-analysis by Wampold et al. who did not find significant differences between CBT and "other therapies" in the treatment of depression [55]. In a small recent RCT, Maina et al. examined the efficacy of STPP and brief supportive therapy in the treatment of minor depressive disorders (dysthymic disorder, depressive disorder not otherwise specified, or adjustment disorder with depressed mood) [56]. Both treatments were superior to a waiting list condition at the end of treatment. At 6-month follow-up, STPP was superior to brief supportive therapy.

## STPP Plus Medication in Depressive Disorders

Clinicians sometimes consider combining psychotherapy with psychopharmacological treatment. In two RCTs, the efficacy of STPP combined with psychopharmacological medication was examined. In the first study, Burnand et al. reported that STPP plus clomipramine was superior to clomipramine alone [57]. In another RCT by de Jonghe et al., STPP was compared with a combination of STPP and antidepressant medication [58]. The advantages of the combined treatment were equivocal. While there were no differences in the ratings of independent observers, differences in self-report measures of depression in favor of the combined treatment were found. Taking a broader perspective, including studies of other forms of psychotherapy (e.g., CBT), there is some evidence that the combined treatment is more effective than psychotherapy alone or pharmacotherapy alone in chronic and severe depression [59–61]. However, evidence is not strong enough to unequivocally recommend the routine combination of psychotherapy and pharmacotherapy in the treatment of depression [59–61].

## Pathological Grief

In two RCTs by McCallum et al. and Piper et al., the treatment for prolonged or complicated grief by short-term psychodynamic group therapy was studied [36, 62]. In the first study, short-term psychodynamic group therapy was significantly superior to a waiting list [62]. In the second study, a significant interaction was found. With regard to grief symptoms, subjects with higher quality object relations improved more in interpretative therapy than those with lower quality object relations, who improved more in a supportive therapy. For general symptoms, changes that are clinically significant favored interpretive therapy over supportive therapy [36].

## Anxiety Disorders

For anxiety disorders, four RCTs are presently available (Table 1.1). With regard to *panic disorder* (with or without agoraphobia), Milrod et al. showed in a recent RCT that STPP was more successful than applied relaxation [63]. For *social phobia*, two RCTs of psychodynamic therapy exist. In the first study [64], short-term psychodynamic group treatment for generalized social phobia was superior to a credible placebo control. In the second RCT, LTPP proved to be as effective as CBT in the treatment of generalized social phobia [65]. In a randomized controlled feasibility study of *generalized anxiety disorder*, STPP was equally effective as a supportive therapy with regard to continuous measures of anxiety, but significantly superior on symptomatic remission rates [66]. However, the sample sizes of that study were relatively small ($N = 15$ vs.

$N = 16$), and the study was not sufficiently powered to detect more possible differences between treatments. In another RCT that is presently being completed, STPP was compared to CBT in the treatment of *generalized anxiety disorder* [67]. From the results that are presently available, STPP and CBT are equally effective with regard to the primary outcome measure. However, in some other secondary outcome measures, CBT seems to be superior. The results of the 1-year follow-up are not yet available. Thus, it is not clear if the differences persist long term.

## STPP Combined with Psychopharmacological Medication in Anxiety Disorders

Also in anxiety disorders, psychotherapy may be combined with psychopharmacological treatment. Wiborg and Dahl examined the efficacy of STPP combined with clomipramine in the treatment of panic disorder [68]. Treatments lasted for 9 months. At follow-up, STPP plus clomipramine was superior to clomipramine alone. However, including studies of other treatments such as CBT, data do not support the general superiority of a combination of psychotherapy and pharmacotherapy in anxiety disorders [59]. Some studies of panic disorder and obsessive-compulsive disorder, however, have found combined treatment superior to monotherapy [59, 69]. For obsessive-compulsive disorder, the superiority of the combined treatment was found in patients with obsessions and in patients with compulsions and a severe comorbid depression [70]. Clinicians have to take the specific conditions of a patient into account in deciding if a combined treatment is useful to a specific patient.

## Posttraumatic Stress Disorder

In an RCT by Brom, Kleber and Defares [71] the effects of STPP, behavioral therapy and hypnotherapy in patients with PTSD were studied. All of the treatments proved to be equally effective and were superior to a waiting list control group. Results of STPP were not only maintained, but continued to improve at the 3-month follow-up. However, further studies of psychodynamic psychotherapy in PTSD are required.

## Somatoform Disorders

At present, four RCTs of STPP in somatoform disorders, which fulfill the inclusion criteria are available (Table 1.1). In the RCT by Guthrie et al. [38] patients with irritable bowel syndrome, who had not responded to standard medical treatment over the previous 6 months, were treated with STPP in addition to standard medical treatment. This treatment was compared to standard medical treatment alone. According to the results, STPP was effective in two thirds of the patients. In another RCT, STPP was significantly more effective than routine care and as effective as medication (paroxetine) in the treatment of severe irritable bowel syndrome [72]. During the follow-up period, however, STPP, but not paroxetine was associated with a significant reduction in health care costs compared with treatment as usual (TAU). In an RCT by Hamilton et al. [39], STPP was compared to supportive therapy in the treatment of patients with chronic intractable functional dyspepsia, who had failed to respond to conventional pharmacological treatments. At the end of treatment, STPP was significantly superior to the control condition. Effects were stable in the 12-month follow-up. Monsen and Monsen [73] compared psychodynamic psychotherapy of 33 sessions with a control condition (no treatment or TAU) in the treatment of patients with chronic pain. Psychodynamic psychotherapy was significantly superior to the control group on measures of pain, psychiatric symptoms, interpersonal problems, and affect consciousness. The results remained stable or even improved in the 12-month follow-up. Thus, specific forms of psychodynamic psychotherapy can be recommended for the treatment of somatoform disorders.

## Bulimia Nervosa

For the treatment of bulimia nervosa, three RCTs of STPP are available (Table 1.1). Significant and stable improvements in bulimia nervosa after STPP were demonstrated in the RCTs by Fairburn et al. [74, 75] and Garner et al. [37]. In the primary disorder-specific measures (bulimic episodes, self-induced vomiting), STPP was as effective as CBT [37, 74, 75]. Apart from this, CBT was superior to STPP in some specific measures of psychopathology [42, 87]. However, in a follow-up of the study of Fairburn et al. [74] using a longer follow-up period, both forms of therapy proved to be equally effective and were partly superior to a behavioral form of therapy [75]. Accordingly, for a valid evaluation of the efficacy of STPP in bulimia nervosa, longer-term follow-up studies are necessary. In an RCT of Bachar et al., STPP was significantly superior to both a TAU group (nutritional counseling) and cognitive therapy [76]. This was true of patients with bulimia nervosa and a mixed sample of patients with bulimia nervosa or anorexia nervosa.

## Anorexia Nervosa

For the treatment of anorexia nervosa, however, evidence-based treatments are barely available [77]. This applies to both psychodynamic psychotherapy and CBT. In an RCT by Gowers et al. [78], STPP combined with four sessions of nutritional advice yielded significant improvements in patients with anorexia nervosa (Table 1.1). Weight and body mass index (BMI) changes were significantly more improved than in a control condition (TAU). Dare et al. [79] compared psychodynamic psychotherapy with a mean duration of 24.9 sessions to cognitive-analytic therapy, family therapy and routine treatment in the treatment of anorexia nervosa (Table 1.1). Psychodynamic psychotherapy yielded significant symptomatic improvements, and STPP and family therapy were significantly superior to the routine treatment with regard to weight gain. However, the improvements were modest, several patients being undernourished at the follow-up. Thus, the treatment of anorexia nervosa remains a challenge and more effective treatment models are required.

## Borderline Personality Disorder

Munroe-Blum and Marziali [80] report that STPP yielded significant improvements on measures of borderline-related symptoms, general psychiatric symptoms, and depression, and was as effective as an interpersonal group therapy (Table 1.1). Bateman and Fonagy studied psychoanalytically oriented partial hospitalization treatment for patients with borderline personality disorder [81, 82]. The treatment lasted a maximum of 18 months, representing LTPP by the definition applied in this review. According to the results, LTPP was significantly superior to standard psychiatric care, both at the end of therapy and at the 18-month follow-up. Giesen-Bloo et al. [83] compared LTPP (transference-focused psychotherapy, TFP) with CBT (schema-focused therapy, SFT). Treatment duration was 3 years with two sessions a week. The authors reported statistically and clinically significant improvements for both treatments. However, SFT was found to be superior to TFP in several outcome measures. Furthermore, a significantly higher dropout risk for TFP was reported. This study, however, seems to be methodologically seriously flawed. The authors used scales for adherence and competence for both treatments for which they adopted an identical cutoff score of 60 indicating competent application. According to the data published by the authors [83, p. 651], the median competence level for applying SFT methods was 85.67. For TFP, a value of 65.6 was reported. While the competence level for SFT clearly exceeded the cutoff, the competence level for TFP just surpassed it. Furthermore, the competence level for SFT is clearly higher than that for TFP. Accordingly, both treatments were not equally competently applied. Thus, the results of that study are questionable. The difference in competence was not taken into account by the authors, neither with regard to the analysis of resulting data nor in the discussion of the results. Thus, this study raises serious concerns about an investigator allegiance effect [84]. On a rigorous methodological level, another RCT comparing psychodynamic psychotherapy (TFP [41]), dialectical behavior therapy (DBT) and psychodynamic supportive psychotherapy was conducted [85]. According to the results, TFP and DBT were equally effective [86]. With regard to the increase of secure attachment and improvements in reflective functioning, TFP was superior to DBT and supportive psychotherapy [87]. A meta-analysis by Leichsenring et al. addressing the effects of psychodynamic psychotherapy and CBT in personality disorders reported that psychodynamic psychotherapy yielded large effects sizes not only for comorbid symptoms, but also for core personality pathology [88]. This was true especially for BPD.

## Cluster C Personality Disorders

There is evidence for the efficacy of psychodynamic psychotherapy in the treatment of Cluster C personality disorders. In an RCT of by Svartberg et al. [89], psychodynamic psychotherapy of 40 sessions was compared to CBT (Table 1.1). Both psychodynamic psychotherapy and CBT yielded significant improvements in patients with DSM-IV Cluster C personality disorders (i.e., avoidant, compulsive, or dependent personality disorder). The improvements refer to symptoms, interpersonal problems and core personality pathology. The results were stable at 24-month follow-up. No significant differences were found between psychodynamic psychotherapy and CBT with regard to efficacy. Muran et al. compared the efficacy of psychodynamic therapy, brief relational therapy, and CBT in the treatment of Cluster C personality disorders and personality disorders not otherwise specified [90]. Treatments lasted for 30 sessions. With regard to mean changes in outcome measures, no significant differences were found between the treatment conditions, neither at termination nor at follow-up. Furthermore, there were no significant differences between the treatments with regard to the patients achieving clinically significant change in symptoms, interpersonal problems, characteristics of personality disorders, or therapist ratings of target complaints. At termination, CBT and brief relational therapy were superior to psychodynamic psychotherapy in one outcome measure (patient ratings of target complaints). However, this difference did not persist at follow-up. With regard to the percentage of patients showing change, no significant differences were found, either at termination or at the follow-up, except in one comparison. At termination, CBT was superior to STPP on the Inventory of Interpersonal Problems [91]. Again, this difference did not persist at the follow-up. The conclusion is that only a few significant differences were found between the treatments that did not persist at follow-up.

## Avoidant Personality Disorder

Avoidant personality disorder (AVPD) is among the above-mentioned Cluster C personality disorders. In a recent RCT, Emmelkamp et al. [92] compared CBT to STPP and a waiting list condition in the treatment of AVPD.

The authors reported CBT as more effective than waiting list control and STPP. However, the study suffers form several methodological shortcomings making the results questionable [93]. Design, statistical analyses, and the reporting of the results again raise concerns about an investigator allegiance effect [84].

## Substance-Related Disorders

Woody et al. [94, 95] studied the effects of STPP and CBT given in addition to drug counseling in the treatment of opiate dependence (Table 1.1). STPP plus drug counseling yielded significant improvements on measures of drug-related symptoms and general psychiatric symptoms. At a 7-month follow-up, STPP and CBT plus drug counseling were equally effective, and both conditions were superior to drug counseling alone. In another RCT, psychodynamic psychotherapy of 26 sessions given in addition to drug counseling was also superior to drug counseling alone in the treatment of opiate dependence [96]. By a 6-month follow-up, most of the gains made by the patients who had received psychodynamic therapy remained. In an RCT by Crits-Christoph et al. [97, 98], psychodynamic psychotherapy of up to 36 individual sessions was combined with 24 sessions of group drug counseling in the treatment of cocaine dependence. The combined treatment yielded significant improvements and was as effective as CBT that was combined with group drug counseling as well. However, both CBT and psychodynamic psychotherapy plus group drug counseling were not more effective than group drug counseling alone. Furthermore, individual drug counseling was significantly superior to both forms of therapy concerning measures of drug abuse. With regard to psychological and social outcome variables, all treatments were equally effective [97, 98]. In an RCT by Sandahl et al. [99], STPP and CBT were compared concerning their efficacy in the treatment of alcohol abuse. STPP yielded significant improvements on measures of alcohol abuse, which were stable at a 15-month follow-up. STPP was significantly superior to CBT in the number of abstinent days and in the improvement of general psychiatric symptoms.

## Effectiveness of Psychoanalytic Therapy in Patients with Complex Psychiatric Disorders: Evidence from Naturalistic Studies

As discussed above, the methodology of RCT is hardly applicable to LTPP lasting several years. Thus, for these long-term treatments, effectiveness studies (naturalistic studies) are the appropriate method of research [9, 12, 13, 15, 100]. The National Institute of Mental Health in the USA (NIMH) has specifically called for more effectiveness research [101].

## Effect Sizes of Psychodynamic Therapy

With regard to psychodynamic therapy, several effectiveness studies that used reliable and valid outcome measures have provided evidence that psychoanalytic therapy yielded large pre–post effect sizes according to the definition given by Cohen [102, 103, 104–109, 110, 111]. These effects refer to symptoms, interpersonal problems, social adjustment, inpatient days and other outcome criteria. In a study aggregating data from several naturalistic studies to allow for disorder-specific evaluations, Jakobsen et al. reported large effect sizes for depressive disorders, anxiety disorders, somatoform disorders, and personality disorders [112].

## Quasi-Experimental Studies of Long-Term Dynamic Therapy: Superiority to Control Groups

As mentioned above, the internal validity of effectiveness studies can be improved by quasi-experimental designs [6, 9]. By definition, quasi-experimental studies do not use random assignment [6]. They use other principles to show that alternative explanations of the observed effect are implausible (for details see Shadish et al.) [6]. For effectiveness studies, levels of evidence must be defined by criteria different from those mentioned above [1–5, 20], which regard RCTs as the gold standard [9]. Recently, a proposal was made to define levels of evidence of effectiveness studies [9].

The criteria of the Task Force on Promotion and Dissemination of Psychological Procedures [19, 20] require that (a) a treatment has proved to be superior to a control condition (placebo or no treatment) or (b) to be as effective as an already established treatment. Several controlled quasi-experimental effectiveness studies showed that psychodynamic therapy meets the criteria (a) and/or (b). These studies included control groups for which comparability with the psychodynamic treatment group was ensured by measures of matching, stratifying, or statistical control of initial differences. In all of these studies, psychodynamic therapy was significantly superior to the respective control condition. These results can be summarized as follows: (1) psychodynamic therapy yielded effect sizes that significantly exceeded the effects of untreated or low-dose-treated comparison groups [104, 109, 111, 113]; (2) longer-term psychodynamic therapy was significantly more effective than shorter forms of psychodynamic psychotherapy [105, 108, 109, 111, 113]; (3) according to the study by Rudolf et al. [105] and Grande et al. [114] psychodynamic therapy was significantly more effective than shorter-term psychodynamic psychotherapy in respect of the very dimension of outcome for which a superiority of long-term psychodynamic therapy is to be expected, that is in respect of structural changes of personality; (4) these results refer to the treatment of multimorbid patients that are not characterized by only one specific mental disorder. Ongoing controlled quasi-experimental studies of psychodynamic therapy are presently being carried out [106, 115, 116].

## Process–Outcome Relationship: Mechanisms of Change

The studies presented above have focused on outcome, not on process variables of psychodynamic psychotherapy. Studies of psychotherapeutic processes provided data regarding mechanisms of change of psychodynamic therapy. First, there is evidence that the outcome of psychodynamic therapy is related to psychotherapeutic techniques and therapist skillfulness [117, 118]: Accuracy of interpretation (Crits-Christoph et al., 1988), adherence of therapists' interventions to the "plan" [119], and competent delivery of expressive, but not of supportive techniques predicted the outcome of STPP and of moderate-length psychodynamic psychotherapy [120]. These findings suggest that specific techniques of psychodynamic psychotherapy as contrasted to nonspecific factors of psychotherapy account for a significant proportion of variance of the outcome of psychodynamic psychotherapy [117]. There is less evidence to suggest that frequency of psychodynamic techniques is related to the outcome [117]. Second, there is evidence for an interaction of technique, outcome, and patient variables: Frequency of transference interpretations seems to be associated with both a poor outcome and alliance in STPP of patients rated low on quality of object relations [36, 121–124]. Although patients with a high quality of object relations may benefit from low to moderate levels of transference interpretations, results suggest that they do not benefit from high levels of transference interpretations [121, 125, 126]. Third, with regard to the therapeutic alliance, there is some evidence that alliance is a modest predictor of treatment outcome [117, 127–130]. Accuracy of interpretation was found to correlate significantly with therapeutic alliance in moderate-length treatments [131]. Thus, one way in which accuracy of interpretation may exert its effect could be by fostering the therapeutic alliance [131]. Fourth, with regard to patient process variables, changes in the focus of psychodynamic psychotherapy were shown to correlate with symptom change [132]. Piper et al. presented results that suggest that expression of affect is a mediating variable of outcome in short-term interpretative group therapy of patients with pathological grief [133]. Fifth, with regard to patients' variables, the following variables were found to predict good outcome of STPP: High motivation, realistic expectations, circumscribed focus, high quality of object relations, and absence of personality disorder [36, 118, 134]. Future research should address the question as to which forms of psychodynamic psychotherapy and for which forms of psychiatric disorders these associations hold and for which they do not. Barber et al., for example, did not find a correlation of alliance to the outcome of psychodynamic psychotherapy for drug-related problems [135]. Furthermore, the caveat of Ablon and Jones – "Brand names of therapy can be misleading" – may also apply to psychodynamic psychotherapy [136, p.780]: The question as to whether the "different" models of psychodynamic psychotherapy differ among each other empirically is open to further research. To answer this question, empirical studies of actual therapy sessions are required that relate process variables to outcome. By this kind of research, empirically supported change processes can be identified [136]. In a review of empirical studies, Blagys and Hilsenroth identified seven features that were significantly more frequently observed in psychodynamic, psychodynamic-interpersonal, or interpersonal psychotherapy than in CBT [137]. With regard to research methodology, dynamic clinicians would not expect individual process items to correlate consistently with outcome across group designs and that more fine-grained single-case analyses are more likely to reveal rich findings.

## Discussion

Under the requirements of the criteria proposed by the Task Force modified by Chambless and Hollon [20, 138], 31 studies were identified that provided evidence for the efficacy of psychodynamic psychotherapy in specific mental disorders. In the 31 studies reviewed here, psychodynamic psychotherapy was either more effective than placebo therapy, supportive therapy, or TAU or as effective as CBT. These results are consistent with the most recent meta-analysis of psychodynamic psychotherapy that reported psychodynamic psychotherapy as superior to waiting list or TAU and as equally effective as other psychotherapies [139]. On the basis of the data of this meta-analysis, it can be shown that the latter is true if psychodynamic psychotherapy is compared directly to CBT only. This meta-analysis found large effects for psychodynamic psychotherapy in target problems, general psychiatric problems and social functioning. These effects were stable at follow-up and tended to increase [139]. On the contrary, it is important to realize for which mental disorders there is not even one RCT of psychodynamic psychotherapy. This is true, for example, for dissociative disorders or for some specific forms of personality disorders (e.g., compulsive or narcissistic). Also, for PTSD further studies are required. For the treatment of children and adolescents, only a few randomized controlled studies providing evidence for the efficacy of specific psychodynamic treatments in specific mental disorders presently exist [21]. Further studies are urgently required.

Several effectiveness studies demonstrated that longer-term psychodynamic therapy yielded large effect sizes and was superior to low/no treatment or to shorter forms of therapy. In these studies, multimorbid patients were treated. Further studies should examine the effectiveness of longer-term psychodynamic therapy in specific, though comorbid mental disorders. A study examining the effectiveness of longer-term psychodynamic therapy in depressive disorders is presently being carried out [115].

According to the results of this review, further research of psychodynamic psychotherapy in specific mental disorders is necessary, including studies of both the outcome and the active ingredients of psychodynamic psychotherapy in these disorders. Measures more specific to psychodynamic psychotherapy should be applied [140]. In many studies, psychodynamic psychotherapy and CBT were equally effective. Future studies should address the common and specific factors of psychodynamic psychotherapy and CBT. They should also examine whether there are gains achieved only by psychodynamic psychotherapy, the question of "added value," due to the treatment having ambitious treatment goals. Furthermore, studies are needed to assess the effectiveness in the community of treatments that have proven efficacious in the laboratory.

# References

1. Clarke, M. & Oxman, A. D. Cochrane reviewer's handbook 4.1.6 (updated January 2003). Oxford: Update Software. Updated quarterly; 2003.
2. Cook, D., Guyatt, G. H., Laupacis, A., Sacket, D. L., & Goldberg, R. J. Clinical recommendations using levels of evidence for antithrombotic agents. Chest 1995; 108 (4 Suppl): 227S–30S.
3. Guyatt, G., Sacket, D. L., Sinclair, J. C., Hayward, R., Cook, D. J., & Cook, R. User's guides to the medical literature. IX. A method for grading health care recommendations. JAMA 1995; 274: 1800–4.
4. Nathan, P. E. & Gorman, J. M. (Eds). A guide to treatments that work, 2nd ed. New York: Oxford University Press; 2002.
5. National Institute for Clinical Excellence. Schizophrenia. Core interventions in the treatment and management of schizophrenia in primary and secondary care. Clinical Guideline 1. London: 2002.
6. Shadish, W. R., Cook, T. D., & Campbell, D. T. Experimental and quasi-experimental designs for generalized causal inference. Boston: Houghton Mifflin Company; 2002.
7. Beutler, L. Identifying empirically supported treatments: What if we didn't? J Consult Clin Psychol 1998; 66: 113–20.
8. Fonagy, P. Process and outcome in mental health care delivery: A model approach to treatment evaluation. Bull Menninger Clin 1999; 63: 288–304.
9. Leichsenring, F. Randomized controlled vs. naturalistic studies: A new research agenda. Bull Menninger Clin 2004; 68: 115–29.
10. Persons, J. & Silberschatz, G. Are results of randomized trials useful to psychotherapists? J Consult Clin Psychol 1998; 66: 126–35.
11. Roth, A. D & Parry, G. The implications of psychotherapy research for clinical practice and service development: Lessons and limitations. J Ment Health 1997; 6: 367–80.
12. Seligman, M. The effectiveness of psychotherapy: The Consumer Reports study. Am Psychol 1995; 50: 965–74.
13. Westen, D., NC., & Thompson-Brenner, H. The empirical status of empirically supported psychotherapies: Assumptions, findings, and reporting in controlled clinical trials. Psychol Bull 2004; 130: 631–63.
14. Rothwell, P. External validity of randomized controlled trials: To whom do the results of this trial apply? Lancet 2005; 365: 82–92.
15. Wallerstein, R. Comment on Gunderson and Gabbard. J Am Psychoanal Assoc 1999; 47: 728–34.

16. Shadish, W. R., Matt, G., Navarro, A., & Phillips, G. The effects of psychological therapies under clinically representative conditions: A meta-analysis. J Consult Clin Psychol 2000; 126: 512–29.
17. Benson, K. & HA. A comparison of observational studies and randomized, controlled trials. N Engl J Med 2000; 342: 1878–86.
18. Concato, J., SN., & Horwitz, R. I. Randomized, controlled trials, observational studies, and the hierarchy of research designs. N Engl J Med 2000; 342: 1887–92.
19. Task Force on Promotion and Dissemination of Psychological Procedures. Training and Dissemination of empirically-validated psychological treatments. Report and recommendations. Clin Psychol 1995; 48: 3–23.
20. Chambless, D. L. & Hollon, S.D. Defining empirically supported treatments. J Consult Clin Psychol 1998; 66: 7–18.
21. Fonagy, P. & Target, M. The psychological treatment of child and adolescent psychiatric disorders. In: Roth, A. & F, P., eds. What works for whom? A critical review of psychotherapy research. New York: Guilford Press; 2005: 385–424.
22. Leichsenring, F. Are psychoanalytic and psychodynamic psychotherapies effective? A review. Int J Psychoanal 2005; 86: 841–68.
23. Gabbard, G. Long-term psychodynamic psychotherapy. Washington, DC: American Psychiatric Publishing; 2004.
24. Gunderson, J. G. & Gabbard, G. Making the case for psychoanalytic therapies in the current psychiatric environment. J Am Psychoanal Assoc 1999; 47: 679–704.
25. Wallerstein, R. The psychotherapy research project of the Menninger Foundation: An overview. J Consult Clinl Psychol 1989; 57: 195–205.
26. Messer, S. B. & Warren, C. S. Models of brief psychodynamic therapy: A comparative approach. New York: Guilford Press; 1995.
27. Shapiro, D. A. & Firth, J. A. Exploratory therapy manual for the Sheffield Psychotherapy Project (SAPU Memo 733). Sheffield, England: University of Sheffield; 1985.
28. Luborsky, L., Mark, D., Hole, A. V., Popp, C., Goldsmith, B., & Cacciola, J. Supportive-expressive psychotherapy of depression, a time-limited version. In: Barber, J. P. & C-C, P., eds. Dynamic therapies for psychiatric disorders (Axis I). New York: Basic Books; 1995: 13–42.
29. Shapiro, D. A., Barkham, M., Rees, A., Hardy, G. E., Reynolds, S., & Startup, M. Effects of treatment duration and severity of depression on the effectiveness of cognitive-behavioral and psychodynamic-interpersonal psychotherapy. J Consult Clin Psychol 1994; 62: 522–34.
30. Mark, D. G., Barber, J. P., & Crits-Christoph, P. Supportive-expressive therapy for chronic depression. J Clin Psychol 2003; 59: 859–72.
31. Crits-Christoph, P., Wolf-Palacio, D., Ficher, M., & Rudick, D. Brief supportive-expressive psychodynamic therapy for generalized anxiety disorder. In: Barber, J. P. & Crits-Christoph, P., eds. Dynamic therapies for psychiatric disorders (Axis I). New York: Basic Books; 1995.
32. Leichsenring, F., Beutel, M., & Leibing, E. Psychodynamic psychotherapy for social phobia: A treatment manual based on supportive-expressive therapy. Bull Menninger Clin 2007; 71: 56–84.
33. Milrod, B., Busch, F., Cooper, A., & Shapiro, T. Manual of panic-focused psychodynamic psychotherapy. Washington, DC: American Psychiatric Press; 1997.
34. Horowitz, M. Stress response syndromes. New York: Aronson; 1976.
35. Horowitz, M. & Kaltreider, N. Brief therapy of the stress response syndrome. Psychiatr Clin North Am 1979; 2: 365–77.
36. Piper, W. E., McCallum, M., Joyce, A. S., & Ogrodniczuk, J. Patient personality and time-limited group psychotherapy for complicated grief. Int J Group Psychother 2001; 51: 525–52.
37. Garner, D., Rockert, W., Davis, R., Garner, M. V., Olmsted, M. P., & Eagle, M. Comparison of cognitive-behavioral and supportive-expressive therapy for bulimia nervosa. Am J Psychiatry 1993; 150: 37–46.

38. Guthrie, E., Creed, F., Dawson, D., & Tomenson, B. A controlled trial of psychological treatment for the irritable bowel syndrome. Gastroenetrology 1991; 100: 450–7.
39. Hamilton, J., Guthrie, E., Creed, F., Thompson, D., Tomenson, B., Bennett, R., Moriarty, K., Stephens, W., & Liston, R. A randomized controlled trial of psychotherapy in patients with chronic functional dyspepsia. Gastroenterology 2000; 119; 661–9
40. Bateman, A. & Fonagy, P. Mentalization-based treatment of BPD. J Personal Disord 2004; 18: 36–51.
41. Clarkin, J., Kernberg, O. F., & Yeomans, F. Transference-focused psychotherapy for borderline personality disorder patients. New York: Guilford Press; 1999.
42. Barber, P., Morse, J. Q., Krakauer, I. D., Chitams, J., & Crits-Christoph, K. Change in obsessive compulsive and avoidant personality disorders following time-limited supportive-expressive therapy. Psychotherapy 1997; 34: 133–43.
43. Luborsky, L., Woody, G. E., Hole, A. V., & Velleco, A. Supportive-expressive dynamic psychotherapy for treatment of opiate drug dependence. In: Barber, J. P. & C-C, P., eds. Dynamic therapies for psychiatric disorders (Axis I). New York: Basic Books; 1995: 131–60.
44. Mark, D. & Faude, J. Supportive-expressive therapy for cocaine abuse. In: Barber J. P. & C-C, P., eds. Dynamic therapies for psychiatric disorders (Axis I). New York: Basic Books; 1995: 294–331.
45. Gabbard, G. O. Psychodynamic psychiatry in clinical practice, 3rd ed. Washington, DC: American Psychiatric Press; 2000.
46. Luborsky, L. Principles of psychoanalytic psychotherapy: Manual for supportive-expressive treatment. New York: Basic Books; 1984.
47. Kernberg, O. A psychoanalytic model for the classification of personality disorders. In: Achenheil, M. BB, Engel, R., Ermann, M. & Nedopil, N. eds. Implications of psychopharmacology to psychiatry. New York: Springer; 1996.
48. Barkham, M., Rees, A., Shapiro, D. A., Stiles, W. B., Agnew, R. M., Halstead, J., Culverwell, A. l., & Harrington, V. Outcomes of time-limited psychotherapy in applied settings: Replication of the second Sheffield Psychotherapy Project. J Consult Clin Psychol 1996; 64: 1079–85.
49. Gallagher-Thompson, D. & Steffen, A. M. Comparative effects of cognitive-behavioral and brief psychodynamic psychotherapies for depressed family caregivers. J Consult Clin Psychol 1994; 62: 543–9.
50. Thompson, L., Gallagher, D., & Breckenridge, J. S. Comparative effectiveness of psychotherapies for depressed elders. J Consult Clinl Psychol 1987; 55: 385–90.
51. Leichsenring, F. Comparative effects of short-term psychodynamic psychotherapy and cognitive-behavioral therapy in depression. A meta-analytic approach. Clin Psychol Rev 2001; 21: 401–19.
52. Leichsenring, F. A review of meta-analyses of outcome studies of psychodynamic therapy. In: Psychodynamic Diagnostic Manual Work Groups of APsaA, IPA, Division 39-APA, AAPDP, NMCOP psychodynamic diagnostic manual (PDM). Bethesda, MD: Alliance of Psychodynamic Organizations; 2006: 819–37
53. Gallagher-Thompson, D., Hanley-Peterson, P., & Thompson, L. W. Maintenance of gains versus relapse following brief psychotherapy for depression. J Consult Clin Psychol 1990; 58: 371–4.
54. Shapiro, D. A., Rees, A., Barkham, M., & Hardy, G. E. Effects of treatment duration and severity of depression on the maintenance of gains after cognitive-behavioral and psychodynamic-interpersonal psychotherapy. J Consult Clin Psychol 1995; 63: 378–87.
55. Wampold, B., Minami, T., Baskin, T. W., & Tierney, S. C. A meta-(re)analysis of the effects of cognitive therapy versus 'other therapies' for depression. J Affect Disord 2002; 68: 159–65.
56. Maina, G., FF., & Bogetto, F. Randomized controlled trial comparing brief dynamic and supportive therapy with waiting list condition in minor depressive disorders. Psychother Psychosom 2005; 74: 3–50.

57. Burnand, Y., Andreoli, A., Kolatte, E., Venturini, A., & Rosset, N. Psychodynamic psychotherapy and clomipramine in the treatment of major depression. Psychiatr Serv 2002; 53(5): 585–90.
58. de Jonghe, F., Kool, S., van Aalst, G., Dekker, J., & Peen, J. Combining psychotherapy and antidepressants in the treatment of depression. J Affect Disord 2001; 64: 217–29.
59. Thase, M. & Jindal, R. Combining psychotherapy and psychopharmacology for treatment of mental disorders. In: Lambert, M., ed. Bergin and Garfields handbook of psychotherapy and behavior change, 5th ed. New York: Wiley; 2004: 743–66.
60. Thase, M. E., Greenhouse, J. B., Frank, E., Reynolds, C. F. 3rd, Pilkonis, P. A., Hurley, K., Grochocinski, V., & Kupfer, D. J. Treatment of major depression with psychotherapy or psychotherapy-pharmacotherapy combinations. Arch Gen Psychiatry 1997; 154: 1009–15.
61. Scott, J. Treatment of chronic depression. N Engl J Med 2000; 342: 1518–20.
62. McCallum, M. & Piper, D. E. A controlled study of effectiveness and patient suitablility for short-term group psychotherapy. Int J Group Psychother 1990; 40: 431–52.
63. Milrod, B., Leon, A. C., Busch, F., Rudden, M., Schwalberg, M., Clarkin, J., Aronson, A., Singer, M., Turchin, W., Klass, E. T., Graf, E., Teres, J. J., & Shear, M. K. A randomized controlled clinical trial of psychoanalytic psychotherapy for panic disorder. Am J Psychiatry 2007; 164: 265–272.
64. Knijnik, D. Z., Kapczinski, F., CE, Margis, R., & Eizirik, C. L. Psychodynamic group treatment for generalized social phobia. Rev Bras Psiquiatr 2004; 26: 77–81
65. Bögels, S., WP, & Sallaerts, S. Analytic psychotherapy versus cognitive-behavioral therapy for social phobia. Paper presented at European Congress for Cognitive and Behavioural Therapies, September 2003, Prague.
66. Crits-Christoph, P., Connolly Gibbons, M. B., Narducci, J., Schamberger, M., & Gallop, R. Interpersonal problems and the outcome of interpersonally oriented psychodynamic treatment of GAD. Psychotherapy: Theory, Research, Practice, Training 2005; 42: 211–24.
67. Leichsenring, F., Winkelbach, C., & Leibing, E. Short-term psychodynamic psychotherapy and cognitive-behavioral therapy in generalized anxiety disorder: A randomized controlled study. 2008 (unpublished manuscript).
68. Wiborg, I. M. & Dahl, A. A. Does brief dynamic psychotherapy reduce the relapse rate of panic disorder? Arch Gen Psychiatry 1996; 53: 689–94.
69. Jenike, M. A. Obsessive-compulsive disorder. N Engl J Med 2004; 3; 350: 259–65.
70. Kuzma, J. M. & Black, D. W. Integrating pharmacotherapy and psychotherapy in the management of anxiety disorders. Curr Psychiatry Rep 2004; 6: 268–73.
71. Brom, D., Kleber, R. J., & Defares, P. B. Brief psychotherapy for posttraumatic stress disorders. J Consult Clin Psychol 1989; 57: 607–12.
72. Creed, F., Fernandes, L., Guthrie, E., Palmer, S., Ratcliffe, J., Read, N., Rigby, C., Thompson, D., & Tomenson, B., & North of England IBS Research Group. The cost-effectiveness of psychotherapy and paroxetine for severe irritable bowel syndrome. Gastroenterology 2003; 124: 303–17.
73. Monsen, K. & Monsen, T. J. Chronic pain and psychodynamic body therapy. Psychotherapy 2000; 37: 257–69.
74. Fairburn, C., Kirk, J., O'Connor, M., & Cooper, P. J. A comparison of two psychological treatments for bulimia nervosa. Behav Res Ther 1986; 24: 629–43.
75. Fairburn, C., Norman, P. A., Welch, S. L., O'Connor, M. E., Doll, H. A., & Peveler, R. C. A prospective study of outcome in bulimia nervosa and the long-term effects of three psychological treatments. Arch Gen Psychiatry 1995; 52: 304–12.
76. Bachar, E., Latzer, Y., Kreitler, S., & Berry, E. M. Empirical comparison of two psychological therapies. Self psychology and cognitive orientation in the treatment of anorexia and bulimia. J Psychother Pract Res 1999; 8: 115–28.
77. Fairburn, C. G. Evidence-based treatment of anorexia nervosa. Int J Eat Disord 2005; 37 (Suppl): 26–30.

78. Gowers, D., Norton, K., Halek, C., & Vrisp, A. H. Outcome of outpatient psychotherapy in a random allocation treatment study of anorexia nervosa. Int J Eat Disord 1994; 15: 165–77.
79. Dare, C. Psychoanalytic psychotherapy (of eating disorders). In: Gabbard, G. O., ed. Treatment of psychiatric disorders. Washington, DC: American Psychiatric Press; 1995: 2129–51.
80. Munroe-Blum, H. & Marziali, E. A controlled trial of short-term group treatment for borderline personality disorder. J Personal Disord 1995; 9: 190–8.
81. Bateman, A. & Fonagy, P. The effectiveness of partial hospitalization in the treatment of borderline personality disorder: A randomized controlled trial. Am J Psychiatry 1999; 156: 1563–69.
82. Bateman, A. & Fonagy, P. Treatment of borderline personality disorder with psycho-analytically oriented partial hospitalization: An 18-month follow-up. Am J Psychiatry 2001; 158: 36–42.
83. Giesen-Bloo, J., van Dyck, R., Spinhoven, P., van Tilburg, W., Dirksen, C., van Asselt, T. , Kremers, I., Nadort, M., & Arntz, A. Outpatient psychotherapy for borderline person-ality disorder: Randomized trial of schema-focused therapy vs transference-focused psychotherapy. Arch Gen Psychiatry 2006; 63: 649–58.
84. Luborsky, L., Diguer, L. Seligman, D. A, Rosenthal, R., Krause, E. D., Johnson, S., Halperin, G., Bishop, M., Berman, J. S., Schweizer, E. The researcher's own allegiances: A 'wild' card in comparison of treatment efficacy. Clin Psychol: Sci Pract 1999; 6: 95–106.
85. Clarkin, J. F., Levy, K. N., Lenzenweger, M. F., & Kernberg, O. F. The Personality Disorders Institute/Borderline Personality Disorder Research Foundation randomized control trial for borderline personality disorder: Rationale, methods, and patient char-acteristics. J Personal Disord 2004; 18: 52–72.
86. Clarkin, J. F., Levy, K. N., Lenzenweger, M. F., & Kernberg, O. F. The Personality Disorders Institute/Borderline Personality Disorder Research Foundation randomized control trial for borderline personality disorder. Am J Psychiatry 2007; 164: 922–928.
87. Levy, K. N., Meehan, K. B., Kelly, K. M., Reynoso, J. S., Weber, M., Clarkin, J. F., & Kernberg, O. F.. Change in attachment patterns and reflective functioning in a rando-mized controlled trial of transference-focused psychotherapy for borderline personality disorder. J Consult Clin Psychol 2006; 74: 1027–40.
88. Leichsenring, F. & Leibing, E. The effectiveness of psychodynamic psychotherapy and cognitive-behavioral therapy in personality disorders: A meta-analysis. Am J Psychiatry 2003; 160: 1223–32.
89. Svartberg, M., Stiles, T., & Seltzer, M. H. Randomized, controlled trial of the effective-ness of short-term dynamic psychotherapy and cognitive therapy for Cluster C person-ality disorders. Am J Psychiatry 2004; 161: 810–7.
90. Muran, J. C., Safran, J. D., Samstag, L. W., & Winston, A. Evaluating an alliance-focused treatment for personality disorders. Psychother Theory, Res, Pract, Train 2005; 42: 532–45.
91. Horowitz, L. M., Alden, L., Wiggins, J. S., & Pincus, A. L. Inventory of interpersonal problems. New York: The Psychological Cooperation; 2000.
92. Emmelkamp, P., Benner, A., Kuipers, A., Feiertag, G. A., Koster, H. C, & van Appeld-dorn, F. J. Comparison of brief dynamic and cognitive-behavioral therapies in avoidant personality disorder. Br J Psychiatry 2006; 189: 60–4.
93. Leichsenring, F. & Leibing, E. Fair play, please! Br J Psychiatry 2007; 190: 80.
94. Woody, G., Luborsky, L., McLellan, A. T., O'Brien, C. P., Beck, A. T., Blaine, Herman, I, & Hole, A. Psychotherapy for opiate addicts: Does it help? Arch Gen Psychiatry 1983; 40: 639–45.
95. Woody, G., Luborsky, L., McLellan, A. T, & O'Brien, C. P. Corrections and revised analyses for psychotherapy in methadone maintenance patients. Arch Gen Psychiatry 1990; 47: 788–9.

96. Woody, G., Luborsky, L., McLellan, A. T., & O'Brien, C. P. Psychotherapy in community methadone programs: A validation study. Am J Psychiatry 1995; 152: 1302–8.
97. Crits-Christoph, P., SL, McCalmont, E., Weiss, R. D., Gastfriend, D. R., Frank, A., Moras, K., Barber, J. P., Blaine, J., & Thase, M. E. Impact of psychosocial treatments on associated problems of cocaine-dependent patients. J Consult Clin Psychol 2001; 69: 825–30.
98. Crits-Christoph, P., SL, Blaine, J., Frank, A., Luborsky, L., Onken, L. S., Muenz, L. R., Thase, M. E., Weiss, R. D., Gastfriend, D. R., Woody, G. E., Barber, J. P., Butler, S. F., Daley, D., Salloum, I., Bishop, S., Najavits, L. M., Lis, J., Mercer, D., Griffin, M. L., Moras, K., & Beck, A. T. Psychosocial treatments for cocaine dependence: National Institute on Drug Abuse Collaborative Cocaine Treatment Study. Arch Gen Psychiatry 1999; 56: 493–502.
99. Sandahl, C., Herlitz, K., Ahlin, G., & Rönnberg, S. Time-limited group psychotherapy for moderately alcohol dependent patients: A randomized controlled clinical trial. Psychother Res 1998; 8: 361–78.
100. de Maat, S., Dekker, J., Schoevers, R., & de Jonghe, F. The effectivenss of long-term psychotherapy: Methodological research issues. Psychother Res 2006; 17: 59–65.
101. Krupnick, J., Sotsky, S. M., Simmens, S., Moyer, J., Elkin, I., Watkins, J., & Pilkonis, P. The role of the therapeutic alliance in psychotherapy and pharmacotherapy outcome: Findings in the National Institute of Mental Health Treatment of Depression Collaborative Research Program. J Consult Clin Psychol 1996; 64: 532–9.
102. Cohen, J. Statistical power analysis for the behavioral sciences. Hillsdale, NJ: Lawrence Erlbaum; 1988.
103. Kazis, L. E., AJ, & Meenan, R. F. Effect sizes for interpreting changes in health status. Med Care 1989; 27 (3 Suppl): S178–89.
104. Dührssen, A. & Jorswieck, E. Eine empirisch-statistische Untersuchung zur Leistungsfähigkeit psychoanalytischer Behandlung [An empirical-statistical study of the effectiveness of psychoanalytic treatment]. Nervenarzt 1965; 36: 166–9.
105. Rudolf, G., Dilg, R., Grande, T., Jakobsen, Th., Keller, W., Krawietz, B., Langer, M., Stehle, S., & Oberbracht, C. Effektivität und Effizienz psychoanalytischer Langzeittherapie: Die Praxisstudie Analytische Langzeitpsychotherapie [Effectiveness and efficiency of long-term psychoanalytic therapy: The practice study of long-term psychoanalytic therapy]. In: Gerlach, A., Springer, A., & Schlösser, A., eds. Psychoanalyse des Glaubens. Gießen: Psychosozial Verlag; 2004.
106. Leichsenring, F., Biskup, J., Kreische, R., & Staats, H. The effectiveness of psychoanalytic therapy. First results of the "Göttingen study of of psychoanalytic and psychodynamic therapy". Int J Psychoanal 2005; 86: 433–55.
107. Luborsky, L., Stuart, J., Friedman, S., Diguer, L., Seligman, D. A., Bucci, W., Pulver, S., Krause, E. D., Ermold, J., Davison, W. T., Woody, G., Mergenthaler, E. The Penn Psychoanalytic Treatment Collection: A set of complete and recorded psychoanalyses as a research resource. J Am Psychoanal Assoc 2001; 49: 217–34.
108. Rudolf, G., Manz, R., & Öri, C. Ergebnisse psychoanalytischer Therapie [Outcome of psychoanalytic therapy]. Z Psychosom Med Psychother, 1994; 40: 25–40.
109. Sandell, R., BJ, Lazar, A., Carlsson, J., Broberg, J., & Schubert, J. Varieties of long-term outcome among patients in psychoanalysis and long-term psychotherapy. A review of findings in the Stockholm Outcome of Psychoanalysis and Psychotherapy Project (STOPP). Int J Psychoanal 2000; 81: 921–42.
110. Brockmann, J., Schlüter, T., & Eckert, J. Die Frankfurt-Hamburg Langzeit-Psychotherapiestudie – Ergebnisse der Untersuchung psychoanalytisch orientierter und verhaltenstherapeutischer Langzeit-Psychotherapien in der Praxis niedergelassener Psychotherapeuten [The Frankfurt-Hamburg study of psychotherapy – results of the study of psychoanalytically oriented und behavioral long-term therapy]. In: Stuhr, U., ML-B, & Beutel, M., eds. Langzeit-Psychotherapie Perspektiven für Therapeuten und Wissenschaftler. Stuttgart, Germany: Kohlhammer; 2001: 271–6.

111. Sandell, R., Blomberg, J., & Lazar, A. Wiederholte Langzeitkatamnesen von Langzeitp-sychotherapien und Psychoanalysen. Z Psychosom Med Psychother 1999; 45: 43–56.
112. Jakobsen, T., Brockmann, J., Grande, T., Huber, D., Klug, G., Keller, W., Rudolf, G., Schlüter, T., Staats, H., & Leichsenring, F. Ergebnisse analytischer Langzeitpsychother-apien: Verbesserungen in Symptomatik und interpersonellen Beziehungen bei spezi-fischen Störungen [Results of psychoanalytic therapy: Improvements in symptoms and interpersonal relations in specific mental disorders]. Z Psychosom Med Psychother 2007; 53: 87–110.
113. Sandell, R., Blomberg, J., Lazar, A., Carlsson, J., Broberg, J., & Schubert, J. Unterschie-dliche Langzeitergebnisse von Psychoanalysen und Langzeitpsychotherapien. Aus der Forschung des Stockholmer Psychoanalyse- und Psychotherapieprojekts. Psyche 2001; 55: 273–310.
114. Grande, T., Dilg, R., Jakobsen, T., Keller, W., Krawietz, B., Langer, M., Oberbracht, C., Stehle, S., Stennes, M., & Rudolf, G. Differential effects of two forms of psychoanalytic therapy: results of the Heidelberg-Berlin study. Psychother Res 2006; 16: 470–85.
115. Huber, D., Klug, G., & von Rad, M. Die Münchner-Prozess-Outcome Studie: Ein Vergleich zwischen Psychoanalysen und psychodynamischen Psychotherapien unter besonderer Berücksichtigung therapiespezifischer Ergebnisse [The München process-outcome study. A comparison between psychoanalyses and psychother-apy]. In: Stuhr, U., ML-B, & Beutel, M., eds. Langzeit- Psychotherapie Perspek-tiven für Therapeuten und Wissenschaftler. Stuttgart, Germany: Kohlhammer; 2001: 260–70.
116. Knekt, P. & Lindfors, O., eds. A randomized trial of the effect of four forms of psychotherapy on depressive and anxiety disorders. Studies in social security and health, 77. Helsinki: Edita Prima, Ltd; 2004.
117. Crits-Christoph, P. & C, B. Alliance and technique in short-term dynamic therapy. Clin Psychol Rev 1999; 6: 687–704.
118. Messer, S. B. What makes brief psychodynamic therapy time efficient. Clin Psychol 2001; 8: 5–22.
119. Messer, S. B., Tishby, O., & Spillman, A. Taking context seriously in psychotherapy research: Relating therapist interventions to patient progress in brief psychodynamic therapy. J Consult Clin Psychol 1992; 60: 678–88.
120. Barber, J. P., Crits-Christoph, P., & Luborsky, L. Effects of therapist adherence and compe-tence on patient outcome in brief dynamic therapy. J Consult Clin Psychol 1996; 64: 619–22.
121. Connolly, M. B., Crits-Christoph, P., Shappell, S., Barber, J. P., Luborsky, L., & Shaffer, C. Relation of transference interpretation to outcome in the early sessions of brief supportive-expressive psychotherapy. Psychother Res, 1999; 9: 485–95
122. Hoglend, P. & P, W. E. Focal adherence in brief dynamic psychotherapy: A comparison of findings from two independent studies. Psychother Res, 1995; 32: 618–28.
123. Ogrodniczuk, J. S., Piper, W. E., Joyce, A. S., & McCallum, M. Transference inter-pretations in short-term dynamic psychotherapy. J Nerv Ment Dis 1999; 187: 572–9.
124. Ogrodniczuk, J. S. & Piper, W. E. Use of transference interpretations in dynamically orientied individual psychotherapy for patients with personality disorders. J Personal Disord 1999; 13: 297–311.
125. Piper, W. E., Azim, H. F. A., Joyce, A. S., & McCallum, M. Transference interpreta-tions, therapeutic alliance, and outcome in short-term individual psychotherapy. Arch Gen Psychiatry 1991; 48: 946–53.
126. Piper, W. E., Azim, H. F. A., Joyce, A. S., McCallum, M., Nixon, G. W. H., & Segal, P. S. Quality of object relations verus interpersonal functioning as predictors of therapeutic alliance and psychotherapy outcome. J Nerv Ment Dis 1991; 179: 432–8.
127. Barber, J. P., Connolly, M. B., Crits-Christoph, P., Gladis, L., & Siqueland, L. Alliance predicts patients outcome beyond in-treatment change in symptoms. J Consult Clin Psychol 2000; 68: 1027–32.

128. Stiles, W. B., A-DR, Hardy, G. E., Barkham, M., & Shapiro, D. A. Relations of the alliance with psychotherapy outcome: Findings in the second Sheffield Psychotherapy Project. J Consult Clin Psychol 1998; 66: 791–802.
129. Beutler, L., Malik, M., Alomohamed, S., Harwood, T.M., Talebi, H., Noble, S., & Wong, E. Therapist variables. In: Lambert, M., ed. Bergin and Garfield's handbook of psychotherapy and behavior change, 5th ed. New York: Wiley 2004: 227–306.
130. Horvath, A. O. The therapeutic relationship, research and theory. An introduction to the special issue. Psychother Res 2005; 15: 3–7.
131. Crits-Christoph, P., Barber, J. P., & Kurcias, J. The accuracy of therapists interpretations and the development of the therapeutic alliance. Psychother Res 1993; 3: 25–35.
132. Crits-Christoph, P. & L, L. Changes in CCRT pervasiveness during psychotherapy. In: LL & Crits-Christoph, P., eds. Understanding transference: The CCRT method. New York: Basic Books; 1990: 133–46.
133. Piper, W. E., OJ, McCallum, M., Joyce, A. S., Rosie, J. S. Expression of affect as a mediator of the relationship between quality of object relations and group therapy outcome for patients with complicated grief. J Consult Clin Psychol 2003; 71: 664–71.
134. Hoglend, P. Suitability for brief dynamic psychotherapy: Psychodynamic variables as predictors of outcome. Acta Psychiatr Scand 1993; 88: 104–10.
135. Barber, J. P., Luborsky, L., Gallop, R., Crits-Christoph, P., Frank, A., Weiss, R. D., Thase, M. E., Connolly, M. B., Gladis, M., Foltz, C., & Siqueland, L. Therapeutic alliance as a predictor of outcome and retention in the National Institute on Drug Abuse Collaborative Cocaine Treatment Study. J Consult Clin Psychol 2001; 69: 119–24.
136. Ablon, S. & Jones, E. Validity of controlled cinical trials of psychotherapy: Findings from the NIMH Treatment of Depression Collaborative Research Program. Am J Psychiatry 2002; 159: 775–83.
137. Blagys, M. & H, MJ. Distinctive features of short-term psychodynamic-interpersonal psychotherapy: A review of the comparative psychotherapy process literature. Clin Psychol Sci Pract 2000; 7: 167–88.
138. Task, Procedures Task Force on Promotion and Dissemination of Psychological Procedures. Training and dissemination of empirically-validated psychological treatments. Report and recommendations. Clin Psychol 1995; 48: 3–23.
139. Leichsenring, F., Rabung, S., & Leibing, E. The efficacy of short-term psychodynamic therapy in specific psychiatric disorders: A meta-analysis. Arch Gen Psychiatry 2004; 61: 1208–16.
140. Siefert, C. J., Defife, J. A., Baity, M. R. Process measures for psychodynamic psychotherapy. In: Levy, R. A. & Ablon, J. S., eds. A handbook of evidence-based psychodynamic psychotherapy. Totowa, NJ: Humana Press; 2008.

# Chapter 2
# Psychodynamic Treatment of Panic Disorder

## Clinical and Research Assessment

Frederic N. Busch and Barbara Milrod

## Introduction

Both pharmacological [1–3] and cognitive-behavioral treatments [4–6] of panic disorder have been found to be effective in treatment. Despite this progress, not all patients respond or are able to tolerate these treatments [4–8]. Relapse is frequent if medication is discontinued before a prolonged maintenance phase [9–12]. Questions remain about the long-term effectiveness of these interventions [4, 13]. In studies of "routine care," generally a poorly defined mix, patients frequently demonstrate persistent symptoms and problems functioning [14]. Little systematic data are available about whether or not these treatments are effective in treating impairments associated with panic disorder, such as occupational dysfunction, relationship difficulties, and diminished quality of life [15, 16]. Given the high morbidity and health costs of this disorder [17–20], it is important to continue to develop the most effective treatments for panic disorder and its related impairments.

Psychodynamic psychotherapy has been a commonly practiced, but poorly studied intervention for panic disorder. The potential value of this treatment is based on the notion that panic patients have a psychological vulnerability to the disorder associated with personality disturbances, relationship problems, difficulties tolerating and defining inner emotional experiences, unconscious conflicts about separation and autonomy, negative emotions such as rage at important loved ones, and conflicted aspects of sexuality. Theoretically,

---

Portions of this chapter are reprinted with permission from Busch FN. Psychodynamic treatment of panic disorder. Prim Psychiatry 2006;13(5):61–66.

Figs 2.1 and 2.2, and Tables 2.1 and 2.2 are reprinted with permission from the American Journal of Psychiatry (Copyright 2007), American Psychiatric Publishing, Inc. from Milrod B, Busch F, Leon AC, et al.: A randomized controlled clinical trial of psychoanalytic psychotherapy for panic disorder. Am J Psychiatry 2007; 164(2):265–272.

F.N. Busch
New York Presbyterian Hospital/Weill Cornell, 10 East 78th Street Apt. 5A, New York, NY 10021, USA
e-mail: FNB80@aol.com

R.A. Levy, J.S. Ablon (eds.), *Handbook of Evidence-Based Psychodynamic Psychotherapy*,     29
DOI: 10.1007/978-1-59745-444-5_2, © Humana Press 2009

psychodynamic treatments could have a greater impact on psychosocial impairment associated with panic, as cognitive-behavioral and psychopharmacological treatments do not focus on this domain. This might in theory lead to a reduction in vulnerability to panic recurrence [21]. The limited research on psychodynamic treatment of panic disorder is described below.

Psychodynamic concepts as they relate to panic disorder will be outlined, followed by a psychodynamic formulation that weaves together neurophysiological and psychological vulnerabilities to panic. Our research group developed this psychodynamic formulation for panic disorder based on psychodynamic theory, systematic psychological assessments, and clinical observations to guide treatment interventions [21–23]. The theory and interventions were used to develop a manualized description of a approach to panic disorder, panic-focused psychodynamic psychotherapy (PFPP) [23], to be employed for clinical and research purposes.

## Psychodynamic Concepts in Panic Disorder

### The Unconscious

According to psychoanalytic theory, symptoms are based at least in part on unconscious fantasies, conflicts, and affects [24]. For instance, clinical and research observations suggest that panic patients have particular difficulty with angry feelings and fantasies toward close attachment figures, such as wishes for revenge [22, 23, 25]. These wishes are felt to represent a threat to attachment figures, which triggers overwhelming anxiety. Oftentimes patients are not fully aware of the intensity of these affects, or of the vengeful fantasies that accompany them. Becoming conscious of these aspects of mental life and rendering them less threatening are important components of psychodynamic psychotherapy for panic disorder.

### Defense Mechanisms

Fantasies and affects that are experienced as dangerous can be avoided through the triggering of defense mechanisms, unconscious mental processes that disguise the fantasies or render them inaccessible to consciousness [26]. Clinical and research observations indicate that panic patients employ particular defenses: reaction formation, undoing, and denial [27]. Reaction formation and undoing play a particular role for panic patients, in that they often unconsciously attempt to convert angry affects to more affiliative ones, diminishing the threat to an attachment figure. In reaction formation, a threatening feeling is replaced by its opposite; oftentimes in panic patients negative feelings are replaced by concern and efforts to help others. In undoing, an unconscious negative affect or fantasy is typically taken back in some way. Denial represents a nonrecognition of the presence of a particular feeling, conflict, or fantasy, such as a patient reporting he was not angry even after someone had done something hurtful to him. In a psychoanalytic treatment, it is helpful to bring these defenses to the patient's attention, as they maintain the patient's avoidance of the emotions that give rise to physiological symptoms. For instance, a patient who follows the statement "I hate him" by "But I really love him," an example of undoing, is often trying to avoid the intensity of his angry feelings.

## Compromise Formation

From a psychoanalytic perspective, psychic symptoms represent a compromise between a conflicted wish and the defense against that wish [24]. Teasing apart the components of this compromise formation can help to elucidate the meaning of the symptom and unconscious elements that trigger it. Thus panic symptoms can include the wish to be dependent and cared for, a denial of negative aspects of core relationships through a focus on anxiety or bodily symptoms, as well as an unconscious expression of anger in the coercive pressure on others to help. Psychoanalytic theory also considers fantasies and dreams, as well as central aspects of people's choices, such as career and sexual partners, to be influenced by compromise formations, encapsulating both wishes and defenses.

For example, Busch et al. [28] describe an 18-year-old girl who had the onset of panic while driving to her eighteenth birthday party celebration. She became unable to drive and had to wait several hours to be picked up by her mother. It emerged in psychotherapy that she associated this birthday with her "independence," and an associated wish to rid herself of her parents and siblings, with whom she was intensely furious. The panic attack was a compromise between several wishes and defenses. It represented her conflicted wish for autonomy in that a heretofore basic skill, driving by herself, was rendered impossible due to intrusion of terrifying fantasies of danger and her own fantasized inadequacy. In addition, her murderous wishes were guiltily redirected toward herself: she was now immobilized and helpless. Panic became a punishment for her aggressive fantasies of autonomy, by tying her evermore to her frustrating family.

## Self and Object Representations

In systematic assessments, patients with panic disorder have been found to have views of their parents as controlling, temperamental, and critical [29, 30]. These become internalized expectations of others' behavior. In addition, because of their temperamental predisposition to fearfulness, panic patients often view others as being essential to their safety and well-being. Recognizing these perceptions of the experience between self and others can help patients understand the irrational dangers they perceive in their relationships.

## Traumatic and Signal Anxiety

Freud distinguished between two types of anxiety: "traumatic" and "signal" anxiety [31]. In traumatic anxiety, related to panic attacks, the ego is overwhelmed by threats from internal dangers. Signal anxiety, on the contrary, can be viewed as an appraisal system in which small doses of anxiety alert the ego to psychologically meaningful dangers, such as potential disruptions in attachment, or threats that might be expected to be experienced from vengeful feelings. Signal anxiety can trigger defenses that act unconsciously to ward off potential dangers. In PFPP, the therapist helps the patient to reappraise the degree of actual danger he is in based on reality, rather than on compelling fantasies.

## Transference

In the course of treatment, conflicts that the patient experiences with others will necessarily reemerge in some form in the relationship the patient develops with the therapist. For example, a panic patient may feel that the therapist would not be able to tolerate her anger and become judgmental or rejecting. This phenomenon, referred to as transference, can provide essential, direct access to intrapsychic conflicts and self and object representations that underlie panic symptoms. The therapist is active in utilizing aspects of the emergence of the transference to help the patient to better grasp his central conflicts.

## Psychodynamic Formulation for Panic Disorder

Busch et al. [21] and Shear et al. [22] developed a psychodynamic formulation for panic disorder based on neurophysiologic predispositions, psychological findings, and psychoanalytic theory. The formulation posits that certain individuals are susceptible to the onset of panic disorder due to a predisposition to anxiety, associated with a fearful temperament described by Kagan et al. [32]. Because of their anxiety, children with this predisposition tend to develop a fearful dependency on others, feeling that parents must be present at all times to provide a sense of safety. In addition, the dependency on others is a narcissistic humiliation for these children, because feelings of safety often require the caregiver's presence. This fearful dependency can develop from a biochemical vulnerability, or from the experience of inadequate and/or traumatic early relationships with significant others, usually parents or other caregivers. In either case, significant others are perceived as "unreliable," prone to abandoning and rejecting the child.

In response to perceived rejection or unavailability, and due to the narcissistic injury of dependency, the child becomes angry at his close attachment figures. This anger is experienced as dangerous, as the associated fantasies could potentially damage the relationship with the people upon whom the child depends, increasing the threat of loss and fearful dependency. Thus, a vicious cycle of fearful dependency and anger can occur. The vicious cycle gets triggered again in adulthood, when the individual experiences or perceives a threat to the integrity of important attachment relationships. Signal anxiety and defenses are triggered, such as undoing, reaction formation and denial, in an attempt to reduce the threat from whatever anger the patient actually experiences. Due to the degree of threat and disorganization engendered by these fantasies, as well as immaturity of the signal anxiety mechanism, the ego becomes overwhelmed and panic levels of anxiety result. Panic attacks further avert conscious acknowledgement of anger and compel attention from others.

This formulation of the origins of fearful dependency is based on limited current knowledge. Although it has been of clinical value in the development of PFPP, further elucidation is necessary to determine the ways in which neurophysiological factors interact with psychological vulnerabilities to panic onset [33]. Gorman et al. [34], for example, describe an oversensitive fear network, with a central role played by the amygdala, stimulation of which has been found to produce panic-like reactions in animals. The amygdala receives input from brainstem structures and the sensory thalamus, pathways likely involved in immediate responses to danger, and cortical regions, which allow for slower processing of data. The authors suggest that psychotherapy may act by increasing the impact of cortical projections over automatic panic responses. Alternatively, Panksepp [35] focuses on a brain PANIC system, linked to separation distress and attachment, with a circuitry that partially overlaps with that described by Gorman et al. [33]. Additional studies (e.g., [36–39]) are providing data to further delineate the neurophysiology of panic and elucidate the relationship between the danger response and attachment systems in the brain and psychological factors.

Relatively recent developments in psychoanalytic theory suggest another component of the process of panic onset and persistence. Mentalization describes the ability to understand oneself and others with regard to motives, desires, and feelings [40]. Panic patients may experience a diminished capacity for aspects of mentalization as regards their anxiety. Rudden et al. [41] have noted a specific lack of access to feelings and fantasies surrounding panic experiences. This lack of mentalization reflects patients' capacity to deny or unconsciously block access to frightening areas of intrapsychic conflict. Greater introspective access to these fantasies and emotional states helps to relieve these dangers.

## Panic-Focused Psychodynamic Psychotherapy

PFPP is a specific manualized form of psychoanalytic psychotherapy [23] that has been subjected to clinical trials and has been found to be efficacious [42]. As opposed to more traditional open-ended psychodynamic psychotherapy and psychoanalysis, PFPP focuses on panic symptoms and the dynamics associated with panic disorder. Material in the sessions other than panic symptomatology is ultimately connected to the dynamics of panic. The treatment follows the overall course of identifying the meanings of panic symptoms, calling attention to defenses that inhibit awareness of panic-specific disavowed feelings, conflicts, and fantasies, and, once made conscious, rendering these feelings less threatening or toxic. Psychoanalytic techniques of clarification, confrontation, and interpretation are employed in this process. Unlike more structured manualized therapies for panic disorder, the three phases of PFPP (Fig. 2.1) are not necessarily sequential, and may occupy differing amounts of time between patients. In outcome studies that have been conducted thus far, PFPP is a twice weekly, 12 week (24 session) time-limited psychotherapy.

### *Phase I*

In phase I of PFPP, the therapist works to identify the specific content and meanings of the panic episodes. In addition, patient and therapist examine the stressors and feelings surrounding the onset and persistence of panic attacks. The patient's developmental history is reviewed to delineate specific vulnerabilities that may have led to panic onset, such as particular representations of parents, traumatic experiences, and difficulty expressing and managing angry feelings. The therapist's nonjudgmental stance aids the patient in articulating fantasies and feelings that may have been unconscious or difficult to tolerate, such as vengeful wishes or abandonment fears. The information is used to identify the presence of intrapsychic conflicts surrounding anger, personal autonomy development, and sexuality. The goal of this phase is reduction in panic symptoms.

### *Phase II*

Phase II seeks to address the dynamics that lead the patient to be vulnerable to panic onset and persistence. As noted, these typically include conflicts surrounding anger recognition and management, ambivalence about autonomy, fears of loss or abandonment (i.e., separation anxiety), and conflicted aspects of sexual excitement. These dynamics are addressed as they emerge in the patient's feelings and fantasies about relationships in their present and past, and in the transference relationship that develops with the therapist. The meanings of symptoms and the employment of defenses also continue to play a role in

**Description of Panic-Focused**
**Psychodynamic Psychotherapy**
**Phase I: Acute Panic:** Panic symptoms carry psychological
meanings and panic-focused psychodynamic psychotherapy
works to uncover unconscious meanings to achieve relief.
Format:
A. Initial evaluation and early treatment:
1) Exploration of circumstances/feelings surrounding
panic onset.
2) Exploration of personal meanings of panic symptoms.
3) Exploration of feelings/content of panic episodes.
B. Common psychodynamic conflicts in panic disorder:
1) Separation and autonomy.
2) Anger recognition; management, and coping with expression.
C. Expected responses to phase I:
1) Panic relief.
2) Reduced agoraphobia.
**Phase II: Panic Vulnerability:** To lessen vulnerability to
panic, core unconscious conflicts must be understood and altered.
These conflicts are often approached through the transference.
Strategy:
A. Addressing the transference.
B. Working through—demonstration that the same conflict
emerges in many settings.
C. Expected responses to phase II:
1) Improved relationships.
2) Less conflicted and anxious experience of separation,
anger, and sexuality.
3) Reduced panic recurrence.
**Phase III: Termination:** Termination permits re-experiencing
of conflicts directly with the therapist so that underlying
feelings are articulated. Patient reaction to termination must
be addressed for minimally the final third (1 month).
A. Re-experiencing central separation and anger themes in
the transference with termination.
Expected responses:
1) Possible temporary recrudescence of symptoms as
feelings are experienced in therapy.
2) New ability to manage separations and autonomy.

**Fig. 2.1** Description of panic-focused psychodynamic psychotherapy

identifying underlying dynamisms. Improved understanding of these conflicts
helps to interrupt the vicious cycle described above, reducing vulnerability to
panic recurrence.

## *Phase III*

The termination phase provides an opportunity to work with the patient's
conflicts about anger and personal autonomy as they emerge in the context of
ending treatment. Patients are actively helped to focus on the experience, and to
articulate their feelings about loss directly with the therapist. Increased awareness and understanding allows for better management of these feelings and the
capacity to avert the development of more severe panic states. An ability to

express anger in ways that feel less threatening is often an important development of the treatment. Increased assertiveness and the capacity to communicate about conflicts in relationships improve psychosocial function and reduce panic vulnerability.

## Treatment Indications

Psychodynamic psychotherapy has typically been thought to be indicated for patients who enter treatment with a particular set of qualities: verbally skilled, psychologically minded, and curious about the origins of their symptoms. These qualities are identical with the qualities that have often been described as being good prognostic indicators for psychoanalysis [43]. Panic patients, however, with their tendency to experience conflicts and affects in their bodies, have limited verbal access to their intrapsychic life and may be frightened to pursue underlying emotional origins of their problems. In our studies, we have found that patients without these skills regularly obtain relief of symptoms from PFPP [44, 45].

## Engaging the Patient

Several factors enable PFPP to work as a short-term treatment, and as an intervention that can help people with little exposure to psychotherapy. In early sessions the therapist focuses on exploring the circumstances and feelings preceding panic onset. This is usually what preoccupies patients most as they start their therapy. Patients become engaged in treatment as they begin to recognize the relationship between their symptoms, the circumstances in which symptoms began, their feelings surrounding panic, and their developmental history.

Ms. A was a 43-year-old married woman with two children who described the onset of panic attacks 1 month prior to consultation. She presented with primary *Diagnostic and Statistical Manual of Mental Disorders* (DSM)-IV panic disorder and mild depressive symptoms not meeting criteria for a specific disorder. She recalled a series of panic attacks just after leaving home for college, but these had resolved spontaneously. At first, Ms. A described her panic as having emerged out of the blue. However, on exploration, the therapist learned that the initial panic attack occurred after an intense conflict with her 15-year-old daughter, the older of two siblings. Ms. A struggled with how to manage her daughter and saw herself as unable to set limits. She experienced limit setting as "too mean." Ms. A quickly grasped that her panic was likely related to these conflicts. She brought up that she was "not very assertive" and always had difficulty confronting others.

Following this initial link of the onset of symptoms to family conflicts, Ms. A became very curious about the sources of her problems. The discussion about her daughter reminded her of her difficulties with her alcoholic father, who was often explosively enraged. The therapist wondered if Ms. A had been frightened of expressing any disagreement with him.

Ms. A responded: "Yes, I think I was scared of that. I'm always trying to be nice to people. I think that will get them to like me. But I'm not sure that it's really helping my daughter to do that." Ms. A was describing reaction formation, in which her anger toward others was converted into becoming "too nice." She then noted: "I realize I should be setting better limits. Yesterday when I stood my ground with her I felt so much better."

This information, presented in the first two sessions of Ms. A's treatment, already provided valuable insights into the origins of her panic disorder: the conflict with her daughter, difficulties with her management of limit setting, and her fears of getting angry, and engaged her interest in exploring the symptoms further.

## The Transference

As treatment progresses, the therapist has more opportunities to explore conflicts as they emerge in the transference. Oftentimes, these occur in the context of angry feelings or separation fears from the therapist.

In a later session, Ms. A complained about an incident with her daughter, in which her daughter had demanded that her family wait for an extended period until she was ready to leave on a family outing. Although the therapist explored the tensions with her daughter in his usual manner, Ms. A left feeling the therapist was unsupportive and viewed her as a "bad mother." She became anxious after the session. That evening she asked her husband to comfort her, but he responded that he had had a stressful day and wanted to read the paper. At that point, she had a panic attack. In the following session, therapist and patient were able to determine that she was quite angry at her therapist and her husband, and that her discomfort with being angry at people she depended on triggered the attack.

## Working Through and Termination

Working through involves identifying the presence of central conflicts in various areas of the patient's life, allowing increased understanding of the ramifications of these central, organizing unconscious conflicts.

For instance, Ms. A realized her unassertiveness was organized around several central developmental experiences: fear of her temperamental father, fear of her sister who was more aggressive and bolder than she, and identification with her mother, who was also unassertive and never confronted her father about problems. Each of these formative developmental situations helped to elucidate the patient's worry that asserting herself would lead to disruptions in her relationships. She felt that being the "nice girl" maintained others' interest in her and was the only way to keep her attachments safe.

As she became more aware of some of the fantasies underlying her fears, Ms. A became more active in "testing" her concerns and behaviors with others. The impact of the shift toward better limit setting with her daughter, and a continued firmer stance on her part, led to a reduction in her daughter's temper tantrums and demanding expectations of her. Ms. A realized that she similarly yielded to her mother's and sister's demands and expectations. She recognized that rather than obtaining the caring and concern she sought, "being nice," allowed others to continue to behave toward her in demanding and hurtful ways. Increased comfort with her anger allowed Ms. A to recognize that her mother was "not a nice person," something that had been difficult for her to tolerate without feeling guilty and anxious. Her criticisms included that her mother was often self-centered, with little actual interest in Ms. A's children.
One day when her sister called and stated in her typical manner: "Mom needs someone to go to the doctor today and I'm working," Ms. A did not respond with her usual ready agreement, but stated that she had plans and could not go. Her sister reacted angrily and hung up on her. Initially Ms. A felt guilty. When her guilt was explored in therapy, it emerged that she feared her anger would damage others in a significant way. And yet she knew that her mother would make some other arrangement to get to the doctor. As her guilt was discussed more openly in therapy, Ms. A felt relieved, freer, and less anxious about being more assertive. She became increasingly aware of her reflexive tendency to be "too nice" and became more assertive in most of her relationships.

Termination provides an important opportunity for examining central conflicts underlying panic directly with the therapist. Anger and fear of losing the relationship with the therapist often intensify at this point, highlighting conflicts that emerged earlier in treatment. In PFPP in research studies, patients were typically pleased about the progress they had made, but often had difficulties expressing disappointment and frustration with the therapist about ending treatment [44, 45].

## Research on Psychodynamic Treatment of Panic Disorder

Few systematic studies using manualized psychoanalytic treatments have been done in populations with panic disorder. Wiborg and Dahl [46] conducted a randomized, controlled trial of a manualized form of psychodynamic psychotherapy in addition to clomipramine, in comparison with clomipramine alone. The 3-month weekly psychotherapy combined with medication reduced relapse rates at 18 months compared to patients treated with clomipramine alone (9 vs. 91%).

An open trial of PFFP was conducted by our research group [44, 45]. Of 21 patients with primary DSM-IV panic disorder who entered the trial, 4 patients dropped out. Of the remaining 17, 16 patients achieved standard remission criteria of their panic and agoraphobia [47]. Significant psychosocial function improvements were noted. All of the therapeutic improvements were maintained at 6-month follow-up. Notably, the eight subjects who also met DSM-IV criteria for major depression at study entry experienced relief of these symptoms as well. Although not a randomized controlled trial, the study suggested that PFPP could provide significant relief of panic disorder.

Recently, our research group completed a randomized controlled trial [42] comparing PFPP to applied relaxation therapy (ART) [48], a treatment for panic disorder that is less active than cognitive-behavioral therapy (CBT) [49], in 49 patients. This study was the first to demonstrate efficacy of a scientifically testable psychodynamic psychotherapy for panic disorder.

Patients entered the study if they met DSM-IV criteria for primary panic disorder with or without agoraphobia, in addition to having at least one panic attack per week. Patients on medication agreed to not change the dose or type of medication throughout the study period (15% of the sample). To gain study entry, patients had to agree to stop all nonstudy psychotherapy. Patients were included if they had severe agoraphobia, comorbid major depression, or personality disorders as comorbid conditions. Exclusion criteria were psychosis, bipolar disorder, and substance abuse (6 months remission necessary).

Patients were symptomatically assessed at baseline, at treatment termination, and at 2, 4, 6, and 12 months after treatment termination by independent raters, blinded to study condition and therapist orientation. The primary outcome measure was the Panic Disorder Severity Scale (PDSS) [50] (Fig. 2.2); other domains monitored were psychosocial function with the Sheehan Disability Scale (SDS) [51], depression, with the Hamilton Depression Rating Scale (HAM-D, [52]) and general nonpanic-related anxiety the Hamilton Anxiety

**Fig. 2.2** Panic Disorder
Severity Scale as primary
outcome measure

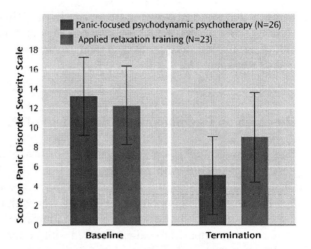

Rating Scale (HAM-A, [53]). Response was defined as a 40% reduction from baseline PDSS score in keeping with standard definitions in the field [47].

PFPP and ART were provided as 24-session, twice-weekly (12 weeks) treatments. ART includes a rationale and explanation about panic disorder, progressive muscle relaxation (PMR) techniques, cue controlled relaxation, and exposure. PMR involves tensing and relaxing particular muscle groups, with therapist suggestions of deepening relaxation. Twice daily homework was assigned. An exposure protocol was included, using relaxation as an active technique to combat emerging panic.

PFPP therapists ($N = 8$) were PhD psychologists or MD psychiatrists who had completed at least 3 years of psychoanalytic training. They received a 12-h course in PFPP, and had at least 2 years of experience with psychodynamic treatment of PD.

ART therapists ($N = 6$), were PhD psychologists or MDs after psychiatric residency, had a 6-h course in ART, and at least 2 years of clinical experience treating panic disorder with ART and CBT. Supervisory experience of both groups of therapists included monthly group supervision and individual supervision as needed.

All psychotherapy sessions were videotaped for adherence monitoring. Adherence to study therapy protocol was assessed based on three videotapes from each treatment using the PFPP Adherence Rating Scale (available from the authors) and the ART Adherence Scale [54]. Both groups demonstrated a high level of adherence to the manualized treatments.

There was a significantly greater proportion of men in the ART group compared to the PFPP group (47 vs. 15%; two-tailed Fisher's exact $p = 0.03$). No other significant demographic or clinical differences were found between the two treatment groups (see Table 2.1). Importantly, no significant baseline differences were observed between randomized groups in severity of PD, PDSS score [50], the SDS [51], the HAM-D, [52], and HAM-A [53] (Table 2.2). PFPP

**Table 2.1** Clinical and Demographic Characteristics

| Variable | Panic-Focused Psychodynamic Psychotherapy ($N = 26$) | | Applied Relaxation Training ($N = 23$) | |
|---|---|---|---|---|
| | Mean | SD | Mean | SD |
| Age at entry (years) | 33.4 | 9.6 | 33.5 | 8.5 |
| Severity of panic disorder (range: 1–8) | 5.7 | 0.8 | 5.8 | 0.8 |
| Comorbid axis I disorders | 2.2 | 1.4 | 2.4 | 1.6 |
| Panic duration (years) | 8.4 | 9.8 | 8.8 | 9.6 |
| | % | | % | |
| Gender (male) | 15 | | 47* | |
| Moderate to severe agoraphobia | 69 | | 86 | |
| Comorbid major depression | 19 | | 26 | |
| Psychotropic use | 19 | | 17 | |
| Axis II diagnosis | 42 | | 56 | |
| Cluster B diagnosis | 11 | | 21 | |

*$p < 0.05$

had a significantly higher response rate than ART (73 vs. 39%; $p = 0.016$) using definitions that are standard in the field (a 40% decrease in the total PDSS score from baseline) [47], and a significantly greater reduction in impairment of

**Table 2.2** Change in clinical severity measures pre- and posttreatment[a]

| Variable | Panic-focused Psychodynamic Psychotherapy ($N = 26$) | | Applied relaxation Training ($N = 23$) | | Analysis | | | Effect Size[b] |
|---|---|---|---|---|---|---|---|---|
| | N | % | N | % | $t$ | df | $p$ | |
| Responder status | 19 | 73 | 9 | 39 | 5.74[c] | 1 | 0.016 | – |
| | Mean | SD | Mean | SD | | | | |
| Panic Disorder Severity Scale baseline | 13.2 | 4.0 | 12.2 | 4.0 | | | | |
| Panic Disorder Severity Scale termination | 5.1 | 4.0 | 9.0 | 4.6 | 3.30 | 47 | 0.002 | 0.95 |
| Sheehan Disability Scale baseline | 14.7 | 8.8 | 14.6 | 6.0 | | | | |
| Sheehan Disability Scale termination | 7.3 | 7.8 | 12.7 | 6.4 | 2.54 | 46 | 0.014 | 0.74 |
| HAM-D baseline | 15.9 | 7.3 | 14.2 | 6.3 | | | | |
| HAM-D termination | 9.0 | 5.6 | 11.5 | 6.7 | 1.84 | 47 | 0.071 | 0.53 |
| HAM-A baseline | 16.0 | 6.9 | 16.0 | 6.0 | | | | |
| HAM-A termination | 8.9 | 5.7 | 11.1 | 6.4 | 0.54 | 47 | 0.588 | 0.16 |

[a]Group comparisons on change in scores pre- and posttreatment. $N$'s vary because of missing data. (One applied relaxation training subject did not complete the Sheehan Disability Scale correctly posttreatment.)
[b]Cohen's d is the between group effect size.
[c]Chi square test.

psychosocial function on the SDS ($p = 0.014$). Significant differences were not observed between the two treatments in the HAM-D ratings of depressive symptoms ($p = 0.07$), or in nonpanic anxiety on the HAM-A ($p = 0.58$).

Thus, in this first randomized controlled trial of a manualized psychoanalytic treatment as a sole intervention for panic disorder, PFPP demonstrated efficacy. Treatment was well tolerated: only two of 26 subjects dropped out of the PFPP condition (7%), in comparison with 8 dropouts from the ART condition (34%). The dropout rate for PFPP was unusually low for an RCT of panic disorder patients in the United States. Patients generally responded well to treatment, even though, due to the inclusion of severe agoraphobia and comorbid depression, they were relatively sicker than panic patients in other major panic outcome studies [47, 49, 55–57]. Although PFPP performed comparably to clinical trials of CBT and medication, these treatments were not directly compared in this study. A study is currently in progress comparing PFPP directly with CBT.

## Conclusion

As panic disorder remains a significant public health problem, it is important to continue to develop and assess therapeutic interventions for this illness. PFPP is a useful alternative treatment for panic and addresses aspects of the disorder that are not likely to be addressed by other, better-tested treatments. Further studies of comparative efficacy of treatments should help to determine which interventions, or series of interventions, are most helpful for panic patients.

## References

1. Otto MW, Tuby KS, Gould RA, McLean RY, Pollack MH: An effect-size analysis of the relative efficacy and tolerability of serotonin selective reuptake inhibitors for panic disorder. Am J Psychiatry 2001;158(12):1989–1992.
2. Bakker A, van Balkom AJ, Spinhoven P: SSRIs vs. TCA's in the treatment of panic disorder: a meta-analysis. Acta Psychiatr Scand 2002; 106(3):163–167.
3. Wilkinson G, Balestrieri M, Ruggeri M, Bellantuono C: Meta-analysis of double-blind placebo-controlled trials of antidepressants and benzodiazepines for patients with panic disorder. Psychol Med 1991;21(4):991–998.
4. Barlow DH, Gorman JM, Shear MK et al.: Cognitive-behavioral therapy, imipramine, or their combination for panic disorder. JAMA 2000;283:2529–2536.
5. Craske MG, Brown TA, Barlow DH: Behavioral treatment of panic: a two-year follow-up. Behav Ther 1991;22:289–304.
6. Craske MG, DeCola JP, Sachs AD et al.: Panic control treatment for agoraphobia. J Anxiety Disord 2003;17:321–333.
7. Marks IM, Swinson RP, Basoglu M et al.: Alprazolam and exposure alone and combined in panic disorder with agoraphobia. Br J Psychiatry 1993;162:776–787.
8. Shear MK, Maser JD: Standardized assessment for panic disorder research: a conference report. Arch Gen Psychiatry 1994;51:346–354.
9. Mavissakalian M, Michelson L: Two year follow-up of exposure and imipramine treatment of agoraphobia. Am J Psychiatry 1986;143:1106–1112.

10. Nagy LM, Krystal JH, Woods SW et al.: Clinical and medication outcome after short-term alprasolam and behavioral group treatment in panic disorder: 2.5 year naturalistic follow-up study. Arch Gen Psychiatry 1989;46:993–999.
11. Noyes R Jr, Garvey MJ, Cook BL: Follow-up study of patients with panic disorder and agoraphobia with panic attacks treated with tricyclic antidepressants. J Affect Disord 1989;16:249–257.
12. Pollack MH, Otto MW, Tesar GE et al.: Long-term outcome after acute treatment with alprasolam and clonazepam for panic disorder. J Clin Psychopharmacol 1993;13:257–263.
13. Milrod B, Busch F: The long-term outcome of treatments for panic disorder: a review of the literature. J Nerv Ment Dis 1996;184:723–730.
14. Vanelli M: Improving treatment response in panic disorder. Prim Psychiatry 2005;12(11): 68–73.
15. Markowitz JS, Weissman MM, Ouellette R et al.: Quality of life in panic disorder. Arch Gen Psychiatry 1989;46:984–992.
16. Rubin, HC, Rapaport, MH, Levine B et al.: Quality of well-being in panic disorder: the assessment of psychiatric and general disability. J Affect Disord 2000;57:217–21.
17. Katon W: Panic disorder: relationship to high medical utilization, unexplained physical symptoms, and medical costs. J Clin Psychiatry 1996;57(Suppl 10):11–18.
18. Swenson RP, Cox BJ, Woszezy CB: Use of medical services and treatment for panic disorder with agoraphobia and for social phobia. J Can Med Assoc 1992;147:878–883.
19. Fyer AJ, Liebowitz MR, Gorman JM et al.: Discontinuation of alprazolam in panic patients. Am J Psychiatry 1987;144:303–308.
20. O'Sullivan G, Marks I: Follow-up studies of behavioral treatment of phobic and obsessive compulsive neurosis. Psychiatr Ann 1991;21:368–373.
21. Busch FN, Cooper AM, Klerman GL, Shapiro T, Shear MK: Neurophysiological, cognitive-behavioral and psychoanalytic approaches to panic disorder: toward an integration. Psychoanal Inq 1991;11:316–332.
22. Shear MK, Cooper AM, Klerman GL, Busch FN, Shapiro T: A psychodynamic model of panic disorder. Am J Psychiatry 1993;150:859–866.
23. Milrod BL, Busch FN, Cooper AM, Shapiro T: Manual of Panic-focused Psychodynamic Psychotherapy. Washington, DC, American Psychiatric Press, 1997.
24. Breuer J, Freud S: Studies on hysteria (1895), in The Standard Edition of the Complete Psychological Works of Sigmund Freud, vol. 2, translated and edited by Strachey J. London, Hogarth Press, 1959, pp 1–183.
25. Kleiner L, Marshall WL: The role of interpersonal problems in the development of agoraphobia with panic attacks. J Anxiety Disord 1987;1:313–323.
26. Freud S: The neuropsychoses of defence (1894), in The Standard Edition of the Complete Psychologic Works of Sigmund Freud, vol. 3, translated and edited by Strachey J. London, Hogarth Press, 1959, pp 45–61.
27. Busch FN, Shear MK, Cooper AM, Shapiro T, Leon A: An empirical study of defense mechanisms in panic disorder. J Nerv Ment Dis 1995;183:299–303.
28. Busch FN, Milrod BL, Singer MB: Theory and technique in the psychodynamic treatment of panic disorder. J Psychother Pract Res 1999;8:234–242.
29. Parker G: Reported parental characteristics of agoraphobics and social phobics. Br J Psychiatry 1979;135:555–560.
30. Arrindell W, Emmelkamp PMG, Monsma A et al.: The role of perceived parental rearing practices in the etiology of phobic disorders: a controlled study. Br J Psychiatry 1983;143:183–187.
31. Freud S: Inhibitions, symptoms and anxiety (1926), in The Standard Edition of the Complete Psychological Works of Sigmund Freud, vol. 20, translated and edited by Strachey J. London, Hogarth Press, 1959, pp 77–174.
32. Kagan J, Reznick JS, Snidman N et al.: Origins of panic disorder, in Neurobiology of Panic Disorder, Ballenger J. (ed.) New York, Wiley, 1990, pp 71–87.
33. Gorman JM., Kent JM, Sullivan G M, Coplan JD: Neuroanatomical hypothesis of panic disorder, revised. Am J Psychiatry 2000;157:493–505.

34. Busch FN, Milrod BL: The nature and treatment of panic disorder, in Textbook of Biological Psychiatry, Panksepp, J. (ed.). Hoboken, NJ, Wiley, 2003, pp. 367–392.
35. Panksepp J: Affective Neuroscience. New York, Oxford, 1998.
36. Neumeister A, Bain E, Nugent AC, Carson RE, Bonne O, Luckenbaugh DA, Eckelman W, Herscovitch P, Charney DS, Drevets WC: Reduced serotonin type 1A receptor binding in panic disorder. J Neurosci 2004;24(3):589–591.
37. Hogg S, Michan L, Jessa M: Prediction of anti-panic properties of escitalopram in the dorsal periaqueductal grey model of panic anxiety. Neuropharmacology 2006;51:141–145.
38. El-Khodor BF, Dimmler MH, Amara DA, Hofer M, Hen R, Brunner D: Juvenile 5HT(1B) receptor knockout mice exhibit reduced pharmacological sensitivity to 5HT(1A) receptor activation. Int J Dev Neurosci 2004;22(5–6):405–413.
39. Rauch SL, Shin LM, Wright CI: Neuroimaging studies of amygdala function in anxiety disorders. Ann NY Acad Sci 2003;985:389–410.
40. Fonagy P: Thinking about thinking: Some clinical and theoretical considerations in the treatment of a borderline patient. Int J Psychoanal 1991;72:1–18.
41. Rudden MG, Milrod B, Aronson A, Target M: Reflective functioning in panic disorder patients: clinical observations and research design. In Mentalization: Theoretical Considerations, Research Findings, and Clinical Implications. New York, The Analytic Press: Taylor & Francis Group 2008, pp.185–206.
42. Milrod B, Busch F, Leon AC et al.: A randomized controlled clinical trial of psychoanalytic psychotherapy for panic disorder. Am J Psychiatry 2007;164(2):265–272.
43. Busch FN, Milrod BL, Singer M: Theory and technique in psychodynamic treatment of panic disorder. J Psychother Pract Res 1999;8:234–242.
44. Milrod B, Busch F, Leon AC et al.: A pilot open trial of brief psychodynamic psychotherapy for panic disorder. J Psychother Pract Res 2001;10:1–7.
45. Milrod B, Busch F, Leon A et al.: An open trial of psychodynamic psychotherapy for panic disorder – a pilot study. Am J Psychiatry 2000;157:1878–1880.
46. Wiborg IM, Dahl AA: Does brief dynamic psychotherapy reduce the relapse rate of panic disorder? Arch Gen Psychiatry 1996;53:689–694.
47. Barlow DH, Gorman JM, Shear MK Woods SW: Cognitive-behavioral therapy, imipramine, or their combination for panic disorder. JAMA 2000;283:2529–2536.
48. Cerny, JA, Vermilyea, BB, Barlow, DH et al.: Anxiety treatment project relaxation treatment manual. 1984. Available from the authors
49. Craske MG, Brown TA, Barlow DH: Behavioral treatment of panic disorder: a two-year follow-up. Behav Ther 1991;22:289–304.
50. Shear MK, Brown TA, Barlow DH et al.: Multicenter collaborative Panic Disorder Severity Scale. Am J Psychiatry 1997;154:1571–1575.
51. Sheehan DV: The Sheehan disability scales. in The Anxiety Disease. New York, Charles Scribner and Sons 1983, p. 151.
52. Hamilton M: A rating scale for depression. J Neurol Neurosurg Psychiatry 1960;23:56–62.
53. Hamilton M: The assessment of anxiety states by rating. Br J Med Psychol 1959;32:50–55.
54. Otto MW, Pollack MH: Adherence ratings for ART. Available from the authors.
55. Marks IM, Swinson RP, Basoglu M, Kuch K, Noshirvani H, O'Sullivan G, Lelliott PT, Kirby M, McNamee G, Sengun S, Wickwire K: Alprazolam and exposure alone and combined in panic disorder with agoraphobia: a controlled study in London and Toronto. Br J Psychol 1993;162:776–787.
56. Clark DM, Salkovskis PM, Hackman A, Middleton H, Anastasiades P, Gelder M: A comparison of cognitive therapy, applied relaxation, and imipramine in the treatment of panic disorder. Br J Psychiatry 1994;164:759–769.
57. Fava GA, Zielezny M, Savron G, Grandi S: Long-term effects of behavioral treatment for panic disorder with agoraphobia. Br J Psychiatry 1995;166:87–92.

# Chapter 3
# A Naturalistic Treatment for Panic Disorder

## The Importance of Emotion-Focused Process

Tai Katzenstein, J. Stuart Ablon, and Raymond A. Levy

## Introduction

Although cognitive-behavior therapy (CBT) has repeatedly demonstrated treatment efficacy for panic disorder [1], establishing the empirical basis for psychodynamic psychotherapy (PD) remains important because CBT is not effective for all panic patients [2, 3]. Busch [4] argues persuasively that diversifying the number of empirically supported psychotherapeutic options available to panic patients is necessary to fully respond to the range of panic patients' clinical needs. As Busch et al. note, while highly effective for many individuals, CBT does not work for all panic patients [2, 3].

Some patients have difficult executing the exposure-based approaches characterizing CBT approaches for panic disorder. Other patients do not engage in the between-session work that functions as a critical cornerstone of CBT approaches. Investigators [3] note that up to 38% of patients experience no symptom relief or relapse subsequent [5] to treatment discontinuation in closely controlled CBT trials. The concern that cognitive-behavioral treatment will not sufficiently facilitate the exploration of the personal meaning of symptoms leads other patients to reject CBT as their modality of choice. For patients who do seek out and receive CBT, questions regarding the long-term efficacy of these treatments remain. Milrod and Busch [5] underscore the problematic lack of evidence supporting the long-term maintenance of short-term treatment gains in CBT. They also underscore the need for treatments that synergistically target symptom reduction as well as broader based changes in personality functioning to maintain treatment gains across time and to effectively address the disruptions across multiple domains that occur for many panic patients [4, 6]. Working to diversify the range of psychotherapeutic treatment options available to panic patients who either do not respond to CBT or who elect to pursue exploratory treatments is

T. Katzenstein
Department of Psychiatry, Massachusetts General Hospital, 15 Parkman Street, WAC 812, Boston, MA 02114-3117, USA
e-mail: tkatzenstein@partners.org

R.A. Levy, J.S. Ablon (eds.), *Handbook of Evidence-Based Psychodynamic Psychotherapy*, 45
DOI: 10.1007/978-1-59745-444-5_3, © Humana Press 2009

critically important in view of the tremendous and incontrovertible psychological, emotional, and social costs of living with panic disorder [7, 8].

Milrod et al. [9] have conducted the first randomized controlled clinical trial of a manualized psychoanalytic psychotherapy for patients with panic disorder. Milrod et al. randomly assigned 49 participants meeting *Diagnostic and Statistical Manual of Mental Disorders* (DSM)-IV criteria for panic disorder to either panic-focused psychodynamic psychotherapy or applied-relaxation training. Both treatments ran twice weekly for 12 weeks. In this study, 3 h per case were rated to ensure adherence to the treatment manual. Patients assigned to the panic-focused psychodynamic psychotherapy condition demonstrated a significantly greater reduction in symptom severity as well as improved psychosocial functioning compared to patients receiving relaxation training. The results of this randomized control trial demonstrate the preliminary efficacy of panic-focused psychodynamic psychotherapy for panic disorder. This study contributes meaningfully to the literature by demonstrating that psychodynamically oriented treatments effectively reduce symptoms and suffering and that these treatments, too, can be empirically examined.

While the use of randomized control trial methodology in the Milrod et al. study is, on the one hand, precisely what facilitates concluding that this psychodynamic treatment for panic disorder influenced positive outcome, this methodology is accompanied by certain limitations [10]. Debate about the best method for empirically validating treatments is ongoing in the clinical research literature. In studies utilizing randomized control methodology, the prioritization of internal validity often comes at the cost of compromised generalizability. This is because treatments that are tested in the artificially controlled settings with atypical patients often bear little resemblance to the patients seen in clinical practice. Also, studies that utilize randomized control methodology tend to compare the outcomes of different interventions as opposed to examining the link between therapy process and outcome [11].

Recently, leading psychotherapy researchers have underscored the potential importance of identifying empirically validated change processes in naturalistic treatment as a fruitful complement to controlled trials [10, 12–14]. These researchers maintain that potentially important clinical information gets overlooked in the development of treatment protocols for controlled trials because of insufficient contact with what actual clinicians and patients are already doing in their treatments in the community. This study represents one attempt to take the focus off prescriptive treatment packages and work first to identify what a group of experienced clinicians did when treating patients with shared diagnoses and presenting problems. We were interested in understanding whether these treatments, which might be best described as "treatment as usual" in the community were associated with positive or negative treatment outcome. We used an empirically derived and clinically relevant measure of treatment process to identify the presence of change processes in a naturalistic treatment so that we could learn how and why patients improved. If empirically validated change processes could be identified, we would have an empirical basis from which to develop or amend clinically relevant treatment.

Previous research [11, 15] has demonstrated the dangers of drawing conclusions about why a treatment is effective without studying process correlates of outcome. When a participant in a controlled clinical trial improves after undergoing psychotherapy, it is assumed that the improvement was caused by the specific interventions that were prescribed by a manual and monitored for adherence. However, this assumption relies heavily on the clinicians' ability to apply certain techniques without using others and to adhere to a particular treatment approach. This line of programmatic research sheds light on the tenuousness of this basic assumption of controlled clinical trials. Even with manualized regimens of psychotherapy, elements "borrowed" from different treatment approaches can be among the active ingredients promoting change. It is impossible to say what factors were associated with improvement after treatment unless the treatment process itself is studied [11]. In treatment research while it is important to know *that* a given treatment is effective, to capitalize on the maximum degree of therapeutic effectiveness as well as design increasingly effective treatments, it is equally important to understand *which* aspects of the underlying process contribute to positive outcome.

In this study, we recruited clinicians who described their primary theoretical orientation as psychodynamic to treat a group of patients with panic disorder as they normally would in their clinical practices. Our goal was to study the process and outcome of the treatments. We were particularly interested in studying how psychodynamic therapists worked with panic disorder patients because psychodynamically oriented clinicians frequently treat panic patients despite the fact that psychodynamic psychotherapy is not an empirically supported therapy (EST) for panic disorder and ESTs that have been well tested in the laboratory do exist for this population (e.g., Panic Control Therapy, see [16]). Another reason for our interest in studying psychodynamic clinicians and panic patients specifically stems from the fact that treatments in controlled trials treatments are typically tested against medication, wait list controls, psychoeducation, or some version of purely supportive treatment. ESTs such as Panic Control Therapy [1] are rarely systematically tested against legitimate alternative psychosocial treatments or treatment as usual in the community. For this reason the true efficacy of CBT approaches relative to psychodynamic and nonprescriptive approaches may be less clear than originally suggested by the American Psychiatric Practice guidelines [17]. The goals of this chapter are to: (1) present and review results issuing from a naturalistic treatment for panic disorder conducted by self-identified psychodynamic clinicians in which attention to patients' emotion emerged as an important predictor of positive outcome and (2) consider the clinical implications suggested by these results. This pilot study utilized the Psychotherapy Process Q-Set (PQS) [18] to empirically describe the psychotherapeutic process characterizing these treatments.

## Aims: Identifying Empirically Supported Change Processes

To empirically identify change processes in these treatments our goals were to
(1) examine the degree of change associated with a naturalistic psychotherapy
for panic disorder in a within subject sample; (2) identify which prototypical
treatment processes best characterized the treatments; (3) identify which prototypical processes were most predictive of positive outcome; and (4) identify
which specific process variables predicted positive outcome. Specifically, we
hypothesized that (1) naturalistic brief psychotherapy for panic disorder would
be a highly effective treatment with gains commensurate with those achieved by
prescriptive treatments; (2) the treatments would be characterized by a high
degree of psychodynamic process and significantly less by elements of interpersonal psychotherapy (IPT) and cognitive-behavioral process; (3) that positive outcome would be predicted by the degree to which psychodynamic (rather
than interpersonal or cognitive-behavioral) process was fostered; (4) that the
specific process variables predicting positive outcome would include focusing
on affect and other process elements consistent with a psychodynamic approach
(e.g., attention to the therapeutic alliance and relationship, interpretation of
defense mechanisms, identification of unconscious feelings and wishes deemed
dangerous, and the linking of current symptoms, behaviors, and feelings to past
experiences).

## Method

### Participants

Participants were 17 patients between the ages of 24 and 55 meeting Structured
Clinical Interview for *DSM-IV* (SCID-IV) criteria for diagnosis of panic disorder at the Massachusetts General Hospital (MGH) outpatient psychiatry
service in Boston. Exclusion criteria for this study included current drug or
alcohol abuse, bipolar disorder, psychosis, suicidality, concurrent psychotherapy or counseling, and any anticipated or actual changes to medication (dosage
or type) less than 8 weeks prior to study entry. Of the 17 patients entering
treatment, 88.2% were female, 11.8% were male. Within the pool of participants, 77.8% identified themselves as Caucasian and 22.4% described themselves as Haitian, Hispanic, or Asian-Indian. In terms of comorbid disorders,
approximately 6% of participants in this sample met diagnostic criteria for
current major depression, 66.7% met criteria for panic disorder with agoraphobia, 38.9% met criteria for current generalized anxiety, 11.1% met criteria
for current social phobia disorder, and 5.6% met criteria for obsessive-compulsive
disorder (OCD). Among study participants, 61.1% reported having previously
taken some form of psychotropic medication. Seventy-six percent of the sample
reported previously pursuing psychotherapy.

Since this was a naturalistic treatment, patients were allowed to continue taking psychotropic medication during the study as long as no changes were made 2 months prior to study enrollment and the patient still met criteria for panic disorder at baseline. While enrolled in the study, 52.9% ($n = 9$) of the participants were concurrently on medication (5 patients taking benzodiazapines, 2 taking a benzodiazapine and antidepressant, 1 patient taking only an antidepressant, and 1 patient taking medications belonging to multiple pharmacological classes). Patients were asked not to make changes in medicine until termination of the study so that changes during the study period would not be confounded by medication changes. During the course of the study, however, one participant changed medication dosage under psychiatric supervision. After consultation with the psychiatrist, this participant was retained because the small change was not believed to represent a serious confound. While receiving treatment, two participants also ceased taking benzodiazapenes on an as needed basis because of improvement in their functioning during the study period.

## Therapists

The seven participating clinicians were all affiliated with the Outpatient Department of Psychiatry at Massachusetts General Hospital. This group included one psychiatrist, one psychiatric resident, two psychologists, and three psychology interns or postdoctoral fellows. Clinicians averaged 12 years of clinical experience. All clinicians identified their primary theoretical orientation as psychodynamic. Therapists were not asked to describe their orientation in any greater specificity because one primary aim of this study was, in fact, to identify empirically the type of treatment processes fostered in actual practice using consensus-based definitions from different theoretical orientations.

## Treatment

To replicate psychodynamic psychotherapy conducted in the community, clinicians were asked to conduct their treatments as they normally would in their clinical practice. As described previously, nonprescriptive therapies including psychodynamic psychotherapy are frequently used to treat panic disorder patients who cannot tolerate or do not respond to medicine or ESTs such as Panic Control Therapy [1]. There were no restrictions about the kind of therapy offered other than treating patients for 22–26 sessions. This range was selected to facilitate clinicians' abilities to decide nonarbitrarily when to end treatment.

## Assessing Outcome

Outcome measures were chosen to assess patient functioning across a number of different domains and from different perspectives (patient, therapist, and independent rater). These measures were administered monthly. Patient follow-up questionnaires were administered 6 months after treatment ended. Independent raters assessed the severity and intensity of patients' panic at baseline and termination using a questionnaire involving one-to-one discussions with patients about their attacks. Several outcome measures in this study were selected because of their assignation as standard instruments to be used in empirical investigations of panic disorder by the 1994 NIH conference report [19]. Other measures were chosen by virtue of their relevance to exploratory psychotherapies.

## Patient Self-Report Measures

The Anxiety Sensitivity Index (ASI) [20] and Panic Disorder Severity Scale (PDSS) [21] were selected to assess panic symptomatology. The Symptom Checklist-90-Revised (SCL-90-R) [22] and Quality of Enjoyment and Satisfaction Questionnaire (Q-LES-Q) [23] were used to assess general psychological and physical functioning.

## Clinician Measures

The Clinical Global Impression Scale (CGI) [24] was selected to assess subjects' panic symptomology. The Global Assessment of Functioning Scale (GAF) [25] was selected to gauge general psychological functioning. The Defensive Functioning Scale (DFS) (DSM-IV) and Social Cognition and Object Relations Scale (SCORS) [Westen, D. (1995). Social Cognition and Objects Relations Scale: Q-Sort for projective stories (SCORS-Q). Unpublished manuscript, Cambridge Hospital and Harvard Medical School, Cambridge, MA; Hilsenroth, M., Stein, M., & Pinsker, J. (2004). Social Cognition and Object Relations Scale: Global Rating Method (SCORS-G). Unpublished manuscript, The Derner Institute of Advanced Psychological Studies, Adelphi University, Garden City, NY] were used to evaluate subjects' defensive styles and object relations.

## Independent Rater Measure

The Multicenter Panic Anxiety Scale (MCPAS) [26] was used to assess the frequency and severity of participants' panic symptoms at baseline and termination. This instrument is identical in content to the previously described patient PDSS. However, it is completed by an independent rater as opposed to the patient.

## Assessing Process

Therapeutic process was examined using the PQS [18]. The PQS is an instrument consisting of 100 items describing actions, behaviors, and thoughts of both therapist and patient in individual as well as dyadic terms. Several characteristics of the PQS speak to its strengths as a measure. It has demonstrated reliability and validity across a variety of different treatment samples including archived treatments of psychodynamic, cognitive-behavioral, client-centered, rational-emotive, and interpersonal therapies [11, 27–30]. See Jones [18] for discussion of the instrument's psychometric properties and more in-depth examination of its defining characteristics. Briefly, the PQSs unique features include utilizing a fixed normal distribution, being ispatively oriented, utilizing the entire therapy hour, and being pantheoretical (i.e., able to be used across multiple orientations).

The PQS has been used to develop prototypes of ideal psychotherapeutic process for a range of theoretical perspectives. Previous research has demonstrated how correlating process ratings with the prototypes can provide an empirical measure of the degree to which a treatment adheres to the theoretical principles of a given orientation (see [11, 15] for more information on the development of the prototypes). Prototypes of psychodynamic, cognitive-behavioral, and interpersonal process were used in this study.

A pool of eight research-oriented psychologists and master's level graduate students in clinical psychology, trained in use of the PQS, completed ratings of audiotapes from this study. Session 12 (the midpoint of most treatments) was selected as the representative hour to be Q-sorted in this study. For each session, independent ratings were completed by at least two judges. The average alpha coefficient reliability for raters completing Q-sorts ($N = 17$) of therapy sessions in this sample was 0.85. This far surpasses the generally acceptable criterion (0.70) used to determine acceptable reliability in therapy process and outcome research [31].

## Results

### Patient Outcome: Did This Naturalistic Psychotherapy Positively Predict Outcome for Patients With Panic Disorder?

Treatment gains across time points were calculated using multiple statistical methods including statistical significance, effect sizes, and clinically significant change [32]. Table 3.1 reports pre- and posttreatment means on patient, clinician, and independent rater questionnaires. Outcome analyses were also calculated after stratifying by medication status. Patients not concurrently taking medication achieved equivalent or better outcome across all measures. Analyses of the 6-month follow-up data revealed no statistically significant changes from

**Table 3.1** Outcome of naturalistic psychotherapy for panic disorder: baseline to endpoint

| | Patient measures | | | Therapist measures | | Rater measure |
|---|---|---|---|---|---|---|
| | SCL-90-R | ASI | PDSS | CGI | GAF | MC-PAS |
| Premean | 0.87 | 30.30 | 10.40 | 4.2 | 59.8 | 5.03 |
| Postmean | 0.54 | 17.60 | 5.88 | 2.60 | 71.60 | 3.3 |
| Statistical significance | 0.01* | 0.00* | 0.00* | 0.01* | 0.00* | 0.00* |
| Effect sizes | 0.74 | 1.30 | 1.10 | 2.4 | 1.8 | 1.1 |

*Note.* Significant pre-/postmeans were determined using within-sample *t*-tests. Effect sizes were calculated using the formula: pretreatment mean − posttreatment mean/pretreatment standard deviation. SCL-90-R = Hopkins Symptom Checklist; ASI = Anxiety Sensitivity Index; PDSS Total = Panic Disorder Severity Scale; CGI = Clinical Global Impression Scale; GAF = Global Assessment of Functioning Scale; MC-PAS = Multicenter Panic Anxiety Scale. *N* = 17.
*p < 0.01.

endpoint to follow-up. In other words, patients maintained treatment gains across all outcome measures 6 months after termination. Thus, our first hypothesis, that naturalistic psychotherapy would be highly effective for treating panic disorder, was confirmed.

**Statistical Significance**

Statistical significance and effect size represent the change between these time points. Paired-sample *t* tests were used to detect statistically significant mean differences between pre- and posttreatment. From pre- to posttreatment, patients reported statistically significant decreases in both the anticipation and experience of anxiety (ASI and PDSS) as well as significant increases in overall functioning (SCL and Quality of Life Enjoyment and Satisfaction Questionnaire). Consistent with the patients' perspectives, clinicians and independent raters reported a statistically significant decrease in panic and anxiety from baseline to endpoint. Clinicians and raters reported decreases in the severity of patients' panic attacks as well as improvement in general functioning (CGI, MCPAS, and GAF). From clinicians' perspectives, patients did not demonstrate a statistically significant change in defensive functioning from pre- to posttreatment. However, clinicians did report statistically significant change (*p* <0.05) in aspects of object relations including patients' emotional investment in values and moral standards (*p* = 0.02) and changes in self-esteem (*p* = 0.02).

**Effect Sizes**

Effect sizes were calculated as another index of change. This was done by subtracting posttreatment from pretreatment means and dividing by the pretreatment standard deviation. The effect sizes suggest substantial improvement in outcome from baseline to endpoint. Fifty-three percent of patients achieved remission according to a criterion used in several other studies in the literature [3, 33].

## Clinically Significant Change

To better understand what the statistical findings meant clinically for this group of patients, clinically significant change was calculated using a stringent method suggested by Jacobson and Truax [34]. When calculating clinical significance, mean scores for the "normal" population (i.e., adults with no Axis I psychiatric disorder) as well as the "dysfunctional population" (i.e., in this case adult patients diagnosed with panic disorder) are referenced. Patient change is considered to be clinically significant only if posttreatment means are closer to the normal mean than the dysfunctional mean. This calculation was completed for the two measures for which population means were available. Sixty-four percent and 70% of patients achieved clinically significant change on the SCL and ASI, respectively.

## *Adherence to Prototypes: Which Theoretical Orientation Most Consistently Characterized the Treatment Process Between Clinicians and Their Patients?*

Our second hypothesis, that the treatments would be best characterized by prototypical psychodynamic process, was not confirmed. To measure adherence to prototypes of ideal therapeutic process as stipulated by expert panels, prototypes were correlated with the Q-sort ratings of the actual treatment sessions. For every patient, the composite Q-rating of each PQS item was correlated with each item's factor score from the corresponding prototype (refer to [11, 15] for a more in-depth discussion of prototype methodology). Pearson correlations were transformed to $z$-scores using Fisher $r$ to $z$ transformations. Figure 3.1 displays the correlations with the three prototypes. The correlations with the CBT prototype ($z$-score $M = 0.50$, SD $= 0.14$) were the strongest followed by the psychodynamic ($z$-score $M = 0.35$, SD $= 0.16$) and

**Fig. 3.1** Adherence to prototypes of ideal treatment process
*Note.* Difference in adherence to the cognitive-behavioral versus other prototypes is statistically significant. The difference in adherence to the interpersonal versus psychodynamic prototype is not statistically significant

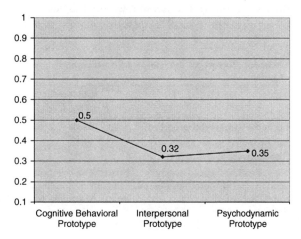

interpersonal prototypes ($z$ score $M = 0.32$, $SD = 0.09$), respectively. There was a statistically significant difference in adherence to the cognitive-behavioral versus psychodynamic and interpersonal prototypes ($t = -2.4$, df $= 16$, $p <$ 0.05; $t = 6.2$, df $= 16$, $p < 0.001$). No statistically significant difference in adherence to the psychodynamic versus interpersonal prototypes emerged ($t = 0.70$, df $= 16$, $p = 0.496$).

## Prototype-Outcome Correlations: Which Theoretical Orientation Was Most Consistently Associated With Positive Outcome?

Our third hypothesis, that the degree of prototypical psychodynamic process fostered would be the best predictor of positive outcome was only partially confirmed. Table 3.2 contains partial correlation coefficients representing the degree to which adherence to each prototype predicted outcome on the main outcome measures (SCL, ASI, and PDSS). Partial correlations were used to control for pretreatment level of severity. Positive correlations reflect outcome in the desired direction. Adherence to the psychodynamic prototype was significantly associated with positive outcome on one (SCL) of the three outcome measures. Adherence to the interpersonal prototype was significantly associated with positive outcome on two (SCL, ASI) of the three outcome measures. Adherence to the cognitive-behavioral prototype was not associated with positive outcome.

## Specific Process Correlates of Outcome: Which Active Ingredients in This Treatment Were Associated With Therapeutic Change?

Our fourth and final hypothesis that the specific process variables most predictive of positive outcome would include focusing on affect/feelings and other elements typical of psychodynamic therapy including attention to the

**Table 3.2** Prototypes correlated with outcome in a naturalistic psychotherapy for panic disorder

|  | Outcome measures | | |
|---|---|---|---|
|  | SCL-90-R | ASI | PDSS |
| Cognitive-behavioral prototype | −0.18 | −0.03 | −0.39 |
| Interpersonal prototype | 0.62** | 0.64** | 0.22 |
| Psychodynamic prototype | 0.50* | 0.22 | 0.03 |

*Note.* Positive correlations reflect favorable associations with outcome. All Pearson correlations are partial correlations controlling for pretreatment scores. $N = 17$. SCL-90-R = Symptom Checklist 90-Revised; ASI = Anxiety Sensitivity Index; PDSS = Panic Disorder Severity Scale.
*$p < 0.05$, **$p < 0.01$.

therapeutic alliance and relationship, interpretation of defense mechanisms, identification of unconscious feelings and wishes deemed dangerous, and the linking of current symptoms, behaviors, and feelings to past experiences, was only partially confirmed. Importantly, nearly half of the top 11 process correlates of outcome reflected patient and therapist attending to affect in some way. These active ingredients in treatment included a focus on helping patients to recognize, experience, and express negative or disavowed emotions, sexual desires, and fears of dependence. This pattern is consistent with psychodynamic theorizing and emotion-focused approaches in the literature, which emphasize attending to panic patients' affect.

To ascertain the specific aspects of the therapeutic process that were strongly associated with positive outcome, partial correlations (controlling for pretreatment) between Q-sort items and patients' outcome scores on the SCL were calculated. Because of the relatively small sample size, effect size rather than significance level was used to identify process correlates of outcome. A moderate correlation of $r > 0.3$ was chosen as a cutoff point to identify robust process correlates of outcome. The importance of decreasing the probability of Type II error at the risk of increasing the probability of Type I error influenced the selection of this value based on Cohen's estimates [35].

Table 3.3 lists the 28 PQS items emerging as process correlates of outcome on the SCL. The same number of items described patient ($N = 11$) and therapist ($N = 10$) within session characteristics, experiences, and qualities. Several items described the nature of the interaction between the two ($N = 7$). Some of the process-correlate items appeared to be thematically related. Interestingly, several items reflecting a focus on feelings and negative emotions by patients and therapists were associated with positive outcome: patient being self-accusatory/expressing shame and guilt (Q 71), verbalizing negative feelings toward the therapist (Q 1), the therapist focusing on patient's feelings of guilt (Q 22), drawing attention to feelings regarded as unacceptable by the patient (Q 50), and emphasizing patients' feelings in an effort to deepen them (Q 81).

Another group of items describing common factors contributing to a strong therapeutic alliance emerged as robust predictors of positive patient outcome on the SCL: humor being used (Q 74), the patient being introspective (Q 97), committed to the therapeutic work (Q 73), and understanding the nature and the expectations of the therapy (Q 72), the therapist accurately perceiving the therapeutic process (Q 28), adopting a supportive stance (Q 45), and being sensitive to the patient's feelings, attuned and empathic (Q 6). Patient's feeling conflicted about dependence on the therapist (Q 8) was an additional item correlating with positive outcome. Two other items generally characteristic of a psychodynamic viewpoint emerged as strongly associated with positive outcome: Sexual feelings are discussed (Q 11), and termination is discussed (Q 75). The following items were also correlates of positive outcome: silences occur during the hour (Q 12), discussion of scheduling or fees occurs (Q 96), and patient has difficulty beginning the hour (Q 25).

**Table 3.3** Individual item process correlates of outcome

| Effect size | Psychotherapy process items | PQS (#) |
|---|---|---|
| 0.70 | T emphasizes P's feelings to deepen them | 81 |
| 0.52 | Humor is used | 74 |
| 0.50 | P verbalizes negative feelings toward T | 1 |
| 0.49 | P is introspective, explores inner thoughts/feelings | 97 |
| 0.49 | P is committed to the work of therapy | 73 |
| 0.49 | P is concerned/conflicted about dependence on the T | 8 |
| 0.47 | P understands the nature of therapy, what is expected | 72 |
| 0.47 | Termination of therapy discussed | 75 |
| 0.43 | T draws attention to feelings P regards unacceptable | 50 |
| 0.42 | T accurately perceives therapeutic process | 28 |
| 0.40 | Sexual feelings and experiences are discussed | 11 |
| 0.38 | Discussion of scheduling or fees | |
| 0.37 | P achieves a new understanding or insight | 32 |
| 0.37 | P is self-accusatory expresses shame, guilt | 71 |
| 0.34 | T focuses on P's feelings of guilt | 22 |
| 0.34 | T is sensitive to the Ps feelings, attuned, empathic | 6 |
| 0.32 | Silences occur during the hour | 12 |
| −0.45 | P's feelings/perceptions are linked to the past | 92 |
| −0.47 | Discussion of activities/tasks to do outside session | 38 |
| −0.37 | P has difficulty beginning the hour | 25 |
| −0.36 | Discussion centers on cognitive themes, ideas, beliefs | 30 |
| −0.34 | T suggests P accept responsibility for problems | 76 |
| −0.33 | T adopts supportive stance | 45 |
| −0.33 | T behaves in a teacher-like (didactic) manner | 37 |
| −0.32 | T encourages independence of action/opinion | 48 |
| −0.54 | P relies upon T to solve his/her problems | 52 |
| −0.62 | P's self-image is focus of discussion | 35 |
| −0.67 | T encourages P to try new ways of behaving with others | 85 |

*Note.* Positive correlations reflect favorable associations with outcome on the SCL-90-R.
PQS = Psychotherapy Process Q-set; T = therapist; P = patient. $N = 17$.

Many of the process correlates associated with negative outcome also shared thematic similarities. Several of these items reflected hallmark aspects of psychodynamic and cognitive-behavioral approaches to treatment: discussion of activities/tasks to do outside session (Q 38), discussion centers on cognitive themes (Q 30), and patient's feelings/perceptions are linked to past (Q 92). Other items associated with negative outcome reflected therapists' prescriptive stances: therapist suggests that patient accept responsibility for problems (Q 76), therapist behaves in a teacher like (didactic) manner (Q 37), therapist encourages independence of action/opinion (Q 48), and therapist encourages patient to try new ways of behaving with others (Q 85). The following items were also correlated with negative outcome: patient relies upon therapist to solve his/her problems (Q 52), and patient's self-image is a focus of discussion (Q 35).

Another group of items not anchored around affect, but also considered to be characteristic of psychodynamic process did not predict outcome (e.g., linking patient's feelings and perceptions to the past or significant focus on defense or transference interpretations). Active ingredients in this treatment characteristic of a psychodynamic approach included a supportive working alliance and the absence of a prescriptive stance taken by the therapist.

## Discussion of the Findings and Their Clinical Implications

Further exploration of naturalistic treatments conducted by self-identified psychodynamic clinicians is warranted. The statistically and clinically significant improvements which patients made in this nonmanualized, naturalistic treatment warrant further exploration of naturalistic treatments conducted by self-identified psychodynamic clinicians. This treatment was associated with patient-reported improvement in the anticipation and experience of anxiety as well as their social and relational functioning. This improvement occurred between baseline and endpoint and baseline to follow-up. Patients' self-reported improvements also extended to the realms of physical health, quality of feelings, quality of social relations, quality of general activities, and overall life satisfaction. Consistent with the improvement reported by patients, independent ratings of patients' severity and frequency of panic attacks were reduced on average by half from baseline to endpoint.

The magnitude of the effect sizes in this pilot study ranged from slightly less to roughly equal those reported in studies employing similar outcome measures [3, 33]. At both endpoint and follow-up, patients' levels of symptomatology and sensitivity toward anxiety were closer to the mean of the normal population than the mean of adults diagnosed with panic disorder. Effect sizes for patient, clinician, and observer completed measures all tended toward the same direction. In line with what has been reported elsewhere in the psychotherapy outcome literature, clinician effect sizes were approximately double those for patients and independent raters. Taken together, the results of this pilot study warrant further exploration of naturalistic treatments conducted by self-identified psychodynamic clinicians.

## *Understanding a Treatment: The Importance of Looking beyond Labels of Theoretical Orientation to Therapy Process in Naturalistic Studies of Psychotherapy*

These treatments practiced by clinicians who self-identified as psychodynamic in orientation were characterized most highly by the presence of cognitive-behavioral process. These treatments also adhered to the psychodynamic and interpersonal prototypes indicating that processes from these orientations were present as well, but to a significantly lesser degree than CBT-oriented treatment process. At first glance, these findings present something of a conundrum. Here were clinicians self-identifying as psychodynamically oriented, fostering process that more closely resembled prototypical CBT than PD practice. And yet, psychodynamic and interpersonal processes were most consistently associated with positive outcome. Upon further reflection, it is not the results themselves but the mutually exclusive way treatment approaches are often viewed that is the source of the conundrum. Clinically speaking, the fact that these psychodynamically oriented clinicians were drawing on processes not typically associated with psychodynamic clinical practice is not surprising. Qualified clinicians do not foster therapeutic process in a patient-proof vacuum. In good treatment, patients' characteristics shape clinicians choices to use certain interventions. As practitioners in the field frequently note, "the reality of what works" with a given patient often requires a mixing of technique, intervention, and therapeutic stance based on the particular patient being treated. In naturalistic settings, where patients present with comorbidities and multiply determined problems, clinicians frequently report drawing on interventions from various schools of thought as the specifics of the case dictate.

Empirical precedence in the literature suggests that psychodynamic (compared to CBT) clinicians employ a particularly diverse range of interventions when conducting brief psychotherapy [15]. In another study of brief psychotherapy, psychodynamic clinicians were found to foster as much cognitive-behavioral as psychodynamic process [15]. In this study, clinicians' decisions to employ the kind of structuring we typically associate with CBT-oriented process may have been linked to the fact that patients were coming in for time-limited treatment of a very specific presenting problem. One implication of these results that stands in contrast to the way treatments are presented in ESTs, is that therapeutic process from multiple orientations can contribute to the process underlying a treatment. The fact that in this study experienced psychodynamic psychotherapists practicing without a manual fostered a treatment of panic that was most highly characterized by cognitive-behavioral process followed by IPT and PD process suggests that the idea of "pure" orientations may be more of a conceptual than a clinical reality.

### The Importance of Emotion-Focused Process in Treating Panic

In terms of predicting outcome, adherence to the interpersonal and psychodynamic prototypes predicted positive outcome more robustly than did adherence to the CBT prototype. This finding is meaningful on two different levels. First, it underscores the mistake inherent in assuming that the prevalence of a therapeutic process equates to positive outcome. In this pilot study, the process characterizing these treatments as a whole (cognitive-behavioral) was not reflected in the aspects of process that predicted positive outcome (interpersonal and psychodynamic) [11, 15]. Importantly, in this study neither the self-described theoretical orientation of the therapists nor the most characteristic elements of the process offered much useful information about what helped patients get better.

The potentially mutative influence of emotion-focused process is supported by the fact that emotion-focused process is represented more saliently on the PD and IPT prototypes than on the CBT prototype. Analysis of the individual PQS items in this study suggests that positive outcome was most robustly predicted by a focus on identifying and expressing (particularly negative) emotion and feelings. The individual process correlates of outcome in this study suggested that effective treatment for panic disorder focused on helping patients recognize, experience, and express negative emotions, sexual desires, and fears of dependency and separation in the context of a supportive working alliance in the absence of a prescriptive stance from the therapist.

Focusing on emotion has played an important role in treatments for panic disorder across a range of theoretical orientations. Shear maintains that the sense of helplessness that unites the subjective experiences of many panic patients stems from poorly articulated emotionality. As a result, Shear urges clinicians and patients to target unexplained emotional reactions by identifying response patterns (shame, guilt, fear, and anger) that emerge in situations eliciting panic attacks. Because clarifying emotional reactions and identifying possible negative emotional triggers decreases patients' sense of helplessness and increase their sense of self-efficacy, these interventions foster mastery and are considered therapeutic.

Milrod et al.'s [6] delineation of unidentified anger as a primary dynamic underlying is another example of the salience that emotions occupy in certain etiological explanations of panic disorder. According to Milrod's conceptualization, the fear and anger that patients experience as a result of conscious and unconscious fantasies can trigger attacks [6]. Milrod emphasizes that the expression/experience of anger for many panic patients is accompanied by an internal experience of losing the love object at whom anger was directed. Additionally, some patients can become quite guilt-ridden and experience retribution anxiety reactive to the expression of anger at important objects or those representing important objects.

The role of emotion in panic disorder has also been considered from cognitive-behavioral perspectives. Barlow, a prominent cognitive-behavioral theoretician and identifies panic patients' tendencies to constrict their range of their emotion to avoid threatening somatic symptoms. This assertion is supported by several studies in the literature examining the connection between alexithymia (characterized by difficulty recognizing and verbalizing feeling, a paucity of fantasy life, concrete speech, and thought closely tied to external events) and panic disorder. In one study [36], panic patients displayed comparatively more alexithymia than did patients with OCD. Similar to Barlow, these investigators concluded that the panic patients' higher alexithymia rates reflected a desire to minimize the range of experienced emotions. The investigators hypothesized that this minimization helped panic patients avoid the standard physiological sensations associated with fear and anxiety they would otherwise catastrophize. The question of whether panic patients' constriction of their emotional experience is a premorbid characteristic or whether it develops as a consequence of the disorder remains.

The finding from this pilot study that cognitive themes emerged as a negative process correlate of outcome may lend further albeit indirect support to the idea that emotion-focused process/interventions are important in the treatment of panic disorder Using Shear's [37] emotion-focused framework, one explanation of this finding may be that cognitive themes were too far removed from the more proximate role of emotions to be associated with positive outcome. In Shear's emotion-focused conceptualization, therapeutic gains are predicated on the identification and exploration of emotional reactions specifically. Another way of understanding the link between cognitive themes and negative outcome is that patients may have used cognitive themes as a way of intellectualizing and defending against troubling thoughts and feelings. Support for this hypothesis exists at a descriptive level as evidenced by the fact that clinicians assigned over half of the patients in the sample to the level of defensive functioning characterized by compromise formation (including intellectualization and isolation of affect).

In summary, for patients in this study, verbalization of negative feelings toward their therapists and exploration of their inner thoughts/feelings were associated with positive outcome. For clinicians, positive outcome was associated with accessing patients' unacceptable feelings, focusing on patients' feelings of guilt, and focusing on patients' feelings to deepen them.

The following excerpt drawn from a clinical hour concretely illustrates the therapist's efforts to help the dyad foster feeling-focused process:

| | |
|---|---|
| P | I don't know what I was feeling. I guess I kind of felt sorry for myself which I hate. I detest it. I don't want to feel that way. I don't want to think about it. It was a busy week at work, so whatever, it's been a stressful week. |
| T | Tell me about feeling sorry for yourself. |
| P | There are 6 million people in world. This is not a unique experience I'm having. I need to move on not just wallow in the past. Feeling sorry for myself is ridiculous. It's complete bullshit. |
| T | I wonder. . .I wonder whether feeling sorry for yourself is standing in for something – whether it's a short-cut for something? |
| P | Being lame and pathetic? |
| T | Hmmm. . .it sounds like it has something to do with feeling sad for the past. |
| P | (silence) I do feel kind of sad for the past. . .actually pretty horribly sad about all that's happened. I hate it. |
| P | This therapy is a lot about how I feel. When do we move on to something else? |

| | |
|---|---|
| *T* | What kinds of things does therapy highlight that you want to move on from? |
| *P* | I don't know...these stupid feelings, I guess. |
| *T* | We're talking about feeling sad for the past. You said something about lame and pathetic? |
| *P* | Well no matter how much we talk, it's not going to change what happened. I hate this. I just feel kind of spoiled complaining like this. |
| *T* | You keep blasting yourself for not "getting over it." But you're not completely moving on. Maybe part of you is needing to feel sad and whatever else you're feeling about what's happened before moving on. |
| *P* | Yeah, I'd give anything to move on. All of this makes me feel weak and petty...like a loser. But it's how I feel. |
| *T* | What does feeling weak and petty and like a loser bring up? |
| *P* | Embarrassed...I feel embarrassed, because I shouldn't complain. And also sad and I think I'm feeling a little angry. |

At the beginning of this excerpt the patient has difficulty knowing his own emotions. As he talks, he identifies feeling sorry for himself. As soon as he identifies this feeling, a feeling he acknowledges not wanting to experience, he changes topic to talking about how busy work has been. The therapist encourages the patient to focus on feeling sorry for himself. The patient has a difficult time doing this. Sticking closely to the patient's feelings, the therapist wonders whether feeling sorry for himself is actually Morse code for a deeper-level feeling. The patient agrees, tentatively at first, and then more emphatically that he does indeed feel sad for the past. This excerpt captures the therapist's efforts to help the patient recognize and more deeply experience feelings that the patient appears to have kept at bay.

## *Limitations*

The methodological limitations inherent in naturalistic research apply to this pilot study. In this study, causal statements about the impact of specific interventions cannot be offered because of the absence of random assignment to a comparison group. Other limitations of this study to target in future studies focus on strengthening the generalizability of these results. This would likely involve utilizing a design with a more even distribution of the number of clinicians per patient, an increased number of patients in the sample, and a greater diversity of patients both in terms of ethnicity and gender. Our sample consisted of 89% women and 78% Caucasian patients. Also, some critics of the prototype method using the PQS have questioned the ability of the 100 Q-set items to comprehensively assess process from certain theoretical perspectives (e.g., [38]) despite the fact that the measure has continued to successfully identify significant predictors of outcome across a range of different treatment modalities.

## Conclusion and Future Directions

The results of this pilot study contribute evidence to a small but growing body of literature suggesting that psychodynamic clinicians can and do treat panic patients effectively [9, 39]. It is important to note that the American Psychiatric Association's relegation of psychodynamic treatments for panic disorder to a low position of clinical confidence [17] follows from the fact that these treatments have not been sufficiently tested as opposed to having been tested and proven ineffective [10]. The psychodynamically oriented clinicians in this study utilized a broad range of treatment approaches including emotion-focused process, elements of CBT process, and psychodynamic elements of process.

In this chapter, emotion-focused process is presented as a potentially significant change process in the effective treatment for panic disorder. Emotion-focused process has been shown to distinguish psychodynamic from cognitive-behavioral psychotherapeutic approaches [40, 41]. The emphasis which a number of contemporary treatment models for brief psychodynamic psychotherapy place on attending to emotion [42, 43], in addition to the synergistic way these approaches target both symptoms and personality functioning, underscores the importance of representing these treatments in the treatment armamentarium for panic disorder.

The results of this study also point to the importance of examining treatment process at multiple levels of analysis. In this pilot study we learned that although clinicians were highly effective, their self-identified primary orientation did not correspond to predominant therapeutic processes fostered in treatment with their patients. We also learned that the most predominant process was not necessarily the most important one. Without careful examination of process at multiple levels, which included both macrolevel (e.g., prototype analyses) and microlevel (e.g., individual item analyses), we might have erroneously labeled the treatment as psychodynamic (because of the clinician's self-reported orientations) or cognitive-behavioral (because this process was most charactersistic). Neither of these labels would have contributed much to our understanding of how to help patients improve. Much like the shortcomings of diagnoses, which often involve an inability to guide treatment, brand names of orientations and therapies leave much to be desired when it comes to understanding what specifically promotes therapeutic change and likely often contribute to faulty assumptions about why patients got better.

This pilot study stands to further contribute to the literature by underscoring an alternative approach to studying treatments that has been proposed in the psychotherapy treatment literature recently. This study utilized an atheoretical empirically grounded approach to identify empirically derived changed processes. Having assumed that clinicians might learn how to conduct effective treatments through experience with hypothesis testing in clinical practice, we studied what experienced clinicians did when left to their own devices to treat patients as they normally do outside research protocol. Although the gold standard procedure currently for evaluating treatment is to test them as packages of intervention under controlled conditions before "exporting" them to clinical practice outside the laboratory, the results of this study also suggest the intriguing possibility that the reverse may make more sense [10]. That is naturalistic study designs could be used to identify what it is that clinicians in the community are doing that appears to be associated with outcome before developing treatments around these processes of change and then testing them empirically. This approach to studying treatments would help afford the additional advantage of narrowing the science–practice chasm and increasing generalizability to the consulting room since treatments constructed around empirically validated change processes practiced by experienced clinicians would likely be embraced by practitioners to a greater degree than manualized treatments developed by researchers in laboratories. This study is an example of a research paradigm that is a useful complement to randomized, controlled trials of ESTs. It exemplifies how process researchers and experienced clinicians can learn from each other by empirically validating change processes in naturalistic treatments.

**Acknowledgment** The authors wish to thank the clinicians from the MGH Psychotherapy Research Program for their willingness to participate in the study and the members of the Berkeley Psychotherapy Research Project for their invaluable help with process ratings

# References

1. Barlow, D. H, Gorman, J. M., Shear, M. K., & Woods, S. W. (2000). Cognitive-behavioral therapy, imipramine, or their combination for panic disorder: A randomized controlled trial. *Journal of the American Medical Association, 283*, 2529–2536.
2. Craske, M. G. & Barlow, D. H. (2001). Panic Disorder and Agoraphobia. In D. H. Barlow (Ed.), *Clinical Handbook of Psychological Disorders: A Step-by-Step Treatment Manual* (pp. 1–60). New York: The Guilford Press.
3. Milrod, B., Busch, F., Leon, A. C., Aronson, A., Roiphe, J., Rudden, M., et al. (2001). A pilot open trial of brief psychodynamic psychotherapy for panic disorder. *Journal of Psychotherapy Practice Research, 10*, 239–244.
4. Busch, F. N. (2008) Psychodynamic Treatment of Panic Disorder: Clinical and Research Perspectives. In R. A. Levy & J. S. Ablon (Eds), *A Handbook of Evidence-Based Psychodynamic Psychotherapy*. Totowa, NJ: Humana Press.
5. Milrod, B. & Busch, F. (1996). Long-term outcome of panic disorder treatment: A review of the literature. *Journal of Nervous and Mental Diseases, 184*, 723–730.
6. Milrod, B., Busch, F., Cooper, A., & Shapiro, T. (1997). *Manual of Panic-Focused Psychodynamic Psychotherapy*. Arlington, VA: Psychiatric Publishing.

7. Markowitz, J. S., Weissman, M. M., & Ouellette, R. (1989). Quality of life in panic disorder. *Archives of General Psychiatry, 46*, 984–992.
8. Swenson, R. P., Cox, B. J., & Woszezy, C. B. (1992). Use of medical services and treatment for panic disorder with agoraphobia and for social phobia. *Canadian Medical Journal. 147*, 878–883.
9. Milrod, B., Leon, A. C., Busch, F., Rudden, M., Schwalberg, M., Clarkin, J., et al. (2006). A randomized controlled clinical trial of psychoanalytic psychotherapy for panic disorder. *American Journal of Psychiatry, 164*, 265–272.
10. Westen, D., Novotny, C. M., & Thompson-Brenner, H. (2004). The empirical status of empirically supported psychotherapies: Assumptions, findings, and reporting in controlled clinical trials. *Psychological Bulletin, 130*, 631–663.
11. Ablon, J. S. & Jones, E. E. (2002). Validity of controlled clinical trials of psychotherapy: Findings from the NIMH treatment of depression collaborative research program. *American Journal of Psychiatry, 159*, 775–783.
12. Garfield, S. L. (1998). Some comments on empirically supported treatments. *Journal of Consulting and Clinical Psychology, 66*, 121–125.
13. Goldfried, M. R. & Wolfe, B. E. (1996). Psychotherapy practice and research: Repairing a strained alliance. *American Psychologist, 51*, 1007–1016.
14. Howard, K. I., Moras, K., Brill P. B., Martinovich, Z., & Lutz, W. (1996). Evaluation of psychotherapy: Efficacy, effectiveness, and patient progress. *American Psychologist, 51*, 1059–1064.
15. Ablon, J. S. & Jones, E. E. (1998). How expert clinicians' prototypes of an ideal treatment correlate with outcome in psychodynamic and cognitive-behavioral therapy. *Psychotherapy Research, 8*, 71–83.
16. Barlow, D. H, Craske, N. G., Cerny, J. A., & Klosko, J. S. (1989). Behavioral treatment of panic disorder. *Behavior Therapy, 20*, 261–282.
17. American Psychiatric Association: Practice Guideline for the Treatment of Patients with Panic Disorder (1998). *American Journal of Psychiatry, 155*, 945–1002.
18. Jones, E. E. (2000). *Therapeutic Action*. Northvale, NJ: Jason Aronson, Inc.
19. Shear, M. K. & Maser, J. D. (1994). Standardized assessment for panic disorder research: A conference report. *Archives of General Psychiatry, 51*, 346–354.
20. Reiss, S., Peterson, R. A., Gursky, D. M., & McNally, R. J. (1986). Anxiety sensitivity, anxiety frequency and the prediction of fearfulness. *Behavior Research and Therapy, 24*, 1–8.
21. Shear, M. K., Brown, T. A., Barlow, D. H., Money, R., Sholomskas, D. E., & Woods, S. W., et al. (1997). Multicenter collaborative panic disorder severity scale. *American Journal of Psychiatry, 154*, 1571–1575.
22. Derogatis, L. R., Lipman, R. S., Rickels, K., Uhlenhuth, E. H., & Covi, L. (1974). The Hopkins symptom checklist: A self-report symptom inventory. *Behavioral Science, 19*, 1–15.
23. Endicott, J., Nee, J., Harrison, W., & Blumenthal, R. (1993). Quality of life enjoyment and satisfaction questionnaire: A new measure. *Psychopharmacology Bulletin, 29*, 321–326.
24. Guy, W. (1976). *Assessment Manual for Psychopharmacology*. Washington, DC: US Government Printing Office.
25. Endicott, J., Spitzer, R. L., Fleiss, J. L., & Cohen, J. (1976). The global assessment scale: A procedure for measuring general severity of psychiatric disturbance. *Archives of General Psychiatry, 33*, 761–777.
26. Barlow, D. H., Gorman, J. M., & Shear, M. K. (1997). *Results from the Multi-Center Comparative Treatment Study of Panic Disorder: Acute and Maintenance Outcome*. Canterbury, England: British Association of Behavioral and Cognitive Psychotherapy.
27. Ablon, J. S. & Jones, E. E. (1999). Psychotherapy process in the NIMH collaborative research program. *Journal of Consulting and Clinical Psychology, 67*, 64–75.
28. Jones, E. E., Cumming, J. D., & Horowitz, M. J. (1988). Another look at the nonspecific hypothesis of therapeutic effectiveness. *Journal of Consulting and Clinical Psychology, 56*, 48–55.

29. Jones, E. E., Hall, S., & Parke, L. A. (1991). The Process of Change: The Berkeley Psychotherapy Research Group. In L. Beutler & M. Crago (Eds), *Psychotherapy Research: An International Review of Programmatic Studies*. Washington, DC: American Psychological Association.
30. Jones, E. E. & Pulos, S. M. (1993). Comparing the process in psychodynamic and cognitive-behavioral therapies. *Journal of Consulting and Clinical Psychology, 61*, 306–316.
31. Orlinsky, D. E. & Howard, K. I. (1986). Process and Outcome in Psychotherapy. In A. E. Garfield & A. E. Bergin (Ed.), *Handbook of Psychotherapy and Behavior Change*, 3rd Edn. New York: Wiley.
32. Lambert, M. J. & Hill, C. E. (1994). Assessing Psychotherapy Outcomes and Processes. In A. E. Bergin & S. L. Garfield (Eds), *Handbook of Psychotherapy and Behavior Change* (pp. 72–113). New York: Wiley.
33. Otto, M. W., Pollack, M. H., Penava, S. J., & Zucker, B. G. (1999). Group cognitive-behavior therapy for patients failing to respond to pharmacotherapy for panic disorder: A clinical case series. *Behavior Research and Therapy, 37*, 763–770.
34. Jacobson, N. S. & Truax, P. (1991). Clinical significance: A statistical approach to defining meaningful change in psychotherapy research. *Journal of Consulting and Clinical Psychology, 59*, 12–19.
35. Cohen, J. (1988). *Statistical Power Analysis for the Behavioral Sciences*. Hillsdale, NJ: Erlbaum.
36. Zeitlin, S. B. & McNally, R. J. (1993). Alexithymia and anxiety sensitivity in panic disorder and obsessive-compulsive disorder. *American Journal of Psychiatry, 150*, 658–660.
37. Shear, M. K., Cloitre, M., & Heckelman, L. (1995). Emotion-focused treatment for panic disorder: A brief, dynamically informed therapy. In J. P. Barber & P. Crits-Christoph (Eds), *Dynamic Therapies for Psychiatric Disorders* (p. 460). New York: Basic Books, Inc.
38. Markowitz, J. C. (2003). Letter to the Ed.: Controlled trials of psychotherapy. *American Journal of Psychiatry, 160*, 186–187.
39. Wiborg, I. M. & Dahl, A. A. (1996). Does brief dynamic psychotherapy reduce the relapse rate of panic disorder? *Archives of General Psychiatry, 53*, 689–694.
40. Blagys, M. D. & Hilsenroth, M. J. (2000). Distinctive features of short-term psychodynamic-interpersonal psychotherapy: A review of the comparative psychotherapy process literature. *Clinical Psychology: Science and Practice, 7*, 167–188.
41. Blagys, M. D. & Hilsenroth, M. J. (2002). Distinctive features of short-term psychodynamic-interpersonal psychotherapy: An empirical review of the comparative psychotherapy process literature. *Clinical Psychology Review, 22*, 671–706.
42. Foscha, D. (2002). The activation of affective changes processes in Accelerated Experiential-Dynamic Psychotherapy (AEDP). In F. W. Kaslow (Editor-In-Chief) & J. J. Magnavita (Volume Editor), *Comprehensive Handbook of Psychotherapy: Vol. 1, Psychodynamic/Object Relations* (pp. 309–343). New York: John Wiley & Sons, Inc.
43. McCullough, L., Kuhn, N., Andrews, S., Kaplan, A., Wolf, J., & Hurley, C. L. (2003). *Treating Affect Phobia: A Manual for Short-term Dynamic Psychotherapy*. New York, NY: Guilford Press.

# Chapter 4
# Empirical Support for Psychodynamic Psychotherapy for Eating Disorders

Heather Thompson-Brenner, Jolie Weingeroff, and Drew Westen

## Introduction: Psychodynamic Psychotherapy for Eating Disorders

The available research suggests that the etiology of eating disorders (EDs) is multifactorial and individually variable, with risk conferred from personality pathology, family history, developmental history, sociocultural phenomena, comorbid disorders, and genetic endowment [1–5]. The treatment of EDs is complicated by characteristic problems in interpersonal relationships, resistance to change in symptomatic behavior, and difficulty in accessing emotional experience [6, 7]. Psychotherapy for EDs must target not only overt symptoms, but also motivation, emotion regulation, insight, and resistance [8]. Among the various forms of "talk therapy," psychodynamic psychotherapy arguably has the most techniques for addressing the complex problems characteristic of individuals with EDs.

Psychodynamic psychotherapies encompass a broad range of techniques and theories. Dynamic therapy focuses on changing individual implicit associative networks, relational patterns (and the internal representations of self and others that accompany them), and ways of regulating impulses and emotions. Patients in dynamic therapy are encouraged to access their implicit feelings, representations, and motives, as well as their characteristic emotion management techniques (defenses), and to learn to better manage the conflicting motivational forces clarified through the psychotherapy process—in other words, to understand and transform their personality. Dynamic therapy may examine the developmental history of these implicit relational and emotional networks, and the relationship between the patient and the therapist may be used as a source of information or transformation regarding the patient's typical relational patterns and disavowed experience [9].

Dynamic therapies have not been adequately tested in treatment trials for EDs, though the recognition that symptom-focused treatments do not fully address these complex disorders is growing. Data from treatment trials for

H. Thompson-Brenner
Boston University, 648 Beacon Street, Boston, MA 02215
e-mail: ht141@hotmail.com

R.A. Levy, J.S. Ablon (eds.), *Handbook of Evidence-Based Psychodynamic Psychotherapy*,
DOI: 10.1007/978-1-59745-444-5_4, © Humana Press 2009

symptom-focused treatments suggest that the majority of patients either drop out or fail to recover [6, 10]. Short-term therapies for bulimia nervosa (BN) such as cognitive–behavioral therapy (CBT) were touted as successful after an early series of randomized controlled trials (RCTs) [11, 12]. It was later noted, however, that these therapies had demonstrated "efficacy" primarily relative to wait-list controls or deliberately inert versions of dynamic therapy [10, 13] and that their success rate was only moderate at best. Naturalistic research suggests that experienced clinicians who treat EDs in the community frequently use psychodynamic psychotherapy, alone or in combination with other interventions, as their main approach [14, 15]. Clinicians note that psychodynamic psychotherapy or integrative therapies are particularly helpful to treat their patients with complex comorbid conditions, with emotion regulation problems, with interpersonal problems, and those who persistently avoid emotional experience [14–16].

The evidence base for psychodynamic psychotherapy for EDs comes from various sources, reviewed in this chapter. The small number of RCTs and pilot studies of psychodynamic psychotherapy for EDs, taken as a whole, suggest that dynamic therapies—when intended by the researchers to perform as active treatments, rather than as largely inert controls—are at least as efficacious as other forms of outpatient psychotherapy for EDs [17–20]. The field clearly needs additional trials of dynamic therapy performing under optional conditions, such as less-constrained treatment length and adequate latitude to focus on personality issues. Additional evidence is provided from naturalistic research, which documents productive change in community samples treated with psychodynamic psychotherapy [8, 14, 15, 21]. Further evidence is provided from studies of related forms of psychotherapy, in most cases adapted from psychodynamic practice but intended as controls in RCTs for EDs. This group of surprisingly efficacious psychodynamic modifications includes interpersonal psychotherapy (IPT) and supportive therapy. Finally, the more extensive research supporting the efficacy of psychodynamic psychotherapy for related conditions, such as personality disorders (PDs), interpersonal problems, and motivation and alliance issues, which characterize groups with EDs, lends some additional evidentiary support to its utility for treating EDs.

## Eating Disorder Diagnoses

Eating disorder classification includes two major diagnoses, anorexia nervosa (AN) and BN, and the category "eating disorder not otherwise specified" (EDNOS), which in fact includes most individuals with EDs [22]. The EDs share the distinctive feature of overconcern with shape, weight, or eating, to a degree that is subjectively distressing and interferes with functioning. Anorexia nervosa is distinguished by low weight—weight below 85% of the ideal for one's height. Anorexia nervosa has two subtypes: "restricting" subtype includes individuals who are low weight through restricting caloric intake and exercise alone, while "binge/purge" subtype includes those who also binge or purge regularly. Bulimia nervosa is characterized by weight above the AN threshold and regular binge eating and purging by vomiting or other compensatory measures, such as driven exercise, fasting, diuretic use, or laxative use. EDNOS is a catch-all category that includes some distinctive eating irregularities, such as binge eating disorder (BED) (binge eating without purging behavior), "chewing and spitting," and night eating syndrome. EDNOS also includes all other patterns in which people experience some of the symptoms of other EDs (body image concerns, purging only, large losses of weight, and strong concern with weight loss and other AN symptoms but not at the 85% weight threshold, etc.).

## Randomized Controlled Trials

The evidence base available from RCTs for EDs in general is not extensive [6, 23]. Recent reviews and meta-analyses have noted that no form of psychotherapy for adult AN has demonstrated an adequate level of efficacy in repeated trials [23]. Only CBT for BN, and to a more limited extent, IPT for BN and family treatment for adolescent AN, has demonstrated efficacy relative to another manualized condition in more than one trial [23]. A recent task force reporting on obstacles to research in EDs noted multiple challenges to conducting full-scale treatment trials, including low base rates of certain EDs in the community, the low motivation or ambivalence about change inherent to the disorders, and the lack of data strongly supporting any form of psychotherapy for use with EDs (AN in particular) [6]. Data for treatments of BN and recently BED are somewhat more available than for AN but still scarce relative to other major mental health disorders.

## Trials of Psychodynamic Psychotherapy for Eating Disorders

Though CBT and behavioral therapies are the most cited randomized trials in the literature, more trials of psychodynamic psychotherapy do exist than are commonly noted or cited in reviews. It is difficult to identify these studies, however, due to a lack of transparency regarding the researchers' intent to (a) truly examine the psychodynamic (or dynamically inspired) treatment group for its potential for success or (b) use the seemingly psychodynamic group primarily as a minimal-intervention control group. In the latter set of studies, the seemingly dynamic (or supportive) treatment approach does not highlight active components of psychodynamic treatment (e.g., active pursuit of denied or disavowed affect and discussion of possible origins of difficulties in relational history). Instead, the manualized approach prioritizes inactive elements (e.g., "neutrality"), by refusing to answer questions, discuss ED symptoms directly, or suggest topics of discussion. These minimal control groups deliberately do not accurately represent psychodynamic practice, and their failure to stand up to more active treatments does not reflect on psychodynamic psychotherapy as it is normally practiced by well-trained clinicians. In addition, the identification of more relevant studies, in which a psychodynamic psychotherapy was intended as an active treatment, is further complicated by the chosen names of these treatment approaches, which—given the breadth of the field at this point—often focus on one or another specific theory of psychodynamic practice (e.g., "self-psychology"). We were able to identify three RCTs for AN using active psychodynamic approaches, one active study of psychodynamic psychotherapy for BN, and one for BED. In addition, one pilot study of integrative psychodynamic psychotherapy for BN and BED produced outcomes worthy of notice.

The three trials of psychodynamic psychotherapy for AN showed consistently positive results. Treasure and colleagues [20] randomly assigned 30 adult patients with AN to either a dynamic intervention termed cognitive analytic therapy (CAT) or educational behavioral therapy (EBT). Cognitive analytic therapy closely focuses on interpersonal relationships, including both the relationship between the therapist and the patient (the transference) and the development of current maladaptive interpersonal patterns in the context of the patient's relational history [24]. Cognitive analytic therapy is based on the theory that anorexic symptoms function as part of repetitive interpersonal schemas, such as avoidance of abandonment or competition as assertion of worth [24]. In the treatment trial for CAT, both the CAT and the EBT groups performed comparably to other treatment trials for outpatient adult with AN: 63% had good or intermediate recovery overall. The CAT and EBT groups did not show significant differences from one another on posttreatment body mass index (BMI); however, individuals in the CAT group reported significantly better self-rated outcome [20]. Dare and colleagues [18] included both CAT and another dynamic treatment, focal psychoanalytic therapy, in an AN trial, which also included family therapy and a minimal contact control group. Focal psychoanalytic therapy was based on short-term dynamic treatment as proposed by Malan [25], who emphasized active interpretation of the unconscious meaning of symptoms in the context of intrapsychic conflicts. In this study of $N = 84$ adult outpatients ($N = 54$ completers) in four groups, both psychoanalytic psychotherapy and family therapy were significantly superior to the control treatment [18]. Finally, Bachar and colleagues [17] included eight individuals with AN in their larger trial of Self Psychology for mixed ED groups (reviewed in more detail below). Though the AN group was obviously too small for separate comparison, Self Psychology produced significantly greater improvement in objective rating of ED outcome overall [17].

The trial of Self Psychology mentioned above [17] is the only truly psychodynamic psychotherapy tested to date in an RCT for BN, according to our review. The trial therapy was based on the work of Kohut, and psychotherapists viewed binge eating as a self-object function, meant to serve emotional needs that were not served well historically in relationships. In accordance with self-psychological technique, the psychotherapy emphasized the mutative nature of the transferential relationship to the therapist, as well as the need for narcissistic support. In addition, the trial included a cognitive orientation and a minimal-intervention nutritional control group. As noted, subjects with both AN ($N = 8$) and BN ($N = 25$) were combined for comparison. Statistical analysis indicated that Self Psychology was efficacious compared to the control group [17], though the trial was too small to allow for strong comparisons between the Self Psychology and cognitive orientation groups.

A larger trial was conducted for patients with BED, comparing group psychodynamic interpersonal psychotherapy (GPIP) to CBT delivered in groups [26]. The psychodynamic intervention in this study was based on the premise that binge eating is a symptom of negative moods that are triggered by interpersonal interactions. Negative interactions are thought to generate and perpetuate cyclical relational patterns [27] and, as theorized by Benjamin and Bowlby, support negative internal representations of self and others [26]. Group psychodynamic interpersonal psychotherapy is also influenced by Yalom's work and is delivered in group form in order to best observe and address in vivo social relational patterns [26]. In the RCT of $N = 135$ total subjects, both GCBT and GPIP produced improvements in ED symptoms relative to a wait-list control, but neither was more efficacious than the other. Group psychodynamic interpersonal psychotherapy was shown to significantly reduce depressive symptoms, including aspects of mood and self-esteem, relative to GCBT at follow-up time points [26, 28].

Multiple authors have suggested that psychodynamic psychotherapy can be usefully integrated with cognitive–behavioral interventions [29–31], and in fact the majority of clinicians practicing in the community choose to integrate approaches with their ED clients [8]. One notable, recent pilot study of subjects with BN ($N = 14$) and BED ($N = 7$) examined a time-limited integrative approach incorporating self-monitoring, prescribed eating, and weekly weighing from CBT for EDs, combined with the examination of key focal conflicts, unconscious and dynamic meaning of symptoms, and the development of insight into the relationship between developmental difficulties and current ED symptoms from typical psychodynamic practice [19]. Though the pilot study had no comparison group, end-of-treatment statistics indicated that all subjects completed the trial, and only 3 of 14 subjects with BN continued to binge and 4 of 13 to purge—a recovery rate between 70 and 80%. Compared to a general recovery rate closer to 40% for individual CBT (albeit a much more stable estimate) [10], the integrative approach seems to hold promise and certainly deserves additional research attention.

## Cognitive–Behavioral Therapy for Eating Disorders: Symptom-Focused Interventions

It is worthwhile to review theory and data concerning CBT for EDs, both as a contrast to the dynamic data and as a source of symptom-focused interventions that might usefully be integrated with psychodynamic approaches. As noted earlier, the most extensive RCT data concern CBT, as Fairburn and colleagues [32, 33] have tested their manualized version of individual CBT for BN in multiple large-scale trials, and data have been published from at least nine other smaller trials of individualized CBT [10]. Cognitive–behavioral therapy for BN as standardized by the Fairburn manual involves structured interventions administered over 20 weeks [34]. Psychotherapists require patients to record all eating, binge eating, and purging episodes and to bring records to sessions. The protocol version of the therapy first requires patients to eat on a normal schedule and then to normalize portions and content of meals, reducing restriction and reintroducing feared foods to the diet [34]. Patients weigh themselves weekly, to reduce both overweighing (which has obsessional and compulsive elements, which increase anxiety over weighing) and underweighing (which as a form of avoidant behavior is also thought to increase anxiety over weight) [35]. Normalized eating and weighing behavior together is observed in CBT to reduce binge eating and purging behavior to some extent. Further interventions involve close observation of the context and precipitants of residual binge eating and purging behaviors, and targeted, semiindividualized interventions around cognitive, behavioral, and emotional triggers to binge eat and to purge [34, 36]. Additional interventions added to the manual more recently target body image disturbances, particularly through the reduction of "checking" and avoiding behaviors, such as frequently checking (or avoiding) mirrors and checking body shape by touch [35, 37].

Though CBT for BN has the most extensive RCT research base, the limitations of CBT for BN are now widely noted. Meta-analysis of CBT RCT data indicates that only 40% of those patients who enter the protocols successfully complete the treatment and recover by the posttreatment evaluation [10]. Symptom levels for those patients who do not recover remain significant, indicating that nonrecovered individuals continue to binge eat and purge several times per week [10]. In addition, careful examination of the relatively strict inclusion and exclusion criteria imposed in the first generation of RCTs of CBT for BN suggests that they likely excluded many potentially severe, difficult-to-treat patients. For example, patients with borderline personality disorder (BPD) and BN have been observed to commonly abuse substances, exhibit self-destructive behavior, and show irregular manifestation of binge/purge symptoms ("subclinical" BN) [14, 38], behaviors which could have easily excluded most individuals with BPD from most CBT trials published to date. Cognitive-behavioral therapy researchers report that more open trials of more flexible protocols, intended to address cooccurring problems as well as eating symptoms, are now under way [39]. Furthermore, short-term CBT is not intended to address personality pathology, and even the more flexible new generation of CBT approaches, which incorporate optional interventions for mood dysregulation and interpersonal difficulties, does not approach these issues as deep-seated personality issues but rather as obstacles to recovery that can be addressed in the second phase of a short-term treatment [40].

Though manualized CBT for BN may be limited in its application to the wide range of comorbid problems that individuals with this diagnosis can have, the outcomes of these treatment trials suggest a few important lessons for psychodynamic psychotherapists about the utility of structured treatment interventions for reducing symptoms in this population. Cognitive–behavioral therapy for BN is built upon the premise that behavioral symptoms create an interlocking, self-perpetuating trap that is difficult to reverse once set in motion [34]. Cognitive–behavioral therapy for BN posits that the imposition of caloric restriction and strict dietary rules leave individuals vulnerable to binge eating, and binge eating sets the stage for a weight-conscious person to employ compensatory measures such as purging and driven exercise. In turn, the belief that these compensatory measures rid the body of the effects of binge eating further disinhibits future binge eating, and binge eating drives additional restriction, again reciprocally making binge eating more likely. Through careful self-monitoring of eating and bulimic behaviors (as well as emotional and interpersonal contexts), systematic introduction of normalized eating, education about the inefficacy of symptoms to control weight, and support to eliminate compensatory behaviors, it is possible to reduce overtly distressing and disruptive ED behaviors, either as a goal unto itself or to the extent that more insight-oriented work can be attempted [19].

## Naturalistic Research in Eating Disorders and Psychodynamic Psychotherapy

Though RCTs have been privileged of late as the key method of treatment research, naturalistic research can yield essential information that is not accessible within the RCT paradigm [13]. Naturalistic examination of treatment as it takes place in the community is able to access large numbers of clinician/patient pairs, and therefore examines multiple therapy variables (e.g., treatment orientation, individual interventions, and length of treatment) and patient variables (e.g., primary diagnosis and severity, comorbid diagnoses and severity) simultaneously. At best, RCTs have the resources to recruit and treat moderate numbers of patients, while naturalistic research may cast a wider net. Furthermore, RCTs are consistently limited to testing a few manualized assortments of interventions that may have shown some efficacy in pilot studies but are essentially chosen at an investigator's preference from the vast number of possible treatment interventions available to unconstrained clinicians.

Systematic naturalistic research has yielded important results regarding the psychodynamic treatment of patients with EDs in the community. One study of patients with bulimic symptomatology treated by experienced clinicians in the community [14] found that many clinicians use psychodynamic psychotherapy alone or in combination with other approaches when treating ED clients. Of a sample of 145 clinicians (members of the American Psychological and

American Psychiatric Associations with five or more years of experience post-training), 35% reported using dynamic therapy as their primary orientation, while 37% reported using CBT, and the remainder were generally eclectic [8]. Basic outcome data indicated that posttreatment improvement rates, recovery rates, and global functioning levels were not significantly different between patients treated by self-identified psychodynamic and cognitive–behavioral clinicians, though psychodynamic psychotherapies were significantly longer than CBTs [8].

Additional analyses of the therapy intervention questionnaire included in that study (the Comparative Psychotherapy Process Scale for Bulimia Nervosa; see [8, 41]) indicated that dynamic therapy and CBT in ED clients show identifiable distinctions, though there was considerable overlap and integration in actual practice. Factor analysis of the therapy intervention questionnaire identified a multifaceted psychodynamic approach, incorporating interventions aimed at identifying unclear and conflicting emotions, investigating patterns in relationships repeated over time and their origins in family relationship, exploring issues with anger/aggression and sexuality, and use of the patient/therapist relationship as a source of information about relationships or new model of relationships [8]. In distinction, CBT as practiced in the community involves developing strategies to eat regularly and appropriately, cope with specific symptoms inside and outside sessions, and challenge irrational or illogical thoughts about food and eating, using explicit advice and homework, including self-monitoring [8]. Other data analyses indicated that most therapists did not use one approach when treating patients with EDs, but rather that almost all therapists practiced integratively, and that psychotherapy integration (or eclecticism) increased when the patients showed more comorbidity [8]. Multiple regression analyses indicated that ED outcome did not vary significantly as a function of the treatment interventions that were employed but that global functioning was significantly positively related to both the use of the psychodynamic group of interventions and the treatment length [8].

## Personality Pathology in Eating Disorders and Psychodynamic Psychotherapy

Research into the nature of personality disturbance in EDs has important implications for treatment. Prospective studies of personality as a risk factor for the development of EDs are not numerous, though recent reviews suggest that perfectionism and obsessional characteristics are risk factors for both AN and BN [42, 43]. Trait impulsivity has not consistently emerged as a risk factor for EDs overall, though some researchers suggest that behavioral impulsivity (e.g., delinquency) indicates risk, while self-reported impulsivity does not [44, 45]. An increasing number of studies have yielded convergent results suggesting that the ED population can be meaningfully divided into empirically derived *personality subtypes*, characteristic of ED patients in particular (i.e., related to, but not the same as, the DSM-IV PD diagnoses), which indicate particular targets and methods for successful treatment intervention.

Using cluster analytic procedures, multiple subtyping studies have identified between three and five personality groups in EDs. Research has consistently suggested the presence of a *high-functioning* subtype with minimal personality pathology; an *emotionally dysregulated* subtype with borderline and histrionic tendencies (e.g., emotional instability); an *avoidant-insecure* subtype, with anxious, depressed, and socially avoidant tendencies; and a *constricted-obsessional* subtype, with obsessional, compulsive, and rigid tendencies [15, 46–50]. In addition, two studies found a *behaviorally dysregulated* type, which showed stimulus-seeking, antisocial, and impulsive dysregulated behavioral traits, rather than symptoms of affective dysregulation [47, 50].

In the major personality subtyping studies to date, including those by these authors, substantial group differences in adaptive functioning, comorbid diagnoses, possible etiological factors, and treatment outcome are observed. In our studies of adults with mixed EDs and adults with BN, personality subtype has been strongly related to global assessment of functioning (GAF) scores [15, 49, 51]. Mean pretreatment GAF score for high-functioning group is 10–20 points higher than the dysregulated group, a statistically significant difference, with the constricted groups falling between them; histories of hospitalization (for problems other than the ED) were similarly significantly more common for the dysregulated group and in some cases for the avoidant-insecure group as well [15, 49, 51].

These ED personality subtype groups also show distinctions in comorbid diagnoses, possible etiological factors, and general treatment response. Subjects with EDs and dysregulated personality styles have shown distinctive comorbidity with posttraumatic stress disorder and substance use disorders. The dysregulated group also shows distinct potential etiological associations with trauma histories and externalizing disorders in first-degree relatives [8, 14, 15, 48, 49]. In contrast, avoidant-insecure and constricted-obsessional subjects have shown distinctive comorbidity with anxiety disorders and associations with internalizing disorders in first-degree relatives [15, 48, 50]. Subjects with high-functioning personality styles have shown less comorbidity and associations to family-history risk factors overall [8, 15, 48, 49, 51]. The subtypes also show some relation to ED symptoms: subjects in the constricted-obsessional and avoidant-insecure groups tend to demonstrate higher levels of current or historical anorexic features, while subjects in the two dysregulated subtypes typically show binge/purge behaviors [46, 48–50]; however, the ED diagnoses do not map directly onto the personality subtypes. Finally, personality subtypes have shown important differences in treatment response and long-term outcome. Multiple regression analyses from studies of BN show that emotional dysregulation and construction negatively predict variance in both ED and global outcome from treatment, over and above that accounted for by the severity of the ED and major Axis I diagnoses [15]. In addition, recent longitudinal evidence suggests that patients with AN diagnoses at baseline have poor long-term ED outcome when avoidant subtype pathology is present, while both dysregulated/impulsive pathology and avoidant pathology predict poor global outcome [51]. Given the substantial differences between these personality subtype groups, it appears unlikely that the ideal treatment for each group, producing the maximum treatment response, would be the same. As noted earlier, clinicians in the community report using more psychodynamic interventions when personality pathology is present [8], and data suggest that they do so for good reason.

Most importantly, psychodynamic psychotherapy has been associated with the successful treatment of patients with EDs with personality pathology. Naturalistic analyses indicate that a therapeutic approach that integrates psychodynamic psychotherapy with other interventions is significantly associated with the change in GAF score and with the achievement of ED symptom remission in the emotionally dysregulated group in particular. In one study, we examined patients with emotional dysregulation treated by cognitive–behavioral therapists.[1] We assessed the degree to which the therapists integrated dynamic interventions such as a focus on past relationships, a focus on emotion regulation, and a focus on the psychotherapeutic relationship (the transference) into their treatments. Patients with moderate-to-high levels of emotional dysregulation receiving integrative treatment showed a mean change in GAF score of 27 points (SD = 15), while similar patients receiving ED-symptom-focused treatment showed a mean change in GAF score of only 15 points (SD = 10) ($t$ [36] = −3.23; $p$ = 0.003). Emotionally dysregulated patients receiving integrative treatment recovered from their ED in 70% of the cases, while patients receiving ED-symptom-focused treatment recovered from their ED in only 30% of the cases (Pearson's $\chi^2$ = 6.4; $p$ = 0.01; $N$ = 40). In Table 4.1, the "integration factor score" reflects the degree to which the CBT therapist was integrating psychodynamic interventions into his or her practice. The correlation ($r$) between the integration factor score and both global and ED outcomes is surprisingly large and statistically significant.

| Table 4.1 Correlations between integration score and outcome in dysregulated patients treated by CBT therapists | | | Change in GAF score | Abstinent from binge eating and purging |
|---|---|---|---|---|
| Integration factor score | $R$ | | 0.43 | 0.42 |
| | $p$ | | 0.004 | 0.007 |
| | $N$ | | 44 | 40 |

---

[1] We focus here on CBT therapists because they show more variability in the degree to which they integrate psychodynamic psychotherapy into their practice. Psychodynamic psychotherapists are uniformly psychodynamic, and therefore no relationship is seen between the use of these interventions and the outcome.

Similarly, new data on adolescents with EDs suggest that the use of psychodynamic psychotherapy is positively associated with better global outcome for patients with personality pathology [21]. Using a measure that identified distinct CBT, psychodynamic, family treatment, emotion regulation, and trauma-focused sets of interventions, psychodynamic psychotherapy was the only significant treatment correlate of global improvement with the subgroup with personality pathology [21].

In summary, basic science research in ED psychopathology has led to the observation that four or five substantial, naturally occurring personality subtypes exist in the population. Four of these subtypes show distinct patterns of long-term personality dysfunction, evidenced in adolescence as well as adulthood and associated with different patterns of comorbidity and treatment response. The limited evidence to date suggests that psychodynamic psychotherapy may be more helpful for the treatment of some of these subtypes, such as the emotionally dysregulated and avoidant groups.

## Psychodynamic Psychotherapy Treatment Trials

Though the trials of explicitly psychodynamic treatments are limited, a number of RCTs have demonstrated the efficacy of interventions that are related to psychodynamic practice and provide insight into what might be useful in treating EDs other than strictly symptom-focused treatments. These related treatments evidencing promise in RCTs for EDs include supportive psychotherapy, IPT, and dialectical–behavioral therapy (DBT).

### Interpersonal Psychotherapy

Interpersonal psychotherapy originated as an effort to manualize a form of typical practice and as a control for several treatment trials, including studies of depression and BN [33, 34, 52, 53]. Interpersonal psychotherapy for BN is a structured, short-term therapy that assesses the development of ED symptoms in the context of relationships, and subsequently targets one of the four types of relational difficulties: role transitions, grief reactions, interpersonal deficits, and interpersonal conflicts [54, 55]. Along with CBT, IPT is now one of the few forms of psychotherapy considered to have support from RCT data. The history of how this came to be is reviewed more extensively elsewhere [13]. In short, a supportive short-term version of "dynamic" therapy was used as a limited-intervention control group in an early Fairburn trial [56]. In a later trial, IPT was substituted for the focal dynamic treatment; however, therapists were enjoined from speaking about the ED symptoms after the initial assessment phase of IPT [54]. In spite of the intentionally limited nature of the intervention, patients who had received IPT in the trial improved in the treatment and continued to improve after the conclusion of treatment, eventually reaching improvement levels similar to the CBT group and significantly better than the second control [33]. These results were subsequently replicated in a larger BN trial with the same comparison groups [32].

Eating disorder researchers now suggest that IPT is likely efficacious for BN due to the frequency of interpersonal problems in ED groups [57]. Examination of IPT suggests that it shares some features in common with dynamic therapy, namely it focuses on relational functioning and relational patterns. However, process research suggests that it may be more similar to CBT than to most forms of dynamic therapy [58]. One major difference is the "present focus" of IPT, which after the assessment phase does not deal extensively with historical relationships [52]. Our own naturalistic research suggests that therapists who practice IPT with ED clients in private practice tend to use both CBT and dynamic interventions and tend to fall somewhere between self-identified CBT and dynamic therapists in the use of both approaches (Thompson-Brenner and Westen, unpublished data).

### Supportive Psychotherapy

Supportive psychotherapy has recently been identified as a potentially efficacious treatment for AN [59]. Similar to the history of IPT, "supportive clinical management" was intended as a control for CBT and IPT in a recent trial for AN. As described by the authors, supportive clinical management includes the educational components of typical clinical management concerning normal eating and weight restoration, delivered primarily via handouts, in combination with a generally supportive, positive, encouraging, nonconfrontational stance [59]. This approach was not the same as similarly named control groups that were not efficacious in early BN trials [60] but was rather developed specifically for the treatment of AN. Unexpectedly, the supportive, clinical-management intervention produced superior outcomes to IPT across primary ED measures. Cognitive–behavioral therapy and IPT did not differ significantly, and CBT and supportive clinical management did not differ from each other, on ED outcome. Concerning global outcome, supportive clinical management was superior to both CBT and IPT in posttreatment GAF scores; the latter two therapies did not differ from each other [59].

Eating disorder researchers have again produced post hoc theories about the success of supportive therapy in this AN trial. One possibility is that supportive psychotherapy, like psychodynamic psychotherapy, does not include early, active symptom intervention, and instead allows AN patients with low motivation and high ambivalence (the majority) to develop their own motivation for improvement and avoids resistance to therapy. Another possibility is that the actively warm, positive, encouraging (i.e., supportive) stance of the therapist is particularly mutative for AN patients who often have pervasive fears of relationships and low self-esteem [51]. Optimally, the positive findings regarding the utility of supportive psychotherapy will be replicated, and the active ingredients will be identified, combined, and augmented to produce a truly active, supportive treatment. Otherwise, supportive psychotherapy, like IPT, could make its way into the treatment community as a limited treatment that does not maximize the potential of either the main approach or related, active techniques.

### Dialectical–Behavioral Therapy

Several treatment trials have tested abridged versions of Dialectical-behavioral therapy (DBT) [61] for patients with EDs, including BN and BED [62–64]. DBT was originally intended for the treatment of borderline PD, which, as is reviewed below, is often comorbid with EDs. Though the structured interventions included in DBT (e.g., diary cards and homework exercises) are drawn largely from cognitive–behavioral practice, the goals of emotion identification and emotional acceptance are akin to aspects of dynamic practice [61]. Dialectical– behavioral therapy also resembles psychodynamic psychotherapy in its emphasis on the therapeutic relationship and on treating therapy-interfering behaviors, or "transference" [61]. In addition, though DBT is focused primarily with managing aspects of the present day, the dialectical or transactional model of psychopathology posits that relational history is central to the development, and maintenance, of patterns of emotional dysregulation. Thus, DBT emphasizes the harmfulness of invalidating environments and the necessity of emotional validation in treatment [61].

Dialectical–behavioral therapy has been adapted for use with EDs, including expanded diary cards, nutritional education, and the application of distress-tolerance techniques to bodily focused judgments and impulses to binge [65, 66]. Dialectical–behavioral therapy for BN produced substantial improvement in one RCT, though recovery rates were not high relative to the results from trials of CBT for BN [62].

## *Other Evidence Supporting Psychodynamic Treatment: The Personality Disorder Literature*

Though only limited, naturalistic data exist concerning the concurrent psychodynamic treatment of personality issues and EDs, an extensive literature exists documenting the utility of psychodynamic treatment of PDs, as well as their characteristic interpersonal features, including difficulty in engaging in treatment.

### Personality Disorders

Incidence rates for the PDs as defined in the Diagnostic and Statistical Manual (DSM-IV) in ED groups are extremely high. In their extensive, recent review of the available literature on PD incidence rates in EDs, Sansone et al. [67]

concluded that the following personality "trends" exist: among individuals with AN-restricting type, obsessive–compulsive personality disorder (OCPD) co-occurs in approximately 22% of cases, avoidant PD at 19%, and BPD at 10%; among individuals with AN-binge eating/purging type, Cluster B and C PDs also dominate the picture with BPD diagnosable in approximately 25% of cases, avoidant and dependent PDs in approximately 15%. In BN, BPD occurs at an average rate of 26%, but some studies report rates as high as 37 and 42%. Obsessive–compulsive personality disorder and Cluster A PDs are the highest co-occurring PDs among those with BED, both at rates around 15%. Prevalence rates for EDs among the population with PDs are notable as well. Zanarini et al. [68] found that of a sample of 379 male and female borderline inpatients, 21% met DSM-III-R criteria for AN, 26% for BN, and 26% for EDNOS. In the same study, of 125 inpatients with other PDs, 13% met criteria for AN, 17% met for BN, and 9% for EDNOS.

Extensive evidence exists supporting the use of psychodynamic psychotherapy for the treatment of PDs. Though a detailed review of this topic is beyond the scope of this chapter, a few points are worth noting. Leichsenring and Leibing [69] conducted a recent, comprehensive meta-analysis of RCT studies of psychodynamic ($N = 14$) and cognitive–behavioral treatments ($n = 11$) of PDs, between 1974 and 2001, primarily for severe Cluster A and B PDs. Psychodynamic treatments were observed to be longer than CBT across studies. The authors calculated weighted and unweighted effect sizes for treatment outcome of each study, concluding that psychodynamic therapies yielded larger mean effect sizes of overall outcome and observer measures than did cognitive–behavioral therapies. The review also noted a large effect size for personality change, indicating long-term changes in personality pathology from psychodynamic psychotherapy at 15-month average follow-up [69]. From the three studies of psychodynamic psychotherapy, which included remittance rates (no longer meeting criteria for a PD at outcome), a 59% recovery rate of PD was calculated. A systematic literature review by Bateman and Fonagy [70], concerning largely the same literature, concludes that there is evidence supporting the effectiveness of psychodynamic psychotherapy (as well as long-term CBT) with PDs generally, and particularly with borderline PD.

**Interpersonal Problems**

Given the high incidence rate of PDs in ED groups, it is unsurprising that the interpersonal and affective qualities characteristic of PDs are observed in ED groups as well. Patients with EDs are observed to have long-standing difficulty in relationships [71–74]. Some research indicates that interpersonal sensitivity may directly help to maintain bulimic symptoms [75]. Women with BED are also noted to report high levels of interpersonal distress, including long histories of social isolation and extreme difficulty in developing and maintaining intimate relationships [45, 73, 74]. Patients with EDs may show the interpersonal deficits characteristic of avoidant PD, as well as the highly conflictual relationships characteristic of borderline PD [46, 47, 50, 51].

Reviews of the PD literature note that outcome measurement is too inconsistent to compare comorbid or associated problems, such as interpersonal outcome [69, 70]. Naturalistic data reviewed above suggest that psychodynamic psychotherapy for EDs as practiced by experienced clinicians in the community includes a specific focus on relational problems, and the origin of relational problems in family and developmental histories, as well as the relationship between the therapist and the patient [8]. There are no data speaking directly to the question of whether the psychodynamic approach, which incorporates historical and transference foci, is more effective than other (efficacious) approaches such as IPT, which almost exclusively addresses present-day relationships and does not focus extensively on the relational history or the transference. As noted above, transference-based treatments such as CAT and Self Psychology have observed success with AN and BN patients in treatment trials [17, 20], and psychodynamic approaches have observed success in community samples [8], particularly with those patients with personality pathology [21]. However, the history of focus on the interpersonal relationship in psychodynamic object relations theory is far more extensive than any other tradition [76], and could well prove superior to other more limited treatments if tested empirically with EDs.

Transference-focused psychotherapy (TFP) and mentalization-based therapy (MBT) are two dynamic therapies, which have been tailored to the treatment of BPD, structured via manuals, and empirically evaluated, and both have suggested that dynamic attention to the relationship with a personality-disordered individual can yield interpersonal results. In their work, Bateman and Fonagy [77–79] have demonstrated the success of their psychoanalytically oriented mentalization-based treatment in the partial hospitalization treatment of borderline women. Mentalization-based therapy focuses on patients' interpersonal awareness and improvement in the coherence of their mental representations, producing improvements in attachment, emotional regulation, and interpersonal functioning [80]. In their development and evaluation of TFP, Clarkin and colleagues [81, 82] have shown that TFP's emphasis on the transference relationship and continual exploration of the patient's sense of self and others reduces suicidal and self-injurious behaviors, compared to the year prior to treatment [81]. These results from trials of psychodynamic treatments for BPD may indicate that similar approaches for the substantial number of individuals with EDs and interpersonal issues may be useful as well.

**Treatment Resistance**

Patients with EDs present for treatment with several other salient characteristics that complicate their readiness and suitability for any form of "talk therapy," be it insight-oriented or symptom-focused. Extensive research suggests that patients with EDs have particular difficulty in identifying their emotions ("alexithymia"), including both impoverished skills in this area and active discomfort with emotional material [83, 84]. Patients with AN are widely observed to enter treatment with general resistance, as they may be skeptical of the therapeutic relationship and feel ambivalence toward getting better [85]. These patients are often known to experience uncertainty that the therapist will be able to understand their unique suffering, fears of engulfment or control, and a general reluctance to enter into a relationship [85, 86]. Interpreting this resistance and the underlying affect is particularly important in establishing a therapeutic alliance and engaging the patient in therapy, as higher defensiveness has been shown to contribute to lower working alliance in CBT and dynamic therapies for depression [87]. Though the topic is beyond the scope of this review, psychoanalytic psychotherapy is arguably based upon the premise that the resistance is the focus of the therapy, and psychodynamic theorists and clinicians have extensive experience in addressing this aspect of practice. Limited research supports this endeavor; for example, Foreman and Marmar [88] found that therapist interpretations of defenses and resistance predicted improvements in alliance and better outcome. Psychodynamic psychotherapies may lend themselves more naturally to dealing with these issues than do more symptom-focused interventions, and therefore may again prove useful if these interventions were standardized and tested empirically with EDs.

## Case Vignette: Dynamic Psychotherapy for Bulimia Nervosa

Ruth is a 30-year-old married woman with one child, who works as a homemaker and part-time freelance writer. Ruth meets criteria for BN and has features of borderline PD. She has a 15-year history of BN, which began with an episode of adolescent AN that was untreated. She has a history of alcohol abuse in college, from which she recovered in Alcoholics Anonymous. She experiences emotional dysregulation, including very strong and labile affect as well as frequent rage and sensitivity to criticism. Like many individuals with EDs, she is a perfectionist; however her perfectionism has borderline features and is better described as a tendency to split her self-representations—she finds it extremely difficult to hold in mind that she might still be a good person if she does anything that she believes is "bad." This pattern of self-criticism and anger in response to her own devaluation (or perceived devaluation by others) applies both to her relationship with food and her relationship with other issues and people in her life. She has been in an integrative psychotherapy for 6 months. She is trying to overcome food rules, and also to react to "breaking" a food rule not by purging and/or restricting, but to be empathic to her own lapses and resume regular eating. She is also trying to accept and express patterns of self-criticism; we are working slowly toward being able to understand the feeling of being judged, and her reactive anger, as dimensions of projections and complex interactions around projective identifications, i.e., she believes others are as critical as she is of herself, and through her own actions, she can cause people to feel and express this judgment that is really a dimension of her relationship to herself and her personal history. Ruth reports that she was always very sensitive and very emotional, and that her large family criticized her for this. She also reports that her mother was extremely self-involved and overwhelmed by the demands of a large family, and that she was emotionally and at times physically neglected. The following text is from the last 15 min of a session.

## Session Excerpt

| | |
|---|---|
| T | How have things been around food this week? |
| P | I had a terrible day yesterday. But I can't handle that right now. I am trying to look only at the good. I am trying to do like you would do. Okay. I have a fear . . . okay. On Wednesday I went to a party. And I ate the bread. I felt really bad about it. Then, yesterday was a snow day. And two rambunctious kids arrived for a ride to school, and then they called school off. Oh, no! Two more rambunctious kids! I was panicking. So I made them English muffins. And we had this gourmet bread in the kitchen—it was calling me. So I had bread—toast, a bowl of oatmeal, yogurt. That was it. But during the day I wanted to be bad. I just wanted to be *bad*. I had already eaten just enough to make me feel bad. But then, I had a normal lunch! I just resumed my day! And I had stew for dinner. |
| T | Hey, how about that! It sounds like you were feeling overwhelmed, and eating bread was a part of that overwhelmed and maybe put-upon feeling. But then instead of getting too mad, or too much into feeling *bad*, you let yourself have a normal day. |
| P | Not terrible! I reviewed the good things. Which you would do for me, I did for myself. Over the past 2 weeks, I have only purged two times. |
| T | That is great, Ruth. |
| P | I know! It really is! Okay, now this is now. The last 2 weeks have been good overall. But Ben is too hooked in with me, so if I say something in a bitchy way he reacts. "*Okay*, Ruth." It makes me want to cry (starts crying). Now his problem is he doesn't eat healthy. His cholesterol is *really* high. So I was on my way out to go running the other morning, and he was eating a *huge* bowl of oatmeal. I eat a quarter cup—he probably eats a cup. I mean of oats before |

they are cooked. So I tried to say, you know, Ben you should really eat healthily. And he was like *"Okay, Ruth!!"* And I wanted to cry.

*T*  I wonder—certainly Ben's health is very important. But you have to worry about food because you have an ED, and you feel you have to measure everything, and you are on your way out running at 6:30 in the morning on a winter day; of course it might also drive you crazy on a personal level that Ben isn't worrying about these things. And that might cause you to snap at him a little bit.

*P*  No, that's not it. I love running. But, he would say I was too compulsive; I have to admit, I am too compulsive, it is just too important to me. And I get irritated. But any time there is resentment toward me—it's like an old family pain—it feels like everyone is always criticizing me—my family would say, "You are too big! You are too loud!" Ben, you asshole! I'm not bad! It's not bad of me to want to take care of you (yelling)!"

*T*  Oh, Ruth, that's such a complicated situation you are describing, so complicated and taking place in a flash. Can we take a few minutes to take apart the pieces?

*P*  Sure.

*T*  It sounds to me—and maybe it's different to you, but consider my perspective for a second—it sounds to me like you are worried about his health, and maybe the issue has a little extra heat for you because it is about food, or maybe not, but your worry comes out in a way that you think maybe sounds bitchy. And if everything were very calm, you might be able to say to yourself, okay, maybe that wasn't the nicest tone of voice. But as soon as Ben snaps back at you all of a sudden, it's like your sisters and mother and everyone is a chorus of harpies screaming that you are bad in your ears, and you just have to scream back at Ben to drown them out.

*P*  Yeah. I know what I feel is fear. So I get controlling. We are both very controlling. I wanted to make a schedule for the kids, because the mornings are so stressful for me, and if I get off to a bad start with food, it is so hard for me to reclaim my day. And Ben was like, "It's impossible, the kids can't get out by 8:30." "It's impossible, they can't get to bed by

|   |   |
|---|---|
|   | whenever. I'll do my best but it's impossible." And then of course he doesn't follow through. |
| T | I can see that if he goes into it with that orientation, like it's impossible, that's a set up for it not to happen. But I wonder if there is a symbolic level. Like he's saying it's impossible for it to happen *perfectly*. In some perfectly stress-free way. |
| P | Yes, I see. That's true. But I'm not trying to deny my part of it! |
| T | I hear you, Ruth. You are really trying to see all the pieces, including yours. |
| P | I don't *want* to be controlling. |
| T | Right. You want to find a way to deal with your fear without being controlling. And it's very hard to hold onto that when people react to you by being angry or passive, aggressive, or whatever. |
| P | It reminds me of the fourth step of AA. The fourth step is to identify your resentments, but then *all* the follow-up questions are about *you*, and what *you* do to contribute and perpetuate and hold on to those resentments. And I'm working so hard on me. But sometimes I don't want to let go of my resentments. |
| T | I think because then it seems like it is *all* you, all your fault. |
| P | Yes (crying). There are so many ways it can be my fault. |
| T | You might be too angry. |
| P | I might be too crazy. And *fat*. And a *liar*. And *IRRITABLE*. |
| T | A crazy, fat, irritable, liar. |
| P | (crying and laughing) you know, I loved AA. In AA, you can just stand up in front of a group of people, and say, you know, "I just farted back there." And someone else will say, not anything about you—that's called cross talk, and it's not allowed—but they might say, "I've farted before, too. You know, I'm a farter" (both laughing). And that's so reassuring! |
| T | That is so funny. But that is not the thing that really bothers you—it's the other stuff you said. It feels good to admit to what you accuse yourself of. |
| P | Right. I want to be able to stand up and admit to being those things—or whatever it is that I really am. |
| T | And not feel ashamed. Feel understood. |
| P | Right. |

## Discussion

### Case Discussion

In this integrative session, the therapist brings up the issue of food, and the patient refers to several specifically symptom-focused goals the therapist and the patient have together. First, Ruth is trying to eat regularly—she knows that when things go awry and she feels she has broken a rule, the behavioral goal is to get back on track with regular, normal eating rather than either binge eating or compensating by vomiting. Second, she is questioning her attitude toward these behaviors and beginning to observe that the labeling of food as "bad" or her behavior as "bad" leads to additional symptomatic expression. However, from a dynamic point of view, her problems with feeling bad go far beyond the food issues, and she quickly engages in a discussion of how these self-representations cause interpersonal complications. In the interaction with her husband, she discusses, she reports she was critical of his eating, but when he reacted angrily, she became extremely upset because the criticism confirmed her own sense of herself (derived, she believes, from childhood experiences), as "all bad," as "fat," "crazy," "irritable," and "a liar." The therapist here strives to help her find a middle path toward integrated (not split) representation of herself as both good and bad, the first step of which is uncovering the projections, memories, and self-criticism that underlies the fight. As noted in the summary of the research above, clinicians treating patients with EDs in the community report integrating approaches (as in this case), and particularly dynamic therapists report helping to identify unclear and conflicting emotions, investigating patterns in relationships repeated over time and their origins in family relationship, and exploring issues with anger/aggression—all of which are seen here. In addition, the research suggests that therapists in the community use the patient/therapist relationship as a source of information about relationships or new model of relationships—in this case, Ruth alludes to the therapist as a partially internalized voice that is emphasizing her own goodness and also alludes to AA (and possibly the therapy as well) as a new place where she feels comfortable revealing her imperfections. Therapeutic action in these arenas, which are intricately interwoven with eating behaviors, is extremely helpful to patients with intense, confusing emotion, complex identity issues, traumatic histories, and chaotic relationships—namely the dysregulated subtype.

### General Discussion

Psychodynamic psychotherapy for EDs has not been adequately tested in RCTs, but data from various sources suggest that active dynamic interventions may be extremely useful for EDs, particularly for the large proportion of patients with personality pathology. Active dynamic interventions include the pursuit of denied, disavowed, or unconscious affect and motivation; the description and acceptance of previously unacceptable self-representations; the discussion of patterns of relationships from childhood and repeated over time; and the examination of the relationship between the patient and the therapist. Psychotherapy trials conducted by nondynamic researchers used largely inert forms of dynamic therapy that emphasized therapist *inactivity* as a control for symptom-focused interventions such as CBT. The few psychotherapy trials conducted by dynamic researchers suggest that various active versions of dynamic therapy, emphasizing factors such as the transference relationship, symptom symbolism, key conflicts, narcissistic vulnerabilities, and relational dynamics, can produce large improvements in ED symptoms. Naturalistic research suggests that these types of interventions may assist in symptom and global change particularly for patients with personality pathology, especially of a dysregulated or borderline type.

Future research might fruitfully focus on psychodynamic interventions for EDs, and various methods might again produce complementary results. Randomized controlled trials for manualized psychodynamic treatments of EDs might produce specific results most palatable to efficacy reviewers. However, interventions that have been to date considered the purview of behavioral and cognitive–behavioral treatments—such as careful monitoring and discussion of eating symptoms, nutritional deprivation, and food rules—have proved so useful that their integration with dynamic interventions and foci are justified. Though "dismantling" strategies for controlled trials, which minimize overlap of brand-name treatments compared in a trial, produce very specific results concerning individual interventions, they miss potential synergistic effects and reduce each form of psychotherapy to stereotyped practices that do not represent psychotherapy as practiced in the community. Integrative treatments—though they may prove equally effective as one another—have been observed to be the standard among experienced clinicians practicing without the constraints of a treatment manual and should be examined by researchers as well. Furthermore, naturalistic research in EDs provides important information to both clinicians and researchers. Before the next generation of dynamic RCTs is developed, naturalistic research should be carefully considered for indications of the most effective dynamic interventions, and the best indications of treatment match between therapy and patient.

# References

1. Bulik, C.M. (2005). Exploring the gene–environment nexus in eating disorders. *J Psychiatry Neurosci, 30*, 335–339.
2. Cassin, S.E., and von Ranson, K.M. (2005). Personality and eating disorders: a decade in review. *Clin Psychol Rev, 25*, 895–916.
3. Gowers, S.G., and Shore, A. (2001). Development of weight and shape concerns in the aetiology of eating disorders. *Br J Psychiatry, 179*, 236–242.

 4. Polivy, J., and Herman, C.P. (2002). Causes of eating disorders. *Annu Rev Psychol*, **53**, 187–213.
 5. Westen, D., Thompson-Brenner, H., and Peart, J. (2006). Personality and eating disorders. *Annu Rev Eat Disord*, **2**, 97–112. Abingdon, UK: Radcliffe Publishing.
 6. Agras, W.S., Brandt, H.A., Bulik, C.M., et al. (2004). Report of the National Institutes of Health workshop on overcoming barriers to treatment research in anorexia nervosa. *Int J Eat Disord*, **35**, 509–521.
 7. Troop, N.A., Schmidt, U.H., and Treasure, J.L. (1995). Feelings and fantasy in eating disorders: a factor analysis of the Toronto Alexithymia Scale. *Int J Eat Disord*, **18**, 151–157.
 8. Thompson-Brenner, H., and Westen, D. (2005). A naturalistic study of psychotherapy for bulimia nervosa, Part 2: therapeutic interventions in the community. *J Nerv Ment Dis*, **193**, 585–595.
 9. Blagys, M.D., and Hilsenroth, M.J. (2000). Distinctive features of short-term psychodynamic interpersonal psychotherapy: a review of the comparative psychotherapy process literature. *Clin Psychol: Sci Pract*, **7**, 167–188.
10. Thompson-Brenner, H., Glass, S., and Westen, D. (2003). A multidimensional meta-analysis of psychotherapy for bulimia nervosa. *Clin Psychol: Sci Pract*, **10**, 269–287.
11. Compas, B.E., Haaga, D.A.F., Keefe, F.J., Leitenberg, H., and Williams, D.A. (1998). Sampling of empirically supported psychological treatments from health psychology: smoking, chronic pain, cancer, and bulimia nervosa. *J Consult Clin Psychol*, **66**, 89–112.
12. Wilson, G.T., and Fairburn, C.G. (1998). Treatments for eating disorders. In: P.E. Nathan and J.M. Gorman (eds) *A guide to treatments that work*. New York: Oxford University Press, 501–530.
13. Westen, D., Novotny, C.M., and Thompson-Brenner, H. (2004). The empirical status of empirically supported psychotherapies: assumptions, findings, and reporting in controlled clinical trials. *Psychol Bull*, **130**, 631–663.
14. Thompson-Brenner, H., and Westen, D. (2005). A naturalistic study of psychotherapy for bulimia nervosa, Part 1: comorbidity and therapeutic outcome. *J Nerv Ment Dis*, **193**, 573–584.
15. Thompson-Brenner, H., and Westen, D. (2005). Personality subtypes in eating disorders: validation of a classification in a naturalistic sample. *Br J Psychiatry*, **186**, 516–524.
16. Haas, H.L., and Clopton, J.R. (2003). Comparing clinical and research treatments for eating disorders. *Int J Eat Disord*, **33**, 412–420.
17. Bachar, E., Latzer, Y., Kreitler, S., and Berry, E.M. (1999). Empirical comparison of two psychological therapies self psychology and cognitive orientation in the treatment of anorexia and bulimia. *J Psychother Pract Res*, **8**, 115–128.
18. Dare, C., Eisler, I., Russell, G., Treasure, J., and Dodge, L. (2001). Psychological therapies for adults with anorexia nervosa randomised controlled trial of out-patient treatments. *Br J Psychiatry*, **178**, 216–221.
19. Murphy, S., Russell, L., and Waller, G. (2005). Integrated psychodynamic therapy for bulimia nervosa and binge eating disorder: theory, practice and preliminary findings. *Eur Eat Disord Rev*, **13**, 383–391.
20. Treasure, J., Todd, G., Brolly, M., Tiller, J., Nehmed, A., and Denman, F. (1995). A pilot study of a randomised trial of cognitive analytical therapy vs educational behavioral therapy for adult anorexia nervosa. *Behav Res Ther*, **33**, 363–367.
21. Thompson-Brenner, H., Boisseau, C.L., Satir, D.A., Eddy, K.T., Weingeroff, J, and Westen, D. (2007). Treatment approach and outcome for adolescent EDs. Presentation at the International Conference for the Academy of Eating Disorders, Baltimore.
22. American Psychiatric Association. (1994). *Diagnostic and Statistical Manual of Mental Disorders*. 4th edition, Washington, D.C.: American Psychiatric Association.
23. National Institute for Clinical Excellence (2004). *Eating Disorders: core interventions in the treatment and management of anorexia nervosa, bulimia nervosa, and related eating disorders*. Retrieved 10/21/2004 from http://www.nice.org/uk/cg009NICEguideline.

24. Treasure, J., Schmidt, U., and Troop, N. (2000). Cognitive analytical therapy and the transtheoretical framework. In: Miller, K.J. and Mizes, J.S. (eds) *Comparative treatments for eating disorders*. New York: Springer Publishing Company, 283–308.
25. Malan, D.H. (1976). *Toward the validation of dynamic psychotherapy*. New York: Plenum.
26. Tasca, G.A., Ritchie, K., Conrad, G., Balfour, L., Gayton, J., Lybanon, V., et al. (2006). Attachment scales predict outcome in a randomized controlled trial for binge eating disorder: an aptitude by treatment interaction. *Psychother Res, 16*, 106–121.
27. Strupp, H.H., and Binder, J.L. (1984). *Psychotherapy in a new key: a guide to time-limited dynamic psychotherapy*. New York: Basic Books.
28. Tasca, G.A., Mikai, S.F., and Hewitt, P.L. (2005). Group psychodynamic interpersonal psychotherapy: summary of a treatment model and outcomes for depressive symptoms. In: Abelian, M.E. (ed.) *Focus on psychotherapy research*. Hauppauge, NY: Nova Science Publishers, 159–188.
29. Johnson, C.L., Connors, M.E., and Tobin, D.L. (1987). Symptom management of bulimia. *J Consult Clin Psychol, 55*, 668–676.
30. Steiger, H. (1989). An integrated psychotherapy for eating-disordered patients. *Am J Psychother, 43*, 229–237.
31. Tobin, D.L., and Johnson, C.L. (1991). The integration of psychodynamic and behaviour therapy in the treatment of eating disorders: clinical issues versus theoretical mystique. In: Johnson, C.L. (ed.) *Psychodynamic treatment of anorexia nervosa and bulimia*. New York: Guilford.
32. Agras, W.S., Walsh, B.T., Fairburn, C.B., Wilson, G.T., and Kraemer, H.C. (2000). A multicenter comparison of cognitive–behavioral therapy and interpersonal psychotherapy for bulimia nervosa. *Arch Gen Psychiatry, 57*, 459–466.
33. Fairburn, C.G., Jones, R., Peveler, R.C., Carr, S.J., Solomon, R.A., O'Connor, M.E., Burton, J., and Hope, R.A. (1991). Three psychological treatments for bulimia nervosa: a comparative trial. *Arch Gen Psychiatry, 48*, 463–469.
34. Fairburn, C.G., Marcus, M.D., and Wilson, G.T. (1993). Cognitive–behavioral therapy for binge eating and bulimia nervosa: a comprehensive treatment manual. In: Fairburn, C.G., and Wilson, G.T. (eds) *Binge eating: nature, assessment, and treatment*. New York, NY: Guilford Press, 361–404.
35. Shafran, R., Fairburn, C.G., Robinson, P., and Lask, B. (2004). Body checking and its avoidance in eating disorders. *Int J Eat Disord, 35*, 93–101.
36. Fairburn, C.G., Cooper, Z., and Shafran, R. (2003). Cognitive behaviour therapy for eating disorders: a "transdiagnostic" theory and treatment. *Behav Res Ther, 41*, 509–528.
37. Shafran, R., Lee, M., Payne, E., and Fairburn, C.G. (2006). An experimental analysis of body checking. *Behav Res Ther, 45*, 113–121.
38. Marino, M.F., and Zanarini, M.C. (2001). Relationship between EDNOS and its subtypes and borderline personality disorder. *Int J Eat Disord, 29*, 349–353.
39. Fairburn, C.G. (2007). Transdiagnostic cognitive behavior therapy: effects and significance. Presentation at the International Conference for the Academy of Eating Disorders, Baltimore.
40. Fairburn, C.G., Bohn, K., and Hutt, M. (2004). EDNOS (Eating Disorder not otherwise specified): why it is important, and how to treat it using cognitive behavior therapy. Workshop Session at the Academy for Eating Disorders Annual Conference, Orlando, FL.
41. Hilsenroth, M.J, Ackerman, S.J., Blagys, M.D., Bonge, D.R., and Blais, M.A., (2005). Measuring psychodynamic-interpersonal and cognitive–behavioral techniques: development of the Comparative Psychotherapy Process Scale. *Psychother: Theory, Res, & Pract, 42*, 340–356.
42. Jacobi, C., Hayward, C., de Zwaan, M., Kraemer, H.C., and Agras, W.S. (2004). Coming to terms with risk factors for eating disorders: application of risk terminology and suggestions for a general taxonomy. *Psychol Bull, 130*, 19–65.

43. Stice, E. (2002). Risk and maintenance factors for eating pathology: a meta-analytic review. *Psychol Bull*, **128**, 825–848.
44. Wonderlich, S.A., Connelley, K.M., and Stice, E. (2004). Impulsivity as a risk factor for eating disorder behavior: assessment implications with adolescents. *Int J Eat Disord*, **36**, 172–182.
45. Bruce, K.R., and Steiger, H. (2005). Treatment implications of axis-II comorbidity in eating disorders. *Eat Disord*, **13**, 93–108.
46. Espelage, D.L., Mazzeo, S.E., Sherman, R., and Thompson, R. (2002). MCMI-II profiles of women with eating disorders: a cluster analytic investigation. *J Pers Disord*, **16**, 453–463.
47. Goldner, E.M., Srikameswaran, S., Schroeder, M.L., Livesley, W.J., and Birmingham, C.L. (1999). Dimensional assessment of personality pathology in patients with eating disorders. *Psychiatry Res*, **85**, 151–159.
48. Thompson-Brenner, H., Eddy, K.T., Satir, D., Boisseau, C.L., and Westen, D. (2008). Personality subtypes in adolescents with eating disorders: validation of a classification approach. *J Child Psychol Psychiatry*, **49**(2), 170–180.
49. Westen, D., and Harnden-Fischer, J. (2001). Personality profiles in eating disorders: rethinking the distinction between axis I and axis II. *Am J Psychiatry*, **158**, 547–562.
50. Wonderlich, S.A., Crosby, R.D., Joiner, T., et al. (2005). Personality subtyping and bulimia nervosa: psychopathological and genetic correlates. *Psychol Med*, **35**, 649–57.
51. Thompson-Brenner, H., Eddy, K., Franko, D.L., Dorer, D., Vaschenko, M., and Herzog, D.B. (2007). A personality classification system for eating disorders: a longitudinal study. Paper presentation at the International Conference for the Academy of Eating Disorders, Baltimore.
52. Tantleff-Dunn, S., Gokee-LaRose, J., and Peterson, R. (2004). Interpersonal psychotherapy for the treatment of anorexia nervosa, bulimia nervosa, and binge eating disorder. In: Thompson, J.K. (ed.) *Handbook of eating disorders and obesity*. New Jersey: John Wiley and Sons, Inc., 163–185.
53. Frank, E., and Spanier, C. (1995). Interpersonal psychotherapy for depression: overview, clinical efficacy, and future directions. *Clin Psychol: Sci Pract*, **2**, 349–369.
54. Fairburn, C.G. (1997). Interpersonal psychotherapy for bulimia nervosa. In: Garner, D.M. and Garfinkel, P. E. (eds) *Handbook for the treatment of eating disorders*, 2nd edition. New York: Guilford Press, 278–294.
55. Wilfley, D.E., Dounchis, J.Z., and Welch, R.R. (2000). Interpersonal Psychotherapy. In: Miller, K.J. and Mizes, J.S. (eds) *Comparative treatments for eating disorders*. New York: Springer Publishing Company, Inc., 128–282.
56. Fairburn, C.G., Kirk, J., O'Connor, M., Anastasiades, P., and Cooper, P.J. (1987). Prognostic factors in bulimia nervosa. *Br J Clin Psychol*, **26**, 223–224.
57. McIntosh, V.V., Bulik, C.M., McKenzie, J.M., Luty, S.E., and Jordan, J. (2000). Interpersonal psychotherapy for anorexia nervosa. *Int J Eat Disord*, **27**, 125–139.
58. Ablon, J.S., and Jones, E.E. (1999). Psychotherapy process in the national institute of mental health treatment of depression collaborative research program. *J Consult Clin Psychol*, **67**, 64–75.
59. McIntosh, V.V., Jordan, J., Carter, F.A., McKenzie, J.M., Bulik, C.M., Frampton, C.M.A., et al. (2005). Three psychotherapies for anorexia nervosa: a randomized, controlled trial. *Am J Psychiatry*, **162**, 741–747.
60. Garner, D.M., Rockert, W., Davis, R., Garner, M.V., Olmsted, M.P., and Eagle, M. (1993). Comparison of cognitive–behavioral and supportive-expressive therapy for bulimia nervosa. *Am J Psychiatry*, **150**, 37–46.
61. Linehan, M.M. (1993). *Dialectical–behavioral treatment of borderline personality disorder*. New York: Guilford Press.
62. Safer, D.L., Telch, C.F., and Agras, W.S. (2001). Dialectical behavior therapy for bulimia nervosa. *Am J Psychiatry*, **158**, 632–634.

63. Telch, C.F., Agras, W.S., and Linehan, M.M. (2000). Group dialectical behavior therapy for binge-eating disorder: a preliminary, uncontrolled trial. *Behav Ther,* **31,** 569–582.
64. Telch, C.F., Agras, W.S., and Linehan, M.M. (2001). Dialectical behavior therapy for binge eating disorder. *J Consult Clin Psychol,* **69,** 1061–1065.
65. Wisniewski, L., and Kelly, E. (2003). The application of dialectical behavior therapy to the treatment of eating disorders. *Cogn Behav Pract,* **10,** 131–138.
66. Wiser, S. and Telch, C.F. (1999). Dialectical behavior therapy for binge-eating disorder. *J Clin Psychol,* **55,** 755–768.
67. Sansone, R.A., Levitt, J.L., and Sansone, L.A. (2005). The prevalence of personality disorders among those with eating disorders. *Eat Disord,* **13,** 7–21.
68. Zanarini, M.C., Frankenburg, F.R, Dubo, E.D., Sickel, A.E., Trikha, A., Levin, A., et al. (1998). Axis I comorbidity of borderline personality disorder. *Am J Psychiatry,* **155,** 1733–1739.
69. Leichsenring, F., and Leibing, E. (2003). The effectiveness of psychodynamic therapy and cognitive behavioral therapy in the treatment of personality disorders: a meta-analysis. *Am J Psychiatry,* **160,** 1223–1232.
70. Bateman, A.W., and Fonagy, P. (2000). Effectiveness of psychotherapeutic treatment of personality disorder. *Br J Psychiatry,* **177,** 138–143.
71. Johnson, C.L., Stuckey, M.K., Lewis, L.D., and Schwartz, D.M. (1982). Bulimia: a descriptive survey of 316 cases. *Int J Eat Disord,* **2,** 3–16.
72. Norman, D.K. and Herzog, D.B. (1984). Persistent social maladjustment in bulimia: a 1-yearfollow-up. *Am J Psychiatry,* **141,** 444–446.
73. Telch, C.F., and Agras, W.S. (1994). Obesity, binge-eating, and psychopathology: are they related? *Int J Eat Disord,* **15,** 53–61.
74. Wilfley, D.E., Agras, W.S., Telch, C.F., Rossiter, E.M., Schneider, J.A., Cole, A.G., et al. (1993). Group cognitive–behavioral therapy and group interpersonal psychotherapy for the nonpurging bulimic individual: a controlled comparison. *J Consult Clin Psychol,* **61,** 296–305.
75. Steiger, H., Gauvin, L., Jabalpurwala, S., Seguin, J.R., and Stotland, S. (1999). Hypersensitivity to social interactions in bulimic syndromes: relationship to binge eating. *J Consult Clin Psychol,* **67,** 765–775.
76. Greenberg, J.R., and Mitchell, S.A. (1983). *Object relations in psychoanalytic theory.* Cambridge: Harvard University Press.
77. Bateman, A., and Fonagy, P. (1999). The effectiveness of partial hospitalization in the treatment of borderline personality disorder: a randomized controlled trial. *Am J Psychiatry,* **156,** 1563–1569.
78. Bateman, A., and Fonagy, P. (2001). Treatment of borderline personality disorder with psychoanalytically oriented partial hospitalization: an 18-month follow-up. *Am J Psychiatry,* **158,** 36–42.
79. Bateman, A.W., and Fonagy, P. (2003). Health service utilization costs for borderline personality disorder patients treated with psychoanalytically oriented partial hospitalization versus general psychiatric care. *Am J Psychiatry,* **160,** 169–171.
80. Fonagy, P., and Bateman, A.W. (2006). Mechanisms of change in mentalization-based treatment of BPO. *J Clin Psychol,* **62,** 411–430.
81. Clarkin, J.F., Foelsch, P.A., Levy, K.N., Hull, J.W., Delaney, J.C., and Kernberg, O.F. (2001). The development of a psychodynamic treatment for patients with borderline personality disorder: a preliminary study of behavioral change. *J Personal Disord,* **15,** 487–495.
82. Clarkin, J.F., Levy, K.N., Lenzenweger, M.F., and Kernberg, O.F. (2004). The personality disorders institute/borderline personality disorder research foundation randomized control trial for borderline personality disorder: rationale, methods, and patient characteristics. *J Personal Disord,* **18,** 52–72.

83. Carano, A., De Berardis, D., Gambi, F., Di Paolo, C., Campanella, D., Pelusi, L., et al. (2006). Alexithymia and body image in adult outpatients with binge eating disorder. *Int J Eat Disord,* **39,** 332–340.
84. Gilboa-Schechtman, E., Avnon, L., Zubery, E., and Jeczmien, P. (2006). Emotional processing in eating disorders: specific impairment or general distress related deficiency? *Depress Anxiety,* **23,** 331–339.
85. Strober, M. (2004). Managing the chronic, treatment-resistant patient with anorexia nervosa. *Int J Eat Disord,* **36,** 245–255.
86. Garner, D.M., Garfinkel, P.E., and Bemis, K.M. (1982). A multidimensional psychotherapy for anorexia nervosa. *Int J Eat Disord,* **1,** 3–46.
87. Gaston, L., Marmar, C.R., Thompson, L.W., and Gallagher, D. (1988). Relation of patient pretreatment characteristics to the therapeutic alliance in diverse psychotherapies. *J Consult Clin Psychol,* **56,** 483–489.
88. Foreman, S.A., and Marmar, C.R. (1985). Therapist actions that address initially poor therapeutic alliances in psychotherapy. *Am J Psychiatry,* **142,** 922–926.

# Chapter 5
# Empirical Evidence for Transference-Focused Psychotherapy and Other Psychodynamic Psychotherapy for Borderline Personality Disorder

**Kenneth N. Levy, Rachel H. Wasserman, Lori N. Scott, and Frank E. Yeomans**

## Psychodynamic Psychotherapy for Borderline Personality Disorder

Writing about psychodynamic psychotherapy for borderline personality disorder (BPD) is difficult because it is not a unified approach. In fact, it is often said that psychoanalysis, although frequently used singularly, is in actuality a plural noun representing an array of theoretical ideas and technical applications. These schools broadly include ego psychology, object relations theory, self-psychology, and attachment theory.

These psychodynamic models can be contrasted with and complemented by other models for treating BPD, such as the behavioral [1], cognitive [2–4], interpersonal [5], and integrative (e.g., dialectical behavior therapy, DBT) [6]. What distinguishes a psychodynamic approach is an explicit focus on both the conscious and unconscious aspects of mental functioning and the implications of these experiences in interaction with biological forces and interpersonal influences.

It is generally concluded that those trained psychoanalytically or dynamically are not interested in research for a host of reasons ranging from the challenges of designing a randomized controlled trial (RCT) that would demonstrate the efficacy of a psychoanalytic approach to epistemological and philosophical disagreements about the nature of science (see [7–9] debates for an illustration). Although many in the psychoanalytic community in the past have been cautious regarding the value of research, some of the earliest psychotherapy research was performed by psychoanalysts [10–18]. Additionally, psychoanalyst and psychodynamic clinicians are increasingly becoming interested in testing psychodynamic hypotheses and establishing a stronger evidence base for treatments based on psychodynamic ideas [8, 9, 19–25]. This increased interest in psychotherapy outcome research has been particularly fruitful with regard to

K.N. Levy
Department of Psychology, Pennsylvania State University, 521 Moore Bldg., University Park, PA 16802, USA
e-mail: klevy@psu.edu

R.A. Levy, J.S. Ablon (eds.), *Handbook of Evidence-Based Psychodynamic Psychotherapy*,
DOI: 10.1007/978-1-59745-444-5_5, © Humana Press 2009

the study of BPD. Severe personality disorders such as BPD are increasingly seen as the mainstay of psychoanalytic clinical work.

A number of these psychodynamic treatments may be quite effective in treating patients with BPD; however, for the purpose of this chapter, we focus primarily on Otto Kernberg's [26, 27] transference-focused psychotherapy (TFP). Before examining the empirical evidence for the efficacy and effectiveness of TFP, we will chronicle findings from the Menninger Foundation Psychotherapy Research Project (MFPRP) and review the evidence for the effectiveness of Russell Meares's [28] interpersonal psychodynamic psychotherapy and Peter Fonagy and Anthoney Bateman's [29] mentalization-based therapy (MBT). We will begin by framing the issues in conceptualizing empirical evidence in psychotherapy studies and we will finish with a summary of conclusions that can be drawn from the literature.

## What Constitutes Empirical Evidence?

Although RCTs are generally considered the gold standard and have important methodological strengths [30], they also suffer from a number of important limitations [24, 30–34]. The focus on RCTs has had the unintended consequence of overlooking other evidence that is relevant for assessing the empirical support of treatments. The numerous limitations of efficacy studies have led many investigators to recommend searching for empirically supported principles (ESPs) of treatment, or evidence-based explanations of treatment, rather than credentialed, trademarked, brand-name, or evidence-based treatment packages [31, 35–37].

Gabbard and colleagues [38] and others [34, 39] have discussed a stage model, or hierarchy, of treatment evidence as a function of considering both internal and external validity. They have suggested that evidence from multiple sources within this model is necessary in order to build an empirically grounded framework for specific forms of psychotherapy. In ascending levels of internal validity and descending levels of external validity, the hierarchy of treatment evidence starts with the provision of an argument or the articulation of clinical innovation and proceeds through clinical case studies, clinical case series, pre–post designs without comparison groups, quasi-experimental designs that include comparisons but without randomization, and then RCTs. Within the RCT category, there is a hierarchy with regard to the control group employed ranging from the use of wait-list controls through treatment as usual groups, placebos, and finally comparison with established, well-delivered alternative treatments. Levy and Scott [34] suggested that this hierarchy, in combination with the examination of evidence for specific techniques and mechanisms of action [40, 41], provides better breadth of evidence and better validity than focusing on RCTs alone. Others have noted that naturalistic studies may be necessary to help bridge the gap between practice and research [42, 43]. Limiting research, practice, and training exclusively to treatments that have been validated in RCTs could impede reasonable avenues of study in the treatment of BPD and obstruct access to treatments that might be better suited to specific patient subgroups.

## Evolving Early Psychodynamic Psychotherapy Research on Borderline Personality Disorder

One of the first systematic attempts at studying psychotherapy outcome of severely disturbed patients was the MFPRP, initially directed by Robert Wallerstein and completed under the stewardship of Otto Kernberg. The Menninger Study [44, 45] began in 1954 and follow-up assessments spanned almost 30 years. In this study, 42 patients were treated, half in classical psychoanalysis and half in supportive and expressive psychodynamic psychotherapies. They were assessed at baseline termination and had multiple follow-ups (100% were followed-up at 2–3 years post-termination). Using detailed case histories from all 42 patients, Wallerstein concluded that supportive techniques "infiltrated" all therapies, including psychoanalysis, and that these techniques accounted for more of the outcome than initially anticipated. This finding has lead to the integration of supportive and expressive techniques seen in many psychodynamic psychotherapies [46–48]. Based on separate analyses of the data from the MRPRP, Kernberg [45] concluded that patients with borderline personality treated by skilled therapists who focused their interventions on the transference showed a significantly better outcome than those treated with a more supportive approach. Although Wallerstein and Kernberg's conclusions appear at odds, they are not mutually exclusive. Supportive techniques could have been used in all treatments to varying degrees, but in Kernberg's, interpretations were less related to outcome with the subset of patients with BPD. Nevertheless, because these conclusions did not come from an RCT, many skeptics remained unconvinced on both sides.

The MFPRP was a landmark study; however, it is also difficult to interpret not only because patients were not randomized to treatment conditions but also because of uncertainty regarding patient diagnoses.[1] Nevertheless, there are some clear lessons and conclusions that can still be drawn from the MFPRP: (1) classical psychoanalysis is most likely not that helpful for BPD patients (particularly the more severely disturbed borderline patient or what Kernberg calls the low-level borderline patient); (2) to the extent that the psychodynamic psychotherapy was supportive, supportive psychotherapy (SPT) appears less effective for low-level BPD patients; (3) one size does not have to fit

---

[1] Although, many of the patients referred after multiple treatment failures and it appears that these patients could be classified as BPD, diagnoses were not made using criteria consistent with a contemporary nosological framework.

all – psychoanalysis can be modified to patients' pathology. This last point is particularly important given that clinical techniques should be tied to the specific developmental psychopathology being addressed (see [49] for elaboration of this point).

## Contemporary Psychotherapy Research on Borderline Personality Disorder

One hypothesis that was confirmed in the MFPRP is that long-term psychodynamic psychotherapy research is difficult to perform. Many in the field believed that such research was so difficult as to render it unfeasible. However, in 1991, Marsha Linehan published the results of her year-long RCT for BPD in which she examined an integrative cognitive–behavioral therapy (CBT) treatment called DBT as compared to treatment as usual. This seminal study has been highly influential on current training and treatment trends. However, one of the most important aspects of this study was that it showed that RCTs of a long-term treatment could be accomplished and thus stimulated a revival in the rigorous study of long-term psychodynamic treatments for BPD.

## Interpersonal Self-Psychological Approach

Russell Meares developed an interpersonal self-psychological (IP) approach for the treatment of BPD guided by the conversational model of Hobson [50], the main aim of which is to foster the emergence of reflective consciousness that William James called *self-consciousness* [51]. A basic tenet of this approach is that self-consciousness is achieved through a particular form of conversation and reflects a specific kind of relatedness. The nearest North American equivalent to this approach comes from Kohut [52] and his followers [53]. Shortly after Linehan published the results of her initial RCT, Meares and colleagues [28] published the results of a pre–post-study examining this approach for patients with BPD. They found that patients at the end of treatment showed an increase in time employed and a decrease in number of medical visits, number of self-harm episodes, and number and length of hospitalizations. Although the inferences that can be drawn from this study are limited by the lack of a control group, these findings supported development and study of psychodynamic treatments for BPD. In a later study [54], researchers compared BPD patients treated twice weekly for 1 year with those in a treatment-as-usual wait-list control group (all wait-listed patients received their usual treatments, which consisted of SPT, crisis intervention only, cognitive therapy, and pharmacotherapy). Thirty percent of IP-treated patients no longer met criteria for a *DSM-III* [55] BPD diagnosis at the end of the treatment year, whereas all of the treatment as usual (TAU) patients still met criteria for the diagnosis. These results demonstrated that psychotherapy based on psychodynamic principles is generally beneficial to patients with BPD in a naturalistic setting, having strong ecological validity. A follow-up of all patients in this cohort 5 years after the treatment found maintained improvements [56]. At the 5-year follow-up, 40% of the patients no longer met criteria for BPD. In addition, there was a progressive reduction in time spent in hospital (although no decrease in hospitalizations) and an increase in time employed. A recently completed second study of similar design [57] replicated these findings. Clearly the findings from these studies suggest the value of their approach and call for the more stringent testing of an RCT.

## Mentalization-Based Therapy

Bateman and Fonagy [58] developed MBT based on the developmental theory of mentalization, which integrates philosophy (theory of mind), ego psychology, Kleinian theory, and attachment theory. Fonagy and Bateman [58] posit that the mechanism of change in all effective treatments for BPD involves the capacity for mentalization – the capacity to think about mental states in oneself and in others in terms of wishes, desires, and intentions. This involves both implicit, unconscious mental processes that are activated along with the attachment system in affectively charged interpersonal situations and coherent integrated representations of mental states of self and others. The concept of mentalization has been operationalized in the reflective function (RF) scale (Fonagy, P., Target, M., Steele, H., & Steele, M. (1998). Reflective Functioning Manual: Version 5.0, for Application to Adult Attachment Interviews. Unpublished Manuscript).

In a randomized clinical trial, Bateman and Fonagy [29] compared the effectiveness of 18 months of a psychoanalytically oriented day hospitalization program to routine general psychiatric care for patients with BPD. Patients randomly assigned to the psychoanalytic day hospital program, now called MBT [59], showed statistically significant improvement in depressive symptoms and better social and interpersonal functioning, as well as significant decreases in suicidal and parasuicidal behavior and number of days in inpatient treatment.

Patients were reassessed every 3 months for up to 18 months postdischarge [60]. Follow-up results indicate that patients who completed the MBT not only maintained their substantial gains but also showed continued steady and statistically significant improvement on most measures, suggesting that BPD patients can continue to demonstrate gains in functioning long after treatment has ended. At 18-month postdischarge follow-up, 59.1% of patients treated with MBT were below the BPD diagnostic threshold, compared to only 12.5% of those treated in routine general psychiatric care. This finding is particularly important because while the overall results of Linehan's studies of DBT are suggestive of its value, naturalistic follow-up of patients in DBT shows variable maintenance of treatment effects, and ongoing impairment in functioning in patients who initially experienced symptom relief. For example, Linehan [61] found no between-group differences in the number of days hospitalized at a 6-month follow-up or in self-destructive acts at the end of a 1-year follow-up (despite the fact that the patients in the DBT group were still receiving DBT therapy, whereas about half the TAU group were not in any therapy). Thus, the durability of the initial gains is unclear; whereas for MBT, there not only is continued improvement, but also seems to be a sleeper effect with increased improvement over time.

An 8-year follow-up of MBT has recently been completed, and the results of that study should be available soon. At this point, the most important tests remaining for MBT are to examine its putative mechanisms of change. Bateman and Fonagy hypothesize that changes in RF underlie the improvements seen in MBT; however, to date findings have not been published regarding changes in levels of RF in MBT-treated BPD patients.

## Transference-Focused Psychotherapy

Since the early 1980s, the Borderline Psychotherapy Research Project at New York Presbyterian Hospital-Weill Cornell Medical Center, headed by Drs. John Clarkin and Otto Kernberg, has been systematizing and investigating an object relations treatment of patients with BPD. This group has generated treatment manuals [26, 27, 62] that describe key strategies and techniques of a highly structured, modified dynamic treatment of patients with borderline personality organization called TFP.

Central to TFP are mental representations derived through the internalization of attachment relationships with caregivers. The degree of differentiation and integration of these representations of self and other, along with their affective valence, constitutes personality organization [63]. According to Kernberg, borderline personality can be thought of as severely disturbed level of personality organization, characterized by unintegrated and undifferentiated representations of self and other (what Kernberg calls identity diffusion and manifested in inconsistent view of self and others), the use of immature defenses (e.g., splitting, projective identification, and omnipotent control), and variable reality testing (e.g., poor conception of one's own social stimulus value).

The major goals of TFP are to reduce suicidality and self-injurious behaviors, and to facilitate better behavioral control, increased affect regulation, more gratifying relationships, and the ability to pursue life goals. This is believed to be accomplished through the development of integrated representations of self and others, the modification of primitive defensive operations, and the resolution of identity diffusion that perpetuate the fragmentation of the patient's internal representational world. In this treatment, the analysis of the transference is the primary vehicle for the transformation of primitive (e.g., split, polarized) to advanced (e.g., complex, differentiated and integrated) object relations. Thus, in contrast to therapies that focus on the short-term treatment of symptoms, TFP has the ambitious goal of not just changing symptoms, but changing the personality organization, which is the context of the symptoms. In contrast to most manuals for CBT or short-term treatments, the TFP manual could be described as principle-based rather than sequentially based, which requires the clinician to be flexible and use clinical judgment. Using video-taped sessions and supervisor ratings, Kernberg and his colleagues have been able to train both senior clinicians and junior trainees at multiple sites to adherence and competence in applying the principles of TFP.

Transference-focused psychotherapy begins with explicit contract setting that clarifies the conditions of therapy, the method of treatment, and the respective roles of patient and therapist. The primary focus of TFP is on the dominant affect-laden themes that emerge in the relationship between borderline patients and their therapists in the here-and-now of the transference. During the first year of treatment, TFP focuses on a hierarchy of goals: containing suicidal and self-destructive behaviors, addressing ways the patient might undermine the treatment since it challenges the patient's fragile and dysfunctional homeostasis, and identifying and recapitulating dominant object relational patterns, as they are experienced and expressed in the here-and-now of the transference relationship.

Within psychoanalysis, TFP is closest to the Kleinian school [64], which also emphasizes a focus on the analysis of the transference. However, TFP can be distinguished from Kleinian psychoanalysis in that TFP is practiced twice per week and that TFP includes a more highly structured treatment frame by emphasizing the treatment contract and a preestablished set of priorities to focus (e.g., suicidality and treatment-interfering behaviors). The role of both the treatment contract and the treatment priorities go beyond that found in more typical psychoanalytic psychotherapy or psychoanalysis, including Kleinian psychoanalysis. In addition, transference interpretations are consistently linked with both extratransference material and, importantly, long-term treatment goals (e.g., better behavioral control). In contrast to Kleinian approaches, the TFP approach is a highly engaged, more talkative, and an interactive one. Additionally, technical neutrality is modified to the extent required to maintain structure. Transference-focused psychotherapy also differs from other expressive psychodynamic approaches with a persistent focus on the here-and-now, a focus on the immediate interpretation of the negative transference, and the emphasis on interpretation of the defensive function of idealization, as well as a focus on the patients' aggression and hostility.

Some of the more salient differences between TFP and DBT, a cognitive–behavioral therapy developed to treat parasuicidal borderline patients, concern parameter of the treatment frame. For example, to avoid the secondary gain that can be experienced by extra contact with the therapist and to encourage the development of autonomy [65], the TFP therapist is considered unavailable between sessions except in the case of emergencies, whereas in DBT, the patient is encouraged to phone the individual therapist between sessions. Another difference is the emphasis in TFP on technical neutrality versus strategies used in DBT including validation, coaching, and cheerleading. Despite these differences, both TFP and DBT have in common a firm, explicit contract, a focus on a hierarchy of acting out behaviors, a highly engaged therapeutic relationship, a structured disciplined approach, and utilize supervision groups as essential for therapists.

In TFP, hypothesized mechanisms of change derive from Kernberg's [63] developmentally based theory of BPD, which conceptualizes the disorder in terms of unintegrated and undifferentiated affects and representations (or concepts) of self and other. Partial representations of self and other are paired and linked by an affect in mental units called "object relation dyads." These dyads are representational elements of psychological structure. In BPD, the lack of integration of the internal object relations dyads corresponds to a "split" psychological structure in which totally negative dyads are split off or segregated from idealized positive dyads of self and other. The putative global mechanism of change in patients treated with TFP is the integration of these polarized affect states and representations of self and other into a more coherent whole. Through the exploration and integration of these "split-off" cognitive-affective units of self- and other representations, Kernberg postulates that the patient's awareness and experience in life become more enriched and modulated, and the patient develops the capacity to think more flexibly, realistically, and benevolently. The integration of the split and polarized concepts of self and others leads to a more complex, differentiated, and realistic sense of self and others that allows for better modulation of affects and in turn clearer thinking. Therefore, as split-off representations become integrated, patients tend to experience an increased coherence of identity, relationships that are balanced and not at risk of being overwhelmed by aggressive affect, a greater capacity for intimacy, a reduction in self-destructive behaviors, and general improvement in functioning.

Using the triad of clarifications, confrontations, and interpretations, the TFP therapist provides the patient with the opportunity to integrate cognitions and affects that were previously split and disorganized. In addition, the engaged, interactive, and emotionally intense stance of the therapist is typically experienced by patients as emotionally holding (containing) because the therapist conveys that he or she can tolerate the patient's negative affective states. The therapist's expectation of the patient's ability to have a thoughtful and disciplined approach to emotional states (i.e., that the patient is a fledgling version of a capable, responsible, and reflective adult) is thought to be experienced as cognitively holding. The therapist's timely, clear, and tactful interpretations of the dominant, affect-laden themes and patient enactments in the here and now of the transference frequently shed light on the reasons that representations remain split off and thus facilitate integrating polarized representations of self and others.

With regard to the flow of treatment, the structured frame of TFP facilitates the full activation of the patient's distorted internal representations of self and other in the ongoing relationship between patient and therapist; this constitutes the transference. It is expected that the unintegrated representations of self and other will be activated in the treatment setting as they are in every aspect of the patient's life. These partial representations are constantly active in determining the patient's experience of real-life interactions and in motivating the patient's behavior. The difference in the therapy is that the therapist both experiences the patient's representation of the interaction and also nonjudgmentally observes and comments on it (within the psychoanalytic literature, this is known as the "third position"). This is facilitated by the therapist establishing a treatment frame and contract, which in addition to providing structure and holding for the patient and a consensual reality from which to examine acting out behavior. The therapist does not respond to the patient's fragmented partial representation, but helps the patient observe it, as well as the implied other that is paired with it. Such interventions are facilitated by the therapist's having already established a consistent treatment frame and contract. In addition to providing structure and a consensual reality from which to examine a patient's acting out behaviour, the treatment frame and contract assists the therapist in minimizing his or own potential for unconstructive, non-therapeutic interactions.

As these internal object relations unfold in the relation with the therapist, the TFP therapist seeks to explicate the patient's internal experience through clarification and reflection because the patient may not have a clear representation of his or her own experience. However, in most cases, this technique alone will not lead to integration, because clarification alone does not address the conflicts that keep the partial representations separated. Confrontation – the technique of enquiring about the elements of the patient's verbal and nonverbal communications in contradiction to each other – and interpretation of obstacles to integration are needed to get the patient beyond the level of split organization. Interpretation includes helping the patient see that he or she identifies at different moments in time with each pole of the predominant object relation dyads within him or her. Increasing the patient's awareness of his or her range of identifications increases his or her ability to integrate the different parts.

On the practical level, the relationship with the therapist in TFP is structured under controlled conditions in order to allow the patient to experience affects without overwhelming the situation and destroying communication. The negotiation of a treatment frame provides a safe setting for the reactivation of the internalized relation paradigms. The safety and stability of the therapeutic environment permits the patient to begin to reflect about what is going on in the present with another person, in light of these internalized paradigms. Similar to what attachment theorists would describe as a safe haven, which along with the guidance of an attachment figure, allows for the exploration of the content of the mind. With guidance from the therapist, the patient becomes aware of the extent to which his perceptions are based more on internalized representations than on what is realistically going on now. The therapist's help to cognitively structure what at first seemed chaotic also provides a containing function for the patient's affects.

Transference-focused psychotherapy fosters change by inhibiting the vicious circle of setting off reactions in others that often occur when the patient behaves with emotion dysregulation in the "real" world (often eliciting the very responses that the patient fears from others). The objective and nonjudgmental attitude of the therapist assists in the reactivation of the internalized experience patterns, their containment, and their exploration for new understandings. Instead of attempting to deter these behaviors by educative means, TFP brings the patient's attention to the internal mental representations behind them, with the goal of understanding, modifying, and integrating them.

Key to the change process is the development of introspection or self-reflection; the patient's increase in reflection is hypothesized to be an essential mechanism of change. The disorganization of the patient involves not only internal representations of self and others, relationships with self and others, and predominance of primitive affects, but also the processes that prevent reflection and full awareness. These primitive defensive processes that characterize a split psychological structure erase and distort awareness. Thought processes can be so powerfully distorted that affects, particularly the most negative ones, are expressed in action without cognitive awareness of their existence.

As the patient progresses in the course of TFP from split-off contradictory self-states to reflectiveness and integration, from action to reflection, this increase in reflectiveness involves two specific levels. The first level is an articulation and reflection of what one feels in the moment. The patient increases his or her ability to experience, articulate, and contain an affect and to contextualize it in the moment. A second, more advanced, level of reflection is the ability to place the understanding of momentary affect states of self and others into a general context of a relationship between self and others across time. This level reflects the establishment of an integrated sense of self and others – a sense against which momentary perceptions can be compared and put in perspective.

One of the important tactics in TFP is setting up the treatment contracts, before beginning the therapy per se. The function of the contract is to define the responsibilities of patient and therapist, protecting the therapist's ability to think clearly and reflect, provide a safe place for the patient's dynamics to unfold, set the stage for interpreting the meaning of deviations from the contract as they occur later in therapy, and provide an organizing therapeutic frame that permits therapy to become an anchor in the patient's life. The contract specifies the patient responsibilities, such as attendance and participation, paying fee, and reporting thoughts and feelings without censoring. The contract also specifies the therapists' responsibilities, including attending to the schedule, making every effort to understand and, when useful, comment, clarifying the limits of his/her involvement, and predicting threats to the treatment. Essentially, the treatment contract makes the expectations of the therapy explicit [66]. There is some controversy regarding the value of treatment contracting. The APA guidelines recommend that therapist contract around issues of safety. Others [67] have suggested that the evidence contraindicates their use and shows them to be ineffective [68]. However, the Kroll [68] study was designed to determine the extent that no-suicide contracts were employed (which was found to be 57%), and although 42% of psychiatrists who used no-suicide contracts had patients who either committed suicide or made a serious attempt, the design of the study does not allow for the assessment of the efficacy of no-suicide contracts. Other data suggest the utility to contracting around self-destructive behavior and treatment threats [69–73]. For example, Yeomans and colleagues [69] in a pre–post study of 36 patients with BPD found that the quality of the therapist's presentation and handling of the patient's response to the treatment contract correlated with treatment alliance and the length of treatment. In addition, in our earlier work on TFP [70], when we did not stress treatment contracting, our drop-out rates were high (31 and 36% at 3 month and 6 month marks of treatment). However, based on the findings of Yeomans et al. [69], Kernberg and colleagues further systematized and stressed the importance of the treatment contract, and in later studies [71, 73, 74], our group found lower rates of dropout (19, 13, and 25%) over a year-long period of treatment. We suggest that these findings taken together suggest that sensitively but explicitly negotiated treatment contracts may have one of the desired effects: resulting in less dropout and longer treatments. Future research will need to address the issue of treatment contracts more directly, particularly testing the effects on parasuicidality and suicidality.

## Transference-Focused Psychotherapy Case Study

As an example of a TFP treatment contract, we offer the case of a 35-year-old woman, who was referred for TFP after 10 years of multiple outpatient and inpatient treatments for depression. After careful a assessment, her diagnosis disorder was determined to be borderline PD with strong narcissistic features. The contracting phase of treatment involves the therapist's describing a set of preconditions for treatment that are directly tied to the patient's presenting difficulties. The first stage of the contracting process was to discuss with the patient that her depressive moods might stem from underlying ways of thinking of herself and others that were automatic to her, not fully in her awareness and not fully accurate. The patient was interested in exploring this possibility. Discussion of the contract followed this discussion of the diagnosis. The therapist explained that an exploratory treatment could not provide true gains unless the patient was involved in some kind of activity in life. The patient took the position that any kind of activity was so overwhelming to her that it threw her back into the depths of depression. The therapist pointed out that the patient was not presently exhibiting the symptoms of a depressive episode. The patient replied that this was because of her extensive treatment and that she had achieved a fragile equilibrium that would be shattered by any attempt to increase her level of functioning. The therapist was sure enough of the diagnosis of a primary Axis II disorder, and his consequent belief that the patient was capable of taking some responsibility in the area of functioning, to state: "The choice of treatment is entirely up to you. If you find what I'm saying is unreasonable, or simply not something that would interest you, we could look into alternative more supportive treatments that would not ask as much of you, but would likely not lead to as much change. I understand that entering into situations where you are involved with other people is very stressful for you and that you have failed at multiple efforts to function in the past. What I am proposing is that you begin some kind of activity, and when you begin to have those reactions, we can explore here what is going on there that contributes to your anxiety and distress. It will very likely be related to the kind of reactions you have that we will be exploring here and in other settings."

The patient agreed in principle. Then the contracting had to address what activity the patient might realistically engage in at that point. She initially proposed reading stories to children at the local library one afternoon each week. The therapist felt that this did not adequately address the needs of an intelligent adult woman to have some income. He proposed starting with a part-time clerical position while she looked into various training possibilities. The patient responded: "I'd rather die than work at a clerical job." This reaction supported the therapist's diagnostic impression. Their discussion, over two sessions, led to the patient's proposing that she could begin to get training in a paraprofessional area, which she did.

Once the treatment frame is in place, the therapy begins and the central work involves helping the patient recognize and integrate the various split-off representations of self and other that make up the patient's internal world. An example is that of a woman who started TFP at age 32 with problems of depression, chronic suicidal ideation, and an inability to maintain social relations or any job because of chronic arguments with others. The first prominent dyad that emerged in her discourse was the image of a weak, injured self who was constantly berated and put down by others. Yet, the patient's initial interactions with the therapist were characterized by a nonstop discourse on her part that left the therapist feeling controlled and unable to speak freely. Exploration of this revealed a devalued image of self in relation to another who would berate her and eventually abandon her. The patient's primitive defense mechanisms were such that she projected the "bad" critical and abandoning object on the therapist and then felt the need to then control it in him. The following interpretation freed the patient from her use of projective identification to participate in a more open and interactive interchange and to explore further.

Responding to the patient's rapid-fire speech in every session, the therapist commented: "Have you noticed how you fill the sessions with a kind of pressured speech that does not leave me any room to comment? (generally, if the therapist tried to speak, the patient would speak over him.) It is as though you feel the need to control me, to keep me from acting freely."

*Patient [angrily]*          "If I didn't control you, you'd leave me, like every-one else."

Exploration of this fear helped the patient understand that her behavior was rooted in an anxiety stemming from an internal image of the other that determined how she experienced her therapist. The next stage of therapy was marked by the patient's increasing criticism of the therapist, which she did not recognize as such consciously. She felt she was reacting in a justified way to his short-comings and failures toward her (e.g., his going away at times). The therapist helped the patient observe her own identification with and enacting of the devaluing, critical one, helped her see its relation to feeling devalued and criticized, and also helped her understand that neither one of these needed to be the case. The patient gained awareness that the drama she experienced endlessly with others was the enactment of a relationship between two parts of herself and that she was living the contradiction of being both the victim and the critic/attacker, although with less awareness of the latter and usually experiencing this relationship as between her and others (a situation she often created) rather than within herself. This awareness allowed her to begin to tame the harsh critical part within her.

As the therapy advanced, there were signs of the patient's attachment to the therapist's attachment to the therapist: coming on time while protesting that therapy was a waste of time, missing her therapy while angrily proclaiming that her therapist was irresponsible for going away, etc. Her therapist made the interpretation that it must be difficult for her to be attached to him (thus going a step beyond anything she had stated and bringing the positive dyad into their dialogue more explicitly) because of her fear that the kind of longing she experienced for him could never be reciprocated by anyone. The therapist's matter-of-fact mention of this imagined positive relationship freed the patient to begin to discuss her fantasies of an ideal relationship with him as the perfect provider and protector she had never experienced. The patient had been reluctant to express this idealized view of their relation for fear that the negative, rejecting image of the other would prove real and destroy her longing for closeness in a brutally humiliating way. The ability to discuss and observe both sides of the split allowed the patient to achieve an integrated, more balanced view of herself, others, and relationships.

## Empirical Evidence for Transference-Focused Psychotherapy

There is now accumulating evidence for the effectiveness and efficacy of TFP [71, 75, 76]. The initial study [71] examined the effectiveness of TFP in a pre–post design. Participants were recruited from varied treatment settings (i.e., inpatient, day hospital, and outpatient clinics) within the New York metropolitan area.

Participants were all women between the ages of 18 and 50 who met criteria for BPD through structured interviews. All therapists (senior therapists to postdoctoral trainees) selected for this phase of the study were judged by independent supervisory ratings to be both competent and adherent to the TFP manual. Three senior supervisors rated the therapists for TFP adherence and competence. "Findings regarding adherence and competence. After the completion of all treatment in the study, three senior supervisors rank-ordered the therapists for adherence and competence in TFP. The range was purposefully truncated, as all therapists were consistently supervised to adherence during the treatment period. With this limited range of competence, we found no relationship between the rank order and patient outcome." Throughout the study, all therapists were supervised on a weekly basis by Kernberg and at least one other senior clinician.

Overall, the major finding in this pre–post study was that patients with BPD who were treated with TFP showed marked reductions in the severity of parasuicidal behaviors, fewer emergency room visits, hospitalizations, days hospitalized, and reliable increases in global functioning. The effect sizes were large and no less than those demonstrated for other BPD treatments [29, 77]. The one-year drop-out rate was 19.1% and no patient committed suicide. These results compared well with other treatments for BPD: Linehan et al.'s study [77] had 16.7% drop out and one suicide (4%); Stevenson and Meares' study [28] had a 16% drop-out rate and no suicides; and Bateman and Fonagy's study [29] had 21% drop-out rate and no suicides. None of the treatment completers deteriorated or was adversely affected by the treatment. Therefore, it appears that TFP is well-tolerated. Further, 53% of participants no longer met criteria for BPD after 1 year of twice-weekly outpatient treatment [78]. This rate compared quite well with that found by others [28, 60]. In addition, reliable increases in global functioning and a generally low drop-out rate were observed in these patients. These results suggest the potential utility of TFP for treating BPD patients and that more research on TFP is warranted (Table 5.1).

A second study [72] provided further support for the effectiveness of TFP in treating BPD. In this study, 26 women diagnosed with BPD and treated with TFP were compared to 17 patients in a TAU group. There were no significant pretreatment differences between the treatment group and the comparison group in terms of demographic or diagnostic variables, severity of BPD symptomatology, baseline emergency room visits, hospitalizations, days hospitalized, or global functioning scores. The 1-year attrition rate was 19%. Patients treated with TFP, compared to those treated with TAU, showed significant decreases in suicide attempts, hospitalizations, and number of days hospitalized, as well as reliable increases in global functioning. All of the within-subjects and between-subject effect sizes for the TFP-treated participants indicated favorable change. The within-subject effect sizes ranged from 0.73 to 3.06 for the TFP-treated participants, with an average effect size of 1.19 (which is well above what is considered "large" [79]) (Table 5.2).

The only RCT to date that has compared an experimental treatment for BPD to an established alternative treatment has been the RCT conducted by The

**Table 5.1** Results of Clarkin et al.'s [71] TFP pre–post study ($N = 17$)

|  | Means | | p-value |
|---|---|---|---|
|  | Pre-Tx | Post-Tx |  |
| BPD Dx | 100% | 47.10% | – |
| Parasuicidal behavior | 5.18 | 4.24 | 0.45 |
| Medical risk | 1.72 | 1.14 | 0.02 |
| Physical condition | 1.89 | 1.12 | 0.01 |
| Hospitalizations | 1.24 | 0.35 | 0.02 |
| Days hospitalized | 39.21 | 4.53 | 0.06 |
| GAF | 45.57 | 59.85 | <0.001 |

BPD Dx was assessed as the percentage of patients with a DSM-III diagnosis of BPD, from the SCID-II. Parasuicidal behavior, medical risk, and physical condition were all assessed from the suicidality subscale of the Overt Aggression Scale – Modified Version for Outpatients [109] over the previous 12-month period. Medical risk was indicative of the severity of parasuicidal and suicidal behaviors. Physical condition was indicative of the condition following such behaviors. Hospitalizations were assessed by checking medical records and represent the total number of hospitalization in the previous 12-month period. Global Assessment of Functioning (GAF) represents the DSM-III Global Assessment of Functioning scale score.

Personality Disorders Institute, funded in part by the Borderline Personality Disorders Research Foundation, to assess the efficacy of TFP compared with DBT and SPT for patients with BPD. Dialectical behavior therapy, which has received preliminary empirical support for its effectiveness, was selected as the active comparison treatment. The putative mechanisms of change in these two treatments are conceived in very different ways. Dialectical behavior therapy is hypothesized to operate through the learning of emotion regulation skills in the validating environment of the treatment [80]. Transference-focused psychotherapy is hypothesized to operate through the integration of conflicted, affect-laden conceptions of self and others via the understanding of these working models as they are actualized in the here-and-now relationship with the therapist. Supportive psychotherapy [81, 82] was used in contrast to these two active treatments not only as a control for attention and support but also as a component control for TFP.

In this study, the BPD patients were recruited from New York City and adjacent Westchester County. Ninety-eight percent of the participants were clinically referred by private practitioners, clinics, or family members. Ninety patients (6 men and 84 women) between the ages of 18 and 50 were evaluated using structured clinical interviews and randomized to one of the three treatment cells. Results showed that all three groups had significant improvement in both global and social functioning, and significant decreases in depression and anxiety. Both TFP- and DBT-treated groups, but not the SPT group, showed significant improvement in suicidality, depression, anger, and global functioning. Only the TFP-treated group demonstrated significant improvements in verbal assault, direct assault, and irritability [75] (Table 5.3).

In an earlier report on this sample, we [76] examined changes in attachment organization and RF as putative mechanisms of change. Attachment organization

**Table 5.2** Results of TFP vs. TAU study

| | TFP (N = 32) Pre-Tx | Completers Post-Tx | ITT Post-Tx | Change Sig | TAU (N = 17) Pre-Tx | Post-Tx | Change Sig | Between-group comparison |
|---|---|---|---|---|---|---|---|---|
| ER visits | 1.18 | 0.42 | 0.59 | <0.01 | 1.53 | 1.73 | ns | TFP>TAU <0.01 |
| Hospitalizations | 1.72 | 0.46 | 0.91 | <0.001 | 2.47 | 1.93 | ns | TFP>TAU <0.01 |
| Days hospitalized | 61.1 | 7.08 | 25.87 | <0.001 | 48 | 53.4 | ns | TFP>TAU <0.01 |
| No. of BPD criteria met | 7.74 | 4.41 | 5.15 | <0.001 | 7.69 | – | – | TFP>TAU – |
| GAF | 45.57 | 61.0 | 59.85 | <0.001 | 44.8 | 44.66 | – | TFP>TAU <0.01 |

ER visits represent the number of emergency room visits in the previous 12-month period. Hospitalizations represent the total number of hospitalization in the previous 12-month period. No. of BPD criteria was assessed with the SCID-II and provides a dimensional rating of the severity of the disorder. GAF represents the DSM-III Global Assessment of Functioning scale score.

**Table 5.3** Results of Clarkin et al.'s [75] randomized clinical trial

| | Significance of change | | |
|---|---|---|---|
| Symptom-based measures | TFP | DBT | SPT |
| *Primary* | | | |
| Suicidality | <0.05 | <0.05 | *ns* |
| Anger | <0.05 | <0.05 | *ns* |
| Irritability | <0.05 | *ns* | *ns* |
| Verbal assault | <0.05 | *ns* | *ns* |
| Direct assault | <0.05 | *ns* | *ns* |
| Motor Impulsiveness | *ns* | *ns* | *ns* |
| Attentional Impulsiveness | <0.05 | *ns* | *ns* |
| Non-planning Impulsiveness | *ns* | *ns* | <0.05 |
| *Secondary* | | | |
| Anxiety | <0.05 | <0.05 | <0.05 |
| Depression | <0.05 | <0.05 | <0.05 |
| GAF | <0.05 | <0.05 | <0.05 |
| Social adjustment | <0.05 | <0.05 | <0.05 |

Suicidality, anger, irritability, verbal and direct assault were assessed with the Overt Aggression Scale – Modified version [109]. Barratt factors are from the Barratt Impulsivity Scale [110]. Anxiety was assessed with the State-Trait Anxiety Inventory [111]. Depression was assessed with the Beck Depression Inventory [112]. GAF represents the DSM-III Global Assessment of Functioning scale score. Social Adjustment was assessed by the Social Adjustment Scale [113].

was assessed using the Adult Attachment Interview (AAI) (George, C., Kaplan, N., & Main, M. (1985). *The Berkeley Adult Attachment Interview.* Unpublished Manuscript, Department of Psychology, University of California, Berkeley) and the RF coding scale (Fonagy, P., Target, M., Steele, H., & Steele, M. (1998). Reflective Functioning Manual: Version 5.0, for Application to Adult Attachment Interviews. Unpublished Manuscript, University College London, London). After 12 months of treatment, we found a significant increase in the number of patients classified as secure with respect to attachment state of mind for TFP, but not the other two treatments. Significant changes in narrative coherence and RF were found as a function of treatment, with TFP showing increases in both constructs during the course of treatment. Findings suggest that 1 year of intensive TFP can increase patients' narrative coherence and RF. Our findings are important because they show that TFP is not only an efficacious treatment for BPD but also works in a theoretically predicted way and thus has implications for conceptualizing the mechanism by which patients with BPD may change. In addition, patients in TFP did better on those variables than those in DBT and SPT. Our findings are especially important given the literature showing that many treatments do not show specific effects on specific, theory-driven mechanisms [83–91] (Table 5.4).

There are a number of methodological strengths of this study such as the use of multiple domains of change to measure outcome, including behavioral, observer-rated, phenomenological, and structural change (i.e., attachment representations, object relations, and mentalization skills). In addition, this

**Table 5.4** Results of Levy et al.'s [114] randomized clinical trial

| Structural measures | TFP | | DBT | | SPT | | Contrast |
|---|---|---|---|---|---|---|---|
| | Pre-Tx | Post-Tx | Pre-Tx | Post-Tx | Pre-Tx | Post-Tx | |
| Reflective functioning | 2.86 | 4.11 | 3.31 | 3.38 | 2.8 | 2.86 | TFP>DBT = SPT |
| Coherence of narrative | 2.93 | 4.02 | 3.00 | 3.25 | 3.25 | 3.16 | TFP>DBT = SPT |

Reflective functioning was assessed based on Fonagy et al.'s [115] manual for scoring RF. Coherence of narrative was assessed based on the Adult Attachment Interview coding system [116].

study included a broad range of BPD patients and not exclusively those with parasuicidality, representing the full spectrum of BPD manifestations. Further, all therapists were experienced in their respective treatment model, had practice cases prior to beginning the study, and were rated for adherence and competence in their delivery of therapy during the study. Adding to the external validity of this research, treatments were delivered in community mental health settings, including outpatient hospitals and private offices of therapists.

In a study in Amsterdam, Arntz and colleagues [92] compared TFP with Young's Schema-Focused Therapy [93] (SFPT), an integrative approach based on cognitive–behavioral or skills-based techniques along with object relations and gestalt approaches. Their study is unique in examining two active treatments over 3 years. Patients benefited from both treatments; however, at first glance, SFPT appeared more efficacious. A number of serious limitations argue against this conclusion.

First, despite randomization, the TFP condition included twice as many recently suicidal patients [76 vs. 38%; there was also a trend ($p = 0.09$) for the TFP condition having more patients with recent self-injury behavior]. Suicidality influences treatment outcome [94].

Second, the differences between the two groups were apparent only in the intent-to-treat (ITT) analyses but not in the completer analyses. A major factor in this difference appears to have been that patients in the TFP condition were significantly more likely to prematurely drop out of their treatment. Although ITT analyses speak to the external validity (e.g., generalizability), completer analyses speak to the issue of sufficient dose and thus the internal validity or integrity of the study. Differences in outcome between completer analyses and ITT suggest loss of validity due to nonrandom dropout. This can negate the control provided by randomization [95]. Completer analyses did not show any statistically significant advantage for SFPT [4, 96].

Third, the findings suggest inadequate implementation of TFP as indicated by lack of adherence by the TFP therapists. The authors report the median adherence level for TFP was 65.6. Given that a score of 60 is considered adherent, about 50% of TFP therapists are nonadherent. In contrast, the

SFPT group had a median score of 85.6 (again with 60 as adherent), suggesting that 50% of the SFT were not just adherent but exceptionally so. Adherence ratings not only were relatively poor for TFP but also appear to be significantly lower than for SFT. Suffice it to say, the authors are reporting a study that compared an exceptionally well delivered treatment with an inadequately delivered one. There should be no surprise that the exceptionally delivered treatment outperformed the poorly delivered treatment, but it is not a fair test and this fact alone may explain the differential outcome between the two treatments. One of the most potent methodological choices that result in allegiance effects is the selection of therapists who differ in skillfulness that favor the allegiance of the researcher [97].

Fourth, treatment integrity includes having experienced treatment cell leaders, choosing experienced and adherent therapists with a proven track record, providing expert supervision, ongoing monitoring of adherence, and having plans for dealing with nonadherence [98]. Each of these issues was problematic in the current study. Supervision was carried out in the form of a peer supervision, known as intervision [98]. Intervision may work well when carried out by exceptionally adherent therapists as was the case for the SFPT. However, such a model would not work well with nonadherent therapists and would be more akin to the blind leading the blind. The authors indicate that treatment integrity was monitored by means of supervision; however, who was doing that monitoring? Yeomans [99] reports the clinical observation that half the therapists were nonadherent, which is consistent with the authors' own independently rated adherence scores. Most disturbing, however, is that Yeomans [99] reports that he informed the study Principal Investigators (PIs) of the nonadherence problem on numerous occasions, including by email and fax and that no action was taken to deal with this problem.

Fifth, therapists and assessors were not blind to ongoing outcome. Partial results were presented prior to study completion [93, 96, 100, 101], creating another possible confound, which could have caused therapist demoralization in the TFP therapists or enhanced motivation in the SFPT therapists [101]. Given these concerns, it would be premature and irresponsible to conclude that TFP is not as efficacious as SFPT is.

Accumulating evidence indicates that TFP may be an effective treatment for BPD. As more data from the RCT is assessed, we will have a better understanding of how the treatment performs under more stringent experimental conditions. Because the RCT better controls for unmeasured variables through randomization, offers controls for attention and support, and compares TFP to an already established, well-delivered, alterative treatment, its outcome will be a strong indicator of the treatment's efficacy and effectiveness. In addition to the assessment of outcome, the RCT has also generated process-outcome studies designed to assess the hypothesized mechanisms of action in TFP that result in the changes seen in these patients [76].

## Conclusions

In summary, there are a number of conclusions that can be drawn from the data reviewed in this chapter. Most generally, there are a number of different psychodynamic treatment models that are useful and supported empirically for treating BPD. In addition, there may be other models that share similar principles that are also quite effective but remain untested. We would recommend that proponents of these approaches work toward their examination in RCT designs.

Specifically, we have learned that the following:

1. Experienced psychodynamic psychotherapist can have high levels of dropout [69, 70, 103].
2. Unmodified classical psychoanalysis is most likely not that helpful for BPD patients (particularly low-level borderlines) [45].
3. Psychoanalysis can be modified to specific types of pathology and can be modified in different ways successfully [28, 29, 75].
4. The principles and goals of psychodynamic treatments for BPD can be articulated and manualized [27, 58]
5. Psychodynamic psychotherapy can be taught to trainees, early career therapists, experienced therapists, and nurses (not just experienced psychoanalyst) [28, 29, 71].
6. We can video or audio tape sessions without disrupting the treatment [71, 75, 89].
7. There is little evidence that purely supportive psychodynamic psychotherapy is effective with BPD patients, although little is know about the extent to which supportive techniques can be or should be integrated in treatments for BPD [75, 76]. Kernberg would argue for less-supportive techniques particularly for low-level BPD patients, whereas Bateman and Fonagy would argue more integration of supportive techniques.
8. Data suggests that therapists can reduce dropout by increasing the structure and explicitly focusing on frame issues with BPD patient; explicit contracts are particularly helpful but may not be necessary if a solid structure and frame can be established and maintained [71, 75, 76].
9. We can perform RCTs of psychodynamic treatments for BPD [29, 75, 76].
10. Some dynamic treatments for BPD can be considered to have beginning empirical support [29, 75, 76], whereas others appear quite promising [28].
11. We can treat unselected and severely disturbed BPD patients not just those with high IQs, high RF, or good quality of object relations [29, 71, 75, 76, 104].
12. Borderline personality disorder patients can show important change in just 1 year [29, 71, 75, 76].
13. We may have broader outcome, longer-lasting outcome, and show changes in personality than those shown in other treatments [29, 71, 75, 76].

14. Long-term treatment is necessary and important in the treatment of BPD in order to see structural changes in personality organization.
15. Supervision is a critical component for the treatment of BPD. All the empirically supported treatments for BPD, not just the psychodynamic ones, have structured ongoing supervision for therapists [29, 71, 75–77, 92]. Additionally, in some studies, differences between groups [92, 105] appear related to difference in the delivery of adequate supervision [98, 106].
16. All treatments for BPD with empirical support are well-structured, devote considerable effort to enhancing compliance (e.g., attention to contracting and frame), have a clear focus, whether that focus is a problem behavior or an aspect of interpersonal relationship patterns; are highly coherent to both therapist and patient; encourage a powerful attachment relationship between therapist and patient, enabling the therapist to adopt a relatively active rather than a passive stance; and are well-integrated with other services available to the patient.

The next step is the identification of the active ingredients or mechanisms of therapeutic action in these treatments [41]. Effectiveness and efficacy aside, the probative importance of these studies for understanding a treatment's actual mechanisms of action is both indirect and limited [107]. Therefore, despite the support for the effectiveness and efficacy of existing treatments for BPD, clinicians and researchers are still confronted with a high degree of uncertainty about the underlying processes of change. The examination of putative mechanisms of change has the potential to answer theoretical questions and to validate models by showing that theoretically specified mechanisms of change are actually related to the treatments' effectiveness. It is very possible that these treatments may work due to unintended mechanisms such as common factors (e.g., expectancies) [108] or a specific technique factor that is essential for good outcome but not necessarily unique to any one treatment [34]. Finally, there may simply be different avenues to effect change in patients with BPD or that different treatments may be more effective with different types of BPD patients.

Additionally, establishment of the underlying mechanisms of the psychopathology in BPD will help to validate clinical approaches. For example, showing through the use of experimental psychopathology paradigms that identity diffusion or deficits in RF underlie the symptoms in BPD would go a long way to establishing the importance of treatment goals emphasized in TFP.

Finally, given the chronicity of BPD, it is crucial to establish the long-term significance of the changes that occur in our treatments. There is already some preliminary evidence that MBT and IP approaches have long-term effectiveness and that this stability of treatment effects may be unique to psychodynamic treatments. If we can continue and accomplish these goals, we may be able to show the unique added value of our approach and avoid going the way of the dodo bird.

# References

1. Hopko, D. R., Sanchez, L., Hopko, S. D., Dvir S., & Lejuez, C. W. (2003). Behavioral activation and the prevention of suicidal behaviours in patients with borderline personality disorders. *Journal of Personality Disorders, 17,* 460–478.
2. Brown, G. K., Newman, C. F., Charlesworth, S. E., Crits-Christoph, P., & Beck, A. T. (2004). An open clinical trial of cognitive therapy for borderline personality disorder. *Journal of Personality Disorders, 18 (3),* 257–271.
3. Davidson, K., Norrie, J., Tyrer, P., Gumley, A., Tata, P., Murray, H., & Palmer S. (2006). The effectiveness of cognitive behavior therapy for borderline personality disorder: Results from the borderline personality disorder study of cognitive therapy (BOSCOT) trial. *Journal of Personality Disorders, 20,* 450–465.
4. Kellogg, S. & Young, J. (2006). Schema therapy for borderline personality disorder. *Journal of Clinical Psychology, 62,* 445–458.
5. Benjamin, L. S. (1993). *Interpersonal Diagnosis and Treatment of Personality Disorders.* New York: Guilford Press, 11.
6. Linehan, M. M. (1993). *Cognitive-Behavioral Treatment of Borderline Personality Disorder.* New York, NY, USA: Guilford Press.
7. Parron, R. (2006). How to do research? Reply to Otto Kernberg. *International Journal of Psychoanalysis, 87,* 927–932.
8. Kernberg, O. F. (2006). The pressing need to increase research in and on psychoanalysis. *International Journal of Psychoanalysis, 87,* 919–926.
9. Kernberg, O. F. (2006). Research anxiety: A response to Roger Perron's comments. *International Journal of Psychoanalysis, 87,* 933–937.
10 Alexander, F. (1937). *Five Year Report of the Chicago Institute for Psychoanalysis. 1932–1937.*
11. Bordin, E. S. (1948). Dimensions of the counseling process. *Journal of clinical Psychology, 4,* 240–244.
12. Fenichel, O. (1930). *Ten Years of the Berlin Psychoanalytic Institute 1920–1930.* Berlin: Berlin Psychoanalytic Institute.
13. Holt, R. R. & Luborsky, L. B. (1958). *Personality Patterns of Psychiatrists: A Study in Selection Techniques (Vol. 2).* Topeka: The Menninger Foundation.
14. Jones, E. (1936). *Decennial Report of the London Clinic of Psychoanalysis, 1926–1936.*
15. Knight, R. O. (1941). Evaluation of the results of psychoanalytic therapy. *American Journal of Psychiatry, 98,* 434–446.
16. Luborsky, L. B. (1953). Self-interpretation of the TAT as a clinical technique. *Journal of Projective Techniques, 17,* 217–223.
17. Strupp, H. H. (1955). Psychotherapeutic technique, professional affiliation, and experience level. *Journal of Consulting Psychology, 19(2),* 97–102.
18. Wallerstein, R., Robbins, L., Sargent, H., & Luborsky, L. (1956). The psychotherapy research project of the Menninger foundation. *Bulletin Menninger Clinic,* 221–280.
19. Blatt, S. J. (2001). The effort to identify empirical supported psychological treatments and its implications for clinical research, practice, and training. *Psychoanalytic Dialogues, 11,* 633–644.
20. Bornstein, R. F. (2001). The impending death of psychoanalysis. *Psychoanalytic Psychology, 18,* 3–20.
21. Fonagy, P. (2000). Grasping the nettle: Or why psychoanalytic research is such an irritant. *The British Psycho-Analytic Society, 36,* 28–36.
22. Fonagy, P., Jones, E. E., Kächele, H., Krause, R., Clarkin, J., Perron, R., Gerber, A., & Allison, E. (2001). *An Open Door Review of Outcome Studies in Psychoanalysis.* (2nd edn.), London: International Psychoanalytic Association.
23. Gerber, A. J. (2001). A proposal for the integration of psychoanalysis and research. *Psychologist-Psychoanalyst, 21(3),* 14–17.

24. Westen, D. & Morrison, K. (2001). A multidimensional meta-analysis of treatments for depression, panic, and generalized anxiety disorder: An empirical examination of the status of empirically supported therapies. *Journal of Consulting & Clinical Psychology, 69(6),* 875–899.
25. Yeomans, F. E. & Clarkin, J. F. (2001). New developments in the investigation of psychodynamic psychotherapy. *Current Opinions in Psychiatry, 14,* 591–595.
26. Clarkin, J. F., Yeomans, F. E., & Kernberg, O. F. (1999). *Psychotherapy for Borderline Personality.* New York, NY, USA: John Wiley & Sons, Inc.
27. Clarkin, J. F., Yeomans, F., & Kernberg, O. F. (2006). *Psychotherapy of Borderline Personality.* New York: Wiley.
28. Stevenson, J. & Meares, R. (1992). An outcome study of psychotherapy for patients with borderline personality disorder. *American Journal of Psychiatry, 149(3),* 358–362.
29. Bateman, A. & Fonagy, P. (1999). Effectiveness of partial hospitalization in the treatment of borderline personality disorder: A randomized controlled trial. *American Journal of Psychiatry, 156(10),* 1563–1569.
30. Borkovec, T. D. & Castonguay, L. G. (1998). What is the scientific meaning of empirically supported therapy? *Journal of Consulting and Clinical Psychology, 66(1),* 136–142.
31. Ablon, J. S. & Jones, E. E. (2002). Validity of controlled clinical trials of psychotherapy: Findings from the NIMH treatment of depression collaborative research program. *American Journal of Psychiatry, 159,* 775–783.
32. Blatt, S. J. & Zuroff, D. C. (2005). Empirical evaluation of the assumptions in identifying evidence based treatments in mental health. *Clinical Psychology Review, 25(4),* 459–486.
33. Howard, K. I., Orlinsky, D. E., & Lueger, R. J. (1995). The design of clinically relevant outcome research: Some considerations and an example. In M. Aveline & D. A. Shapiro (Eds), *Research Foundations for Psychotherapy Practice* (pp. 3–47). Chichester; New York: Wiley.
34. Levy, K. N. & Scott, L. N. (2007). The 'art' of interpreting the 'science' and the 'science of interpreting the 'art' of treatment of borderline personality disorder. In S. Hoffman & J. Weinburger (Eds), *The Art and Science of Psychotherapy.* London: Brunner-Routledge.
35. Castonguay, L. G. & Beutler, L. E. (2005). Principles of therapeutic change: A task force on participants, relationships, and techniques factors. *Journal of Clinical Psychology, 62(6),* 631–638.
36. National Institute of Mental Health. (2002, December 9–10). Psychotherapeutic interventions: How and why they work. Retrieved April 1, 2003, from: http://www.nimh.nih.gov/scientificmeetings.interventions.cfm
37. Rosen, G. M. & Davison, G. R. (2003). Psychology should list empirically supported principles of change (ESPs) and not credential trademarked therapies or other treatment packages. *Behavior Modification, 27,* 300–312.
38. Gabbard, G. O., Gunderson, J. G., & Fonagy, P. (2002). The place of psychoanalytic treatments within psychiatry. *Archives of General Psychiatry, 59(6),* 505–510.
39. Clarke, M. & Oxman, A. (1999). Cochrane reviews will be in Medline. *BMJ, 319(7222),* 1435.
40. Clarkin, J. F. & Levy, L. N. (2006). Psychotherapy for patients with borderline personality disorder: Focusing on the mechanisms of change. *Journal of Clinical Psychology, 62(4),* 405–410.
41. Levy, K. N., Clarkin, J. F., Yeomans, F. E., Scott, L. N., Wasserman, R. H., & Kernberg, O. F. (2006). The mechanisms of change in the treatment of transference focused psychotherapy. *Journal of Clinical Psychology, 62,* 481–501.
42. Morrison, K. H., Bradley, R., & Westen, D. (2003). The external validity of controlled clinical trials of psychotherapy for depression and anxiety: A naturalistic study. *Psychology & Psychotherapy: Theory, Research & Practice, 76(2),* 109–132.
43. Seligman, M. E. P. (1995). The effectiveness of psychotherapy: The consumer reports study. *American Psychologist, 50(12),* 965–974.

44. Wallerstein, R. (1986). *Forty-Two Lives In Treatment–A Study of Psychoanalysis and Psychotherapy*. New York: Guilford Press.
45. Kernberg, O. F., Burnstein, E., Coyne, L., Appelbaum, A., Horowitz, L., & Voth, H. (1972). Psychotherapy and psychoanalysis: Final report of the Menninger foundation's psychotherapy research project. *Bulletin of Menninger Clinic, 36*, 1–275.
46. Luborsky, L. B., McLellan, A. T., Woody, G. E., O'Brien, C. P., & Auerbach, A. (1985). Therapist success and its determinants. *Archives of General Psychiatry, 42(6)*, 602–611.
47. Rockland, L. H. (1992). *Supportive Therapy for Borderline Patients: A Psychodynamic Approach*. New York: Guilford Press.
48. Gabbard, G. O., Allen, J. G., Frieswyk, S. H., Colson, D. B., Newsom, G. E., & Coyne, L. (1996). *Borderline Personality Disorder Tailoring Psychotherapy to the Patient*. Washington, D.C.: American Psychiatric Press.
49. Kazdin, A. (2001). Progression of therapy research and clinical application of treatment require better understanding of the change process. *Clinical Psychology: Science and Practice, 8*, 143–151.
50. Hobson, R. F. (1985). *Forms of Feeling: The Heart of Psychotherapy*. London: Tavistock.
51. James, William (1890). *The Principles of Psychology*. New York: Holt.
52. Kohut, H. (1971). *The Analysis of the Self*. New York: International University Press.
53. Ornstein, P. H. (1998). Hidden and overt rage: their interpretation in the psychoanalytic treatment process. *Canadian Journal of Psychoanalysis, 6*, 1–14.
54. Meares, R., Stevenson, J., & Comerford, A. (1999). Psychotherapy with borderline patients: I. A comparison between treated and untreated cohorts. *Australian and New Zealand Journal of Psychiatry, 33 (4)*, 467–472; discussion 478–481.
55. American Psychiatric Association. (1980). *Diagnostic and Statistical Manual of Mental Disorders* (3rd edn). Washington, DC: Author.
56. Stevenson, J., Meares, R., & D'Angelo, R. (2005). Five-year outcome of outpatient psychotherapy with borderline patients. *Psychological Medicine, 35(1)*, 79–87.
57. Korner, A., Gerull, F., Meares, R., & Stevenson, J. (2006). Borderline personality disorder treated with the conversational model: A replication study. *Comprehensive psychiatry, 47*, 406–411.
58. Bateman, A. W. & Fonagy, P. (2006). *Mentalization-Based Treatment for Borderline Personality Disorder: A Practical Guide*. Oxford, Oxford University Press.
59. Bateman, A. W. & Fonagy, P. (2004). Mentalization-based treatment of BPD. *Journal of Personality Disorders, 18(1)*, 36–51.
60. Bateman, A. & Fonagy, P. (2001). Treatment of borderline personality disorder with psychoanalytically oriented partial hospitalization: An 18-month follow-up. *American Journal of Psychiatry, 158(1)*, 36–42.
61. Linehan, M. M., Heard, H. L., & Armstrong, H. E. (1993). Naturalistic follow-up of a behavioral treatment for chronically suicidal borderline patients. *Archives of General Psychiatry, 50(12)*, 971–974.
62. Yeomans, F. E., Clarkin, J. F., & Kernberg, O. F. (2002). *A Primer of Transference Focused Psychotherapy for the Borderline Patient*. Northvale, NJ: Jason Aronson.
63. Kernberg, O. F. (1984). *Severe Personality Disorders: Psychotherapeutic Strategies*. New Haven, CT: Yale University Press.
64. Steiner, J. (1993). *Psychic Retreats – Pathological Organisations in Psychotic, Neurotic and Borderline Patients*. London: Routledge.
65. Yeomans, F. E. (1993). When a therapist overindulges a demanding borderline patient. *Hospital and Community Psychiatry, 44*, 334–336.
66. Clarkin, J. (1996). The utility of a treatment contract. *Journal of Practical Psychiatry and Behavioral Health, 2*, 368–369.
67. Sanderson, C., Swenson, C., & Bohus, M. (2002). A critique of the American Psychiatric Practice Guideline for the treatment of patients with borderline personality disorder. *Journal of Personality Disorder, 16*, 122–129.

68. Kroll, J. (2000). Use of no-suicide contracts by psychiatrists in Minnesota. *American Journal of Psychiatry*, *157*, 1684–1686.
69. Yeomans, F. E., Gutfreund, J., Selzer, M. A., & Clarkin, J. F. (1994). Factors related to drop-outs by borderline patients: Treatment contract and therapeutic alliance. *Journal of Psychotherapy Practice & Research, 3(1)*, 16–24.
70. Smith, T. E., Koenigsberg, H. W., Yeomans, F. E., & Clarkin, J. F. (1995). Predictors of dropout in psychodynamic psychotherapy of borderline personality disorder. *Journal of Psychotherapy Practice & Research*, 4 *(3)*, 205–213.
71. Clarkin, J. F., Foelsch, P. A., Levy, K. N., Hull, J. W., Delaney, J. C., & Kernberg, O. F. (2001). The development of a psychodynamic treatment for patients with borderline personality disorders: A preliminary study of behavioral change. *Journal of Personality Disorders*, 16 *(6)*, 487–495.
72. Levy, K. N., Clarkin, J. F., Schiavi, J., Foelsch, P. A., & Kernberg, O. F. (in review). *Transference Focused Psychotherapy for Patients Diagnosed with Borderline Personality Disorder: A Comparison with a Treatment-As-Usual Cohort.*
73. Clarkin, J. F., Levy, K. N., Lenzenweger, M. F., & Kernberg, O. F. (2005). The Personality Disorders Institute/Borderline Personality Disorder Research Foundation randomized control trial for borderline personality disorder: rationale, methods, and patient characteristics. *Journal of Personality Disorders*, 18 *(1)*, 52–72.
74. Levy, K. N., Clarkin, J. F., & Kernberg, O. F. (2006). Change in attachment and reflective function in the treatment of borderline personality disorder with transference focused psychotherapy. *Journal of Consulting and Clinical Psychology*, *74*, 1027–1040.
75. Clarkin, J. F., Levy, K. N., Lenzenweger, M. F., & Kernberg, O. F. (2007). A multiwave RCT Evaluating three treatments for borderline personality disorder. *American Journal Psychiatry*, *164*, 922–928.
76. Levy, K. N., Meehan, K. B., Kelly, K. M., Reynoso, J. S., Weber, M. Clarkin, J. F., & Kernberg, O. F. (2006). Change in attachment and reflective function in the treatment of borderline personality disorder with transference focused psychotherapy. *Journal of Consulting and Clinical Psychology*, *74*, 1027–1040.
77. Linehan, M. M., Armstrong, H. E., Suarez, A., Allmon, D., & Heard, H. L. (1991). Cognitive-behavioral treatment of chronically parasuicidal borderline patients. *Archives of General Psychiatry*, 48 *(12)*, 1060–1064.
78. Clarkin, J. F. & Levy, K. N. (2003). Influence of client variables on psychotherapy. In M. Lambert (Ed.), *Handbook of Psychotherapy and Behavior Change* (5th edn, pp. 194–226). New York: Wiley & Sons.
79. Cohen, J. (1988). *Statistical Power Analysis for the Behavioral Sciences*. Mahwah, NJ: Erlbaum.
80. Lynch, T. R., Chapman, A. L., Rosenthal, M. Z., Kuo, J. R., & Linehan, M. M. (2006). Mechanisms of change in dialectical behavior therapy: Theoretical and empirical observations. *Journal of Clinical Psychology*, 62 *(4)*, 459–480.
81. Applebaum, S. A. (1981). *Effecting Change in Psychotherapy*. London: Aronson.
82. Applebaum, S. A. (2005). *Supportive Psychotherapy*. In J. M. Oldham, A. E. Skodol, & D. S. Bender (Eds), *Textbook of Personality Disorders*. Arlington, VA: The American Psychiatric Publishing, Inc..
83. Ablon, J. S., Levy, R. A., & Katzenstein, T. (2002). Beyond brand names of psychotherapy: Identifying empirically supported change processes. *Psychotherapy: Theory, Research, Practice, Training, 43 (2)*, 216–231.
84. Ablon, J. S. & Jones, E. E. (1998). How expert clinicians' prototypes of an ideal treatment correlate with outcome in psychodynamic and cognitive–behavioral therapy. *Psychotherapy Research, 8*, 71–83.
85. Castonguay, L. G., Goldfried, M. R., Wiser, S., & Raue, P. J. (1996). Predicting the effect of cognitive therapy for depression: a study of unique and common factors. *Journal of Consulting and Clinical Psychology*, 64 *(3)*, 497–504.

86. DeRubeis, R. J. & Feeley, S. (1990). Determinants of change in cognitive therapy for depression. *Cognitive Therapy and Research, 14* (5), 469–482.

87. DeRubeis, R. J., Evans, M. D., Hollon, S. D., Garvey, M. J., Grove, W. M., & Tuason, V. B. (1990). How does cognitive behavioral therapy work? Cognitive change and symptom change in cognitive therapy and pharmacotherapy for depression. *Journal of Consulting and Clinical Psychology, 58,* 862–869.

88. Ilardi, S. S. & Craighead, W. E. (1994). The role of nonspecific factors in cognitive therapy for depression. *Clinical Psychology: Science and Practice,* 1 *(2),* 138–156.

89. Jones E. E. & Pulos, S. M. (1993). Comparing the process in psychodynamic and cognitive-behavioral therapies. *Journal of Consulting and Clinical Psychology,* 61, 306–316.

90. Shaw, B. F., Elkin, I., Yamaguchi, J., Olmstead, M., Vallis, T. M., Dobson, K. S., Lowery, A., Sotsky, S. M., Watkins, J. T., & Imber, S. D. (1999). Therapist competence ratings in relation to clinical outcome in cognitive therapy of depression. *Journal of Consulting and Clinical Psychology,* 67 *(6),* 837–846.

91. Trepka, C., Rees, A., Shapiro, D. A., & Hardy, G. E. (2004). Therapist competence and outcome of cognitive therapy for depression. *Cognitive Therapy and Research, 28,* 143–157.

92. Giesen-Bloo, J., Van Dyck, R., Spinhoven, P., Van Tilburg, W., Dirksen, C., Van Asselt., et al. (2006). Outpatient psychotherapy for borderline personality disorder: A randomized clinical trial of schema focused therapy versus transference focused psychotherapy. *Archives of General Psychiatry, 63,* 649–658.

93. Young, J. E., Klosko, J., & Weishaar, M. E. (2003). *Schema Therapy: A Practitioner's Guide.* New York: The Guildford Press.

94. Oldham, J. M. (2006). Borderline personality disorder and suicidality. *American Journal of Psychiatry, 163,* 20–26.

95. Howard, K. I., Krause, M. S., and Orlinsky, D. E. (1986). The attrition dilemma: Towards a new strategy for psychotherapy research. *Journal of Consulting and Clinical Psychology, 54,* 106–110.

96. Arntz, A. (2004). Borderline personality disorder. In: T. A. Beck, A. Freeman, D. D. Davis and X. Associates (Eds), *Cognitive Therapy of Personality Disorders* (2nd edn, pp. 187–215). New York: The Guilford Press.

97. Luborsky, L., Diguer, L., Seligman, D. A., Rosenthal, R., Krause, E. D., Johnson, S., et al. (1999). The researcher's own therapy allegiances: A "wild card" in comparisons of treatment efficacy. *Clinical Psychology: Science and Practice, 6,* 95–106.

98. Clarkin, J., Levy, K., Lenzenweger, M., & Kernberg, O. (2004). The Personality Disorders Institute/Borderline Personality Disorder Research Foundation randomized control trial for borderline personality disorder: rationale, methods, and patient characteristics. *Journal of Personality Disorders,* 18 *(1),* 52–72.

99. Yeomans, F. E. (2006). Questions concerning the randomized trial of schema focused therapy vs. transference focused psychotherapy. *Archives of General Psychiatry, 64 (5),* 609–610.

100. Giesen-Bloo, J. H., Arntz, A., van Dyck, R., Spinhoven, P., & van Tilburg, W. (2001). Outpatient treatment of borderline personality disorder: Analytical psychotherapy versus cognitive behavior therapy. Paper presented at the World Congress of Behavioral and Cognitive Therapies, July 17–21, Vancouver, Canada.

101. Giesen-Bloo, J. H., Arntz, A., van Dyck, R., Spinhoven, P., & van Tilburg, W. (2002). Outpatient treatment of borderline personality disorder: Analytical psychotherapy versus cognitive behavior therapy. Paper presented at the Transference Focused Psychotherapy for Borderline Personality Symposium, November 16–17, New York, USA.

102. Chalmers, T., Smith, H., Blackburn, B., Silverman, B., Schroeder, B., Reitman, D., & Ambroz, A. (1981). A method for assessing the quality of a randomized control trial. *Controlled Clinical Trials, 2,* 31–49.

103. Waldinger, R. & Gunderson, J. (1984). Completed psychotherapies with borderline patients. *American Journal of Psychotherapy, 38*, 190–202.
104. Hoglend, P., Amlo, S., Marble, A., Bogwald, K. P., Sorbye, O., Sjaastad, M. C., & Heyerdahl, O. (2006). Analysis of the patient-therapist relationship in dynamic psychotherapy: An experimental study of transference interpretations. *American Journal of Psychiatry, 163*, 1739–1746.
105. Linehan, M. M., Comtois, K. A., Murray, A. M., Brown, M. Z., Gallop, R. J., Heard, H. L., et al. (2006). Two-year randomized controlled trial and follow-up of dialectical behavior therapy vs. therapy by experts for suicidal behaviors and borderline personality disorder. *Archives of General Psychiatry, 63 (7)*, 757–766.
106. Levy, K. N. (2006, June 11). RE: New Publication in the Archives on a comparison of Schema (Young) focus. Message posted to psychodynamic research, archived at psychodynamicresearch@yahoogroups.com
107. Garfield, S .L. (1990). Issues and methods in psychotherapy process research. *Journal of Consulting and Clinical Psychology, 58 (3)*, 273–280.
108. Weinberger, J. (1995). Common factors aren't so common: The common factors dilemma. *Clinical Psychology: Science and Practice, 2*, 45–69.
109. Coccaro, E. F., Harvey, P. H., Kupshaw-Lawrence, E., Herbert, J. L., Bernstein, D. P. (1991). Development of neuropharmacologically based behavioral assessments of impulsive aggressive behavior. *J Neuropsychiatry Clinical Neuroscience, 3 (supp 2)*, 44–51.
110. Patton, J. H., Stanford, M. S., Barratt, E. S. (1995). Factor Structure of the Barratt Impulsiveness Scale. *Journal of Clinical Psychology, 51(6)*, 768–774.
111. Spielberger, C. D. & Gorsuch, R. L. (1983). Manual for the state-trait anxiety inventory (form Y): self-evaluation questionnaire. Consulting Psychologists Press, Palo Alto, CA.
112. Beck, A. T., Ward, C. H., Mendelson, M., Mock, J., & Erbaugh, J. (1961). An inventory for measuring depression. *Archives of General Psychiatry, 4*, 561–571.
113. Weissman, M. M. & Bothwell, S. (1976). Assessment of social adjustment by patient self-report. *Archives of General Psychiatry, 33*, 1111–1115.
114. Levy K. N., Meehan K. B., Kelly K. M., Reynoso J. S., Clarkin J. F., Kernberg O. F. (2006). Change in Attachment Patterns and Reflective Function in a Randomized Control Trial of Transference-Focused Psychotherapy for Borderline Personality Disorder. *Journal of Consulting and Clinical Psychology, 74*, 1027–1040.
115. Fonagy, P., Steele, M., Steele, H. & Target, M. (1997). *Reflective-functioning manual: version 4.1. For application to the Adult Attachment Interviews.* Unpublished manuscript, University College London.
116. Main, M. & Goldwyn, R. (1984). Predicting rejection of her infant from mother's representation of her own experience: implications for the abused-abusing intergenerational cycle. *Child Abuse and Neglect, 8* (2), 203–217.

# Chapter 6
# Studying Change in Defensive Functioning in Psychotherapy Using the Defense Mechanism Rating Scales: Four Hypotheses, Four Cases

**J. Christopher Perry, Stephen M. Beck, Prometheas Constantinides, and J. Elizabeth Foley**

**Abstract** Defense mechanisms are one of the original and the most durable theoretical contributions of psychoanalysis to dynamic psychology. Research has shown that there is a hierarchy of the general level of adaptation of defenses, divided into seven levels, which can be summarized as the level of overall defensive functioning (ODF). This chapter examines how the quantitative assessment of defense mechanisms can yield indicators of the progress and outcome in psychotherapy research. Four cases are presented with short- to long-term psychotherapy and one with very long follow-up. Each demonstrates how different aspects of defensive functioning change over different time periods and states (i.e., depressed vs. not depressed) exemplifying four hypotheses about how defenses change. The first is that as individuals change, they increase their overall level of defensive functioning, and at the same time, variability in defensive functioning tends to decrease, indicating increased resilience to stress. The second is that change in defense levels occurs in a stepwise fashion in which individuals trade off defenses lower on the hierarchy for those in the middle and only later developing those at the top of the hierarchy. The third is that individuals and groups have their own rates of change, which may vary across naturalistic and different treatment conditions, yet to be determined. Depressed states may be associated with initially large changes that then decelerate, whereas personality disorders (PDs) may have long initial periods of induction in the therapeutic process ("priming"), before change is initiated and becomes, more or less linear. Treatments that increase this rate of change are likely to be seen as more effective. Finally, in line with most of the research to date, as defensive functioning improves, symptoms will decrease and other aspects of functioning will improve. Although single cases do not prove a hypothesis, these cases offer some empirical support, while clearly demonstrating the value

J.C. Perry
The Institute of Community and Family Psychiatry, Sir Mortimer B. Davis Jewish, General Hospital, 4333 Chemin de la Côte Ste-Catherine, Montréal, Québec H3T 1E4, Canada, and McGill University, Montreal, Québec, Canada; The Erikson Institute for Training and Research at the Austen Riggs Center, Stockbridge, MA 01262-0962, USA

R.A. Levy, J.S. Ablon (eds.), *Handbook of Evidence-Based Psychodynamic Psychotherapy*,      121
DOI: 10.1007/978-1-59745-444-5_6, © Humana Press 2009

of research in this field. Furthermore, the identification of defenses in verbatim interviews and psychotherapy sessions permits the moment-to-moment analysis of the apparent effect of interventions on defensive functioning, also a topic worthy of further research.

One of the earliest observations at the inception of psychoanalysis was that defense mechanisms inhibit, manage, and sometimes redirect the expression of motives and affects in symbolically meaningful ways when psychological conflicts are triggered. Beginning with the publication of *The neuropsychoses of defence*, Freud [1] described repression, reaction formation, displacement, and other defense mechanisms but he never became interested in their systematic study. Later, Anna Freud [2] began to systematize them. In further theoretical development, Waelder [3] posited that defenses could have multiple functions beyond guarding against forbidden wishes, which could include the gratification of wishes. Schafer [4] further expanded this idea suggesting that defenses also seek to increase gratification and to reduce pain, while still defending against forbidden wishes. Hartmann, et al. [5] suggested that some ego functions were neutralized or conflict-free, and not directed against forbidden wishes. They emphasized that defenses and some other ego functions (e.g., reality testing) could be directed either against motives or toward objects and events in the external world to improve the individual's adaptation to reality factors. Norma Haan [6] extended this view by giving separate roles to defenses that deal with intrapsychic conflict and to related mechanisms that help adapt the individual's motives to the demands and constraints of the external world. Thus she separated defense from related coping mechanisms. Subsequently, Lazarus and Folkman [7] rejected most of the views of the defense and drive perspective in favor of studying only coping as conscious mechanisms, which individuals employ to deal with external stress. A plethora of research on conscious coping has followed (see review [8]), while research on defense mechanisms has also proceeded at a slightly slower and less well-funded pace (see review [9]).

In psychoanalytic psychology, defense mechanisms are widely viewed as one constituent in the structure underlying personality or character. For instance, in his description of the difference between psychotic, borderline, and neurotic levels of personality organization, Kernberg [10] noted particular defenses along with identity formation and reality testing as the cornerstones of character. Recognizing the advances in assessing defenses (see below), defenses were added in Appendix B of DSM-IV [11] as a dynamic aspect of personality that could be coded separately from PDs. The presumption is that individuals tend to use the same repertoire of defenses, and these constitute the defensive structure of personality. Structural change over the course of treatment should then result in improvement in defensive functioning, i.e., a change in the defense repertoire toward more adaptive defenses. Advances in assessing defenses now allow us to track changes in defenses so that psychotherapists can see the effects of treatment on their patients during and after treatment. This chapter is devoted to this issue.

This chapter will examine one method of rating defense mechanisms, the Defense Mechanism Rating Scales (DMRS), and demonstrate how it may be used in the study of psychotherapy process and outcome. Using a longitudinal perspective on four cases, we will demonstrate how defenses can be viewed as a dynamic outcome variable, in addition to their usual function as mechanisms operating from moment to moment in real time. Although defensive and coping functioning are currently separated, if not divorced, we will also present some early data suggesting that a reconciliation may be possible based on the commonality of overall level of functioning, allowing defense and coping to relate to one another once again, if not actually remarry.

## What are Defenses?

As noted elsewhere [9, 12–14], there is an approximate consensus among researchers on the following aspects of the defense mechanism construct.

1. A defense mechanism is the individual's automatic psychological response to internal or external stressors or emotional conflict (see DSM-IV, Appendix B Defensive Functioning Scale, pp. 751–757). The action of a defense is triggered by the occurrence of what Freud [15] called *signal anxiety,* arising whenever internal wishes or drives conflict with internalized prohibitions or external reality constraints.
2. Defenses generally act automatically, without conscious effort. Often, the individual is totally unaware of the defensive operation, although in some instances, he or she may have partial awareness.
3. Defenses contribute to character traits that are in part made up of specific defenses that an individual tends to use repetitively in divers situations. Individuals tend to specialize, using a set or repertoire of defenses across various stressors, depending on the motives or conflicts active at the time. The defenses an individual shows at any point in time may vary in degree or specificity with the stressor, making some state effects expectable [16], while the average frequency of using the defense is dispositional. Whether there is specificity between type of stressor and choice of individual defense used is an empirical question.
4. One review tallied 42 different individual defense mechanisms described by various authors [17]. Although there is no clear rationale for selecting a definitive list of defenses [18], a process of consensus has favored those defenses with clear, nonoverlapping definitions, reliable application and demonstrated empirical findings. Although this process is advanced, it is not completed.
5. Defenses affect adaptation [14, 18]. Each defense may be highly adaptive in certain situations. Nonetheless, there is a clear hierarchy of defenses in relation to the overall adaptiveness of each individual defense. Defenses at the lower end are usually maladaptive, save in a few situations, while those at the higher end are adaptive in a broader array of circumstances.

6. When defenses are least adaptive, they protect the individual from awareness of the stressors, anxiety, and/or associated conflicts, but at the price of constricting awareness, freedom to choose ways of responding, and flexibility to maximize positive outcomes. When they are most adaptive, defenses maximize awareness of internal and external motives, stressors and constraints and thereby maximize the expression and gratification of wishes, minimize negative consequences, and enlarge the scope of choices and sense of control. Some individuals label the most adaptive defenses as *coping mechanisms*, after Haan [6], whereas many in the dynamic tradition retain the defense designation, because the so-called coping mechanisms share many characteristics with other defenses. This question of terminology, defense vs. coping, is a mixture of questions of preference, definition, and science.

7. Whether defenses emerge in a certain developmental sequence is an empirically open issue. The usage of developmental terms to describe groups of defenses, such as immature or mature, is done for reasons of history and convenience only. In fact, preverbal toddlers may use high proportions of mature or high adaptive-level defenses [19], which suggests that much more is needed to understand why some adults come to use the lower-level defenses associated with PDs. However, during adulthood, there appear to be sequences in which certain lower-level defenses progress to higher-level defenses on the continuum of adaptiveness [14]. For instance, acting out in early life (e.g., rebelling against authority) may evolve later to reaction formation (taking the side of authority) and eventually to altruism (helping the less powerful obtain fair responses from authority). These sequences deserve study because they may hold important implications for patterns of therapeutic change in personality, both as a patient "trades up" within a therapy session and how he or she develops over time. Our clinical examples address this in particular.

8. Identifying and understanding the function of defenses serves as an aid to understanding the problems and therapeutic challenges in treatment. For instance, defenses in the lower half of the defense hierarchy mediate many of the most maladaptive ways of handling stress and conflict in PDs and depression. Specific defense levels may be associated with certain individual disorders or clusters, which relate to core psychopathology, such as splitting and projective identification in borderline personality [10, 20, 21], or omnipotence and devaluation in antisocial and narcissistic personality disorders (NPDs) [22]. Whenever used, these same defenses serve as instantaneous markers alerting the clinician that a core issue for a given person may be operating.

## The Hierarchy of Defenses

Defenses have been hierarchically ordered based on the empirical relationship to general measures of adaptiveness or psychological health. A number of studies have led to a generally accepted hierarchy [12, 14, 18, 23, 24]. Examples include the Defensive Functioning Scale in DSM-IV [11, 25], and the DMRS

**Table 6.1** DMRS hierarchy of defense levels and individual defense mechanisms

I. Mature

7. *High adaptive level (mature):* affiliation, altruism, anticipation, humor, self-assertion, self-observation, sublimation, and suppression

II. Neurotic

6. *Obsessional level:* intellectualization, isolation of affect, and undoing

5. *Other neurotic level:* (a) repression, dissociation, (b) reaction formation, displacement

III. Immature

4. *Minor image-distorting level (narcissistic):* devaluation of self or object images, idealization of self or object images, and omnipotence

3. *Disavowal level:* denial, projection, rationalization. Although not a disavowal defense, autistic fantasy is scored at this level

2. *Major image-distorting level (borderline):* splitting of other's images, splitting of self-images, and projective identification

1. *Action level:* acting out, hypochondriasis, and passive aggression

IV. Psychotic

0. *Defensive dysregulation level (psychotic):* distortion, psychotic denial, delusional projection, and psychotic dissociation.

*Overall defense maturity (ODF):* 0–7 scale summarizes defensive functioning by taking the mean of all the defense scores, each weighted by the above 0–7 scheme.

hierarchy (Table 6.1). Defenses that have common aims are grouped together in one of the eight levels. For instance, among the so-called immature defenses, the disavowal level includes three defenses – denial, rationalization, and projection. These have a common function of disavowing certain affects, actions, ideas, or motives, which others can identify in the person using them. However, each defense differs in method of handling the disavowed material. Denial actively avoids it altogether, rationalization avoids it by covering it up with something deemed more socially acceptable, while projection avoids it by misattributing it to others and thereby maintaining an interest in it, but at a distance. The defense levels range from the lowest level of defensive dysregulation (so-called psychotic defenses) to the high adaptive level (so-called mature defenses). Healthier individuals use a larger proportion of highly adaptive defenses and a lower proportion of defenses at the low end of the hierarchy. The DMRS does not yet have a complete section of psychotic-level defenses, such as psychotic denial, distortion, and delusional projection [18], as to date the method has mostly been used on nonpsychotic samples.

## The Defense Mechanism Rating Scales Quantitative Rating Method

We currently score defenses according to the quantitative directions of the DMRS, fifth edition [26]. The DMRS is a quantitative, observer-rated method [9], which is almost identical to the qualitative Provisional Defense

Axis in Appendix B of DSM-IV [11, 27]. Each of 30 defenses is identified whenever it occurs in the session. This method differs from other observer-rated methods that are qualitative or semiquantitative ratings (e.g., most prominent defenses as in Vaillant [14]), which yield global ratings for the whole interview [9].

Three levels of scoring are used, all of which are continuous, ratio scales.

1. *Individual defense score.* A proportional or percentage score is calculated by dividing the number of times each defense was identified by the total instances of all defenses for the session.
2. *Defense-level score.* The defenses are arranged into seven defense levels hierarchically arranged by their general level of adaptiveness. Each defense level is represented by a proportional or percentage score.
3. *Overall defensive functioning.* The ODF score is obtained by taking the average of each defense level score, weighted by its order in the hierarchy, yielding a number between 1 (lowest) and 7 (highest).

In addition, the defense-level scores can be divided into several superordinate levels: mature, neurotic, immature, and psychotic, although in most publications using the DMRS, the fourth is not included.

There is good convergent and discriminant validation for the overall hierarchy vis-a-vis other functioning and symptom measures [18, 24, 27–29]. Inter-rater reliability can be quite high at the level of identifying the number of defenses and ODF with intraclass $R$ values above 0.80, while the defense levels and individual defenses are generally somewhat lower (see review [30]). Short-term stability was determined by rating five consecutive weekly psychotherapy sessions [16], which indicated that about half the variance is due to trait, while the other half of variance was due to state effects that varied from session to session. The stability of ODF was intraclass $R$ $(I_R)$ = 0.48, while the stabilities of the individual defense levels had a median of 0.47, range 0.08–0.73. By contrast, the number of defenses used per session varied greatly (stability $I_R$ = .18), indicating that the rate of using defenses (e.g. number per 50-min session) is highly state-dependent.

Studies using the DMRS have indicated the range of defensive functioning from healthy-neurotic to personality-disordered. A community sample of mothers with no recent stressors and no psychiatric-treatment history gave Relationship Anecdote Paradigm (RAP) interviews, which were rated for defenses (unpublished data of the first author). Most healthy individuals had ODF scores ranging from 5.0 to 6.4 with a mean above 5.6. Perry and Hoglend [27] found that depressed individuals had a mean ODF of 4.68 at intake which with treatment rose to 5.11, indicating that they returned to a neurotic level of functioning as the episode diminished. The psychotherapy pilot study [16] indicated that PDs had ODF scores below 5.0 with a mean of 4.32 (range 3.31–4.97) in the early months of psychotherapy. Furthermore within the PD group, those with borderline personality disorder (BPD) had significantly lower ODF than those with non-BPD group (4.07 vs. 4.62), although the samples were small. These data indicate that there is good convergence between an ordering of diagnostic groups and a normative group of nonill women and the level of ODF. This suggests that ODF and possibly specific levels may serve as a dynamic measure of adaptive functioning.

Based on previous work examining defenses common in individuals with depression (both major depression and dysthymic disorder), Hoglend and Perry [31] examined a group of eight so-called depressive defenses, a subgroup immature defenses. These include acting out, passive aggression, help-rejecting complaining, splitting of self-images, splitting of others' images, projective identification, projection, and devaluation. Depressed individuals with major depression who had a greater proportion of these defenses had poorer responses to treatment by 6 months compared to those with fewer of these defenses. This suggested that these defenses may play a particular role in the onset or maintenance of depression, suggesting that they may also serve as a marker of the underlying dynamic vulnerability to depression. This idea is explored in several of our cases below.

## Hypotheses for Psychotherapy and Long-Term Change

1. *Individuals have a general level and range of day-to-day defensive functioning, representing their level of defensive adaptation.* Personality disorders in particular have a general level of defensive functioning lower than neurotic and healthy-neurotic individuals with higher reactivity to stressors. Although most individuals with PDs have a defense repertoire that spans the hierarchy of defenses, depending on occasion, salient stressors may interact with or trigger some of their psychological conflicts, which, in turn, pull for defenses from particular levels. For instance, we previously published [16] a case of a man with passive-aggressive PD who in the early years of treatment had a generally high level of action defenses but with substantial session-to-session variability. The spikes upward in using action and other immature defenses were usually related to issues of authority and invalidation of his point of view. However, whenever these issues were absent, the subject functioned more at a neurotic level. After the third year of treatment, not only had ODF begun to rise significantly, but the week-to-week variability decreased. This stabilizing of the defensive structure, or increased resilience in the face of stress, indicated that defensive functioning was becoming less state-dependent and more trait-like, alongside improvement in the general overall level of functioning.

   Thus we hypothesize that improvement in defensive functioning involves both an increase in the overall level and a decrease in the amount of variability, indicating increased resilience to stress.

2. *Improvement occurs in stages more often than across all levels of defensive functioning.* In the above case example, as the patient improved, the action

level defenses decreased linearly throughout the treatment, while the minor-image-distorting defenses (e.g., idealization) temporarily increased before beginning to decrease after 3 years. As these lower-level defenses decreased, there was an increased reliance on neurotic-level defenses – repression, reaction formation, and displacement – while the already high level of obsessional defenses remained stable. Finally, there was a nonsignificant increase in high adaptive-level defenses. This case illustrates Vaillant's finding that as young adults age, they first trade off immature for neurotic-level defenses, and somewhat later they trade off neurotic for mature-level defenses [18].

Thus we hypothesize that individuals whose defensive functioning involves a large proportion of immature defenses will improve in stepwise fashion with respect to the proportion of defenses at each level. The lowest-level defenses, such as action and major-image-distorting defenses, will begin to decrease earliest, other immature defenses – disavowal and minor-image-distorting defenses – will begin to decrease next – perhaps after a small temporary increase – while the neurotic-level defenses will tend to increase. Finally, after the above improvements are well under way, high adaptive-level defenses will begin to show significant improvement. Although this is the hypothesized complete development cycle, it is of course possible that developmental progression may slow or cease at any point for various reasons.

Individuals who initially have a very high level of neurotic defenses may follow the same general stepwise movement, although the therapy literature suggests that there may be periods of regression in defensive functioning before there is any significant increase in high adaptive-level defenses.

3. *Each person and each class of persons (e.g., a specific disorder) may have unique rates of change under natural history or specific treatment conditions.* For instance, individuals who are in an episode of major depression will show a different rate of change from ill to remission, which may be faster than from the early period of remission until a subsequent follow-up period. Individuals and disorders can be classed by their rates of change, which may be informative about the type and goals of therapy that may be effective. Additional research may then examine differential predictors of these rates of change, such as childhood neglect or abuse, linking developmental experiences with pathology and the natural course or response to treatment.

4. *As defensive functioning improves, symptoms decrease and social role adaptation also improves.* This hypothesis is a general version of the finding of cross-sectional associations between defensive functioning and measures of adaptation (see review [12]). As a general hypothesis, it should hold across a wide variety of measures of symptoms and functioning, indicative of the general underlying psychological role that defenses play in psychopathology and adaptation. As a result, a period of sustained, healthy, defensive functioning should presage sustained improvement in other aspects of psychological functioning. Whether change in defenses mediate the other improvements, or is merely correlated with them, will require further study.

## Case Illustrations

In the remainder of the chapter, we describe four case reports focusing on findings that illustrate how defensive functioning changes over time. These are illustrated graphically by figures of quantitative ratings of dynamic or RAP interviews or psychotherapy sessions.

## *Case A. A Woman with Recurrent Major Depression*

The first case is taken from a pilot study ($n = 12$) of adults with acute, recurrent major depression who entered a comparative treatment trial of antidepressive medications (ADM) and 20 sessions of either cognitive–behavioral therapy or dynamic psychotherapy. The aim of the study was to estimate the proportion of subjects who attained a full recovery from depression, defined as greater than 8 weeks with a Hamilton Rating Scale for Depression-17 (HRSD-17) score below 6, and remained well at 1-year follow-up. A related aim was to examine whether potential psychological mediators of depression – especially defenses – would normalize by termination and remain at healthy levels at 1 year. This explicitly examined whether initially elevated depressive defenses would decrease to below a healthy cutoff (< about 7%), and ODF would reach healthy-neurotic levels (> about 5.64). If short-term psychotherapy and ADM were generally curative, then the median figures for the sample should lie in the recovered ranges at termination and/or follow-up.

The patient was a 29-year-old married special education teacher who sought treatment for a depression following a miscarriage. She felt deeply ashamed of being unable to control her feelings, of which disappointment was the most salient. She did not express anger over the miscarriage but expressed fear that she was not going to be able to have a baby, possibly due to a previous abortion. She had been an only child, often lonely, for whom self-sufficiency and not being a bother to her parents became a hallmark. She had married a very supportive and nice man whom she initially had not been attracted to but came to like as she realized how good he made her feel. After joining the research project, she was randomly assigned to 20 sessions with a senior cognitive–behavioral therapy (CBT) therapist. This therapy has been described in detail elsewhere [32] and was scored on the Analytic Process Scales. Although working in the cognitive–behavioral model, the treatment addressed the patient's reluctance to express her own feelings, clarified some of them, and helped her explore her own emotional life as well as think through her responses. Treatment was considered very successful and the patient returned to work, became pregnant, and worked through her fear that the pregnancy would end badly. Her HRSD-17 score dropped from 24 at intake to 9 (mild depression) at termination and 6 (the cutoff for nondepressed) at 1-year follow-up. Similarly the Beck Depression Inventory (BDI) went from 12 (above the depressed range) to 7 (nondepressed) to 0 at 1 year.

This case was selected because her change in defensive functioning was close to the median of the sample, hence illustrative of the average response of defensive functioning to a 20-session treatment. The patient's dynamic interviews at intake, termination, and 1-year follow-up were scored for defenses, blind to time, and other data. At intake, the patient had 17% immature defenses of which the majority, 9%, were the eight so-called depressive defenses. Her neurotic defenses constituted the bulk of her defensive functioning at 78%, while high adaptive-level defenses were 6%. Illustrated in Fig. 6.1, her depressive defenses dipped to 2% at termination, then rose somewhat to 5% by 1 year. At the same time, neurotic defenses rose to 89% at termination but at one year follow-up they decreased to 78%, about where they started at intake. Finally, Fig. 6.1 also shows that her high adaptive (mature) defenses were largely unchanged, at 7%, at termination, but rose somewhat to 12% by 1 year. Figure 6.2 displays ODF across the three time periods. She began with an ODF of 4.97 in the depressive range just below the neurotic range. It rose to 5.33 at termination and to 5.38 by 1 year, both in the middle of the neurotic range. This constituted a within-condition effect size (ES) of 1.13 equal to the mean and close to the median for the sample (ES = 0.99)

This case improved in line with the above hypotheses. She began in the depressive range and moved to the neurotic range, trading off depressive for

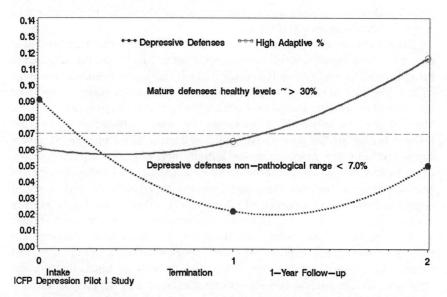

**Fig. 6.1** Depressive defenses decrease to normative levels after 20 sessions, regressing slightly at 1 year. High adaptive (mature)-level defenses begin to improve only after termination at the 1-year follow-up, attaining about one-third of normative levels

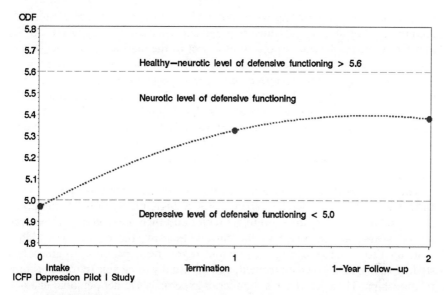

**Fig. 6.2** After 20 sessions of treatment, overall defensive functioning (ODF) rises from depressive to neurotic levels, shy of healthy-neurotic levels at 1-year follow-up

neurotic-level defenses. Only at 1-year did she begin to increase her high adaptive defenses somewhat, at the expense of a decrease in her neurotic-level defenses. Most of her positive changes occurred while she was in treatment and were concurrent with the large decrease in depressive symptoms. The exception was the increase in high adaptive-level defenses at 1 year, which coincided with a further reduction in depressive symptoms. From a defense point of view, the patient was characterologically mildly depressive (depressive defenses) and more strongly obsessional and counter-dependent (reaction formation, displacement, undoing, intellectualization, and isolation). At termination and 1 year, the neurotic defense constellation remained the largest part of her defense repertoire. This is consistent with the conclusion that treatment was very successful for treating the depressive part of her character but, in all likelihood, returned her to the status quo ante of those neurotic-level characterological defenses in place prior to the depressive episode. In the time frame of 1 year, she improved meaningfully but, as was generally true for the sample, she did not attain a healthy-neurotic level of functioning.

## Case B. A Two-and-Half-Year Therapy Episode in a Patient with Borderline Personality Disorder–Narcissistic Personality Disorder

In this case, we will fully describe the changes in defensive functioning across the hierarchy. This was a 24-year-old single woman who was referred after terminating a therapy during which she had become very regressed, suicidal, accompanied by acting out, which required extensive use of hospitalization. At that termination, she sent a poisonous object in the mail to her former therapist's office and was charged with assault. Following this event and subsequent legal proceedings, she was referred elsewhere. By agreement she was seen once weekly in dynamic psychotherapy for a little over 2 years, until the therapist had to terminate due to a change in job. She also had adjunctive CBT during the first year only. At termination, she was referred for further dynamic psychotherapy to another therapist. At intake, her Axis I diagnoses included dysthymic disorder, with a past history of bulimia, while on Axis II she had both BPD and NPD. She was on no medication.

This case was chosen to demonstrate the process of change in a patient with BPD and NPD who, while starting with a high proportion of immature defenses, had strong motivation to get better and then made great strides over several years. At the outset of the current therapy, the patient was highly motivated to avoid repeating her previous regressive experience, to renew her studies, to live in her own apartment, and eventually to be able to tolerate close relationships. There had been a number of experiences in her personal history, which she was aware were important, but she strongly preferred keeping the initial focus on staying in school and avoiding any further hospitalizations.

In her first year of therapy, she attended regularly. The focus was on external current issues, and transference was addressed more to manage it, and understand its immediate impact, than to explore it at deeper genetic levels. There were a number of regressive episodes in the first year, such as a disappointment in an interaction with a teacher following a test. Typically, these disappointments were dealt with by acting out (e.g., getting drunk), passive aggression (e.g., staying in her car overnight at school), projective identification (e.g., blaming the teacher and seeing him as the cause of her actions), and splitting (e.g., seeing herself as all bad when subsequently discussing it). She responded quite well when the therapist and she agreed upon limits to regressive wishes, which sometimes included the threat of increasing the frequency of sessions! Therapy focused on helping her trade up to utilize other defenses already in her repertoire, such as rationalization (e.g., "the test was hard and no one did well") or omnipotence (e.g., "I think I can do better than the others in the class, anyway"). The result was that there were quite wide swings in defensive functioning from session to session in the first year. These are illustrated in Figs 6.3–6.5.

For each defense level, we ran simple linear regression models with time (session number) as the independent variable. Table 6.2 shows the results of individual linear regression models of her defense-level scores over times. Her action and major image-distorting (borderline) defense levels were initially around 13–14% each of her total defensive functioning, while both decreased highly significantly by the end of the 2.5 years of treatment, each ending at less than 2% of defensive functioning (also see Fig. 6.3). The other two immature defense levels, next highest on the defense hierarchy, behaved slightly

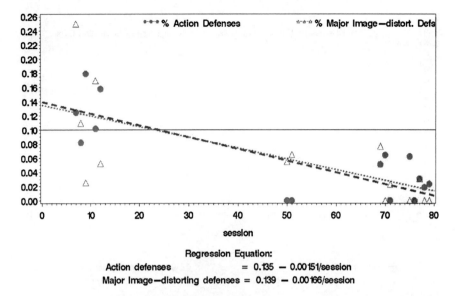

Regression Equation:
Action defenses                = 0.135 − 0.00151/session
Major Image−distorting defenses = 0.139 − 0.00166/session

**Fig. 6.3** High levels of both action and major image-distorting (borderline)-level defenses decrease steadily over 79 sessions (2 + years), attaining levels consistent with no longer having definite borderline personality disorder (BPD)

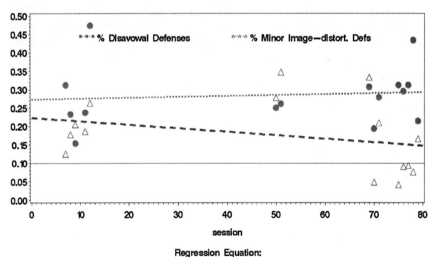

Regression Equation:
Minor Image−distorting defenses = 0.223 − 0.000944/session
Disavowal defenses             = 0.272 + 0.000255/session

**Fig. 6.4** Disavowal-level defenses (e.g., rationalization) increase slightly, while minor image-distorting (narcissistic) defenses increase, then begin to decrease over 79 sessions. As BPD diminishes, the patient relies temporarily on defenses associated with narcissistic personality disorder (NPD)

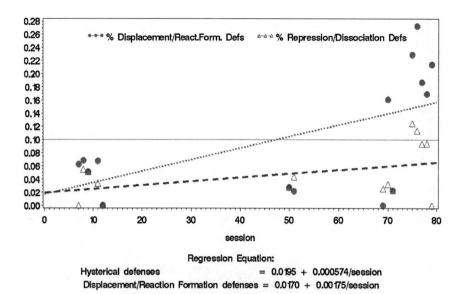

Regression Equation:
Hysterical defenses                          = 0.0195 + 0.000574/session
Displacement/Reaction Formation defenses = 0.0170 + 0.00175/session

**Fig. 6.5** Over the 79 sessions, hysterical (mostly repression) and other neurotic defenses (displacement and reaction formation) increase, reflecting a shift toward neurotic away from personality-disordered-level functioning

differently. Disavowal defenses were almost one-quarter of her defense reper-toire and increased nonsignificantly, while minor image-distorting (narcissistic) defenses initially increased then decreased (nonsignificantly) toward the end of

**Table 6.2** Case A: change in defense levels and ODF over 79 sessions (2 years)

| Defense level | Intercept /final estimate | Slope | $t, df = 14$ | $p$-value | $R^2$/adjusted $R^2$ |
|---|---|---|---|---|---|
| 7 High adaptive | 9.7%, 15.6% | 0.0738% | 0.96 | 0.35 | 0.067/–0.005 |
| 6 Obsessional | 9.1%, 15.7% | 0.0831% | 1.95 | 0.07 | 0.227/0.168 |
| 5a Hysterical | 2.0%, 6.5% | 0.0574 | 1.71 | 0.11 | 0.184/0.122 |
| 5b Displace-RF | 1.7%, 15.5% | 0.175% | 2.59 | 0.02 | 0.340/0.289 |
| 4 Minor image-distorting | 22.3%, 14.8% | –.0944% | 1.11 | 0.29 | 0.086/0.016 |
| 3 Disavowal | 27.2%, 29.2% | 0.0255% | 0.34 | 0.74 | 0.009/–0.07 |
| 2 Major image-distorting | 13.9%, 0.8% | –0.166% | 3.61 | 0.003 | 0.499/0.462 |
| 1 Action | 13.4%, 1.6% | –0.151% | 4.58 | 0.0005 | 0.617/0.588 |
| *Summary Scores* | | | | | |
| II. Neurotic | 12.8%, 37.7% | 0.316 | 2.87 | 0.01 | 0.389/0.342 |
| III. Immature | 77.5%, 46.7% | –0.390 | 3.41 | 0.005 | 0.472/0.431 |
| No. of defenses | 40.5, 45.2 | 0.0585 | 0.43 | 0.67 | 0.014/–0.067 |
| ODF | 3.55, 4.64 | 0.0138 | 3.88 | 0.002 | 0.537/0.501 |

the second year (see Fig. 6.4). Meanwhile the subject showed increases in three neurotic defense levels, significantly with displacement/reaction formation and nonsignificant trends with repression/dissociation (hysterical) and obsessional defenses (see Fig. 6.5). Finally, the correlated changes in the tripartite defense levels are shown in Fig. 6.6. As the immature defenses decreased highly significantly, the neurotic defenses increased significantly, while the high adaptive (mature) defense level increased nonsignificantly. As a result, ODF improved highly significantly, beginning at an ODF estimated by the model at 3.55, increasing 1.09 points to 4.64 estimated at session 79. In addition, the variability in ODF, as represented by the range, decreased from a high of 1.21 points after intake to 1.00 after 1 year and 0.72 points after the second year. The final result was that by the foreshortened end of the treatment, the subject had reached a level of ODF consistent with narcissistic personality, still somewhat below the level of neurotic character functioning. This indicates that the goal of stabilizing the patient had been achieved with an extensive reduction in the lowest-level defenses, trading up to higher immature and neurotic levels, but not yet to high adaptive defenses within the time frame of the therapy.

These results are consistent with the hypotheses. As the subject improved, her ODF increased and the session-to-session variability in ODF decreased. The patient had consolidated her defensive functioning to a level common with narcissistic personality but no longer borderline. Further work was still necessary to develop healthy-neurotic functioning. As to her life goals, by the end of therapy, she had completed her program of studies and was contemplating her

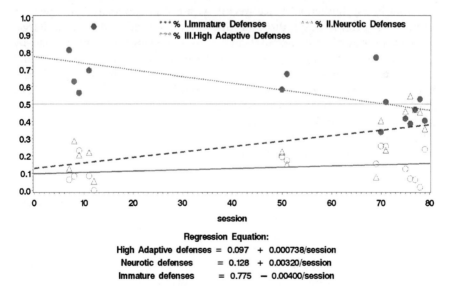

Regression Equation:
High Adaptive defenses = 0.097 + 0.000738/session
Neurotic defenses       = 0.128 + 0.00320/session
Immature defenses       = 0.775 − 0.00400/session

**Fig. 6.6** With all defense levels divided into three categories, as immature defenses decrease, neurotic defenses increase at very similar rates, while high adaptive (mature) defenses increase more slowly

next career move. She had successfully kept a job and had begun a somewhat superficial relationship with a boyfriend, albeit one whom she found somewhat disappointing. She did not have any significant regressions in the year prior to termination, nor had there been any emergency room visits or hospitalizations over the treatment course. She was uncertain as to her next career move, as she was concerned about parental pressures on her to follow a certain career path. No regression in functioning occurred at termination as she transferred treatment to a subsequent therapist. Thus she exemplified the third hypothesis as well that improvement in ODF is associated with improvement in other measures of functioning and social role adaptation.

## Case C. A Woman Entering Residential Treatment and Followed for 13.25 Years

This woman in her early twenties entered residential, intensive dynamic treatment at the Austen Riggs Center following a series of life stressors leading to a suicide attempt. She had recently married someone about whom she was highly ambivalent while on the rebound from a previous relationship. She was working and going to college part-time and became highly symptomatic. On Axis I she had major depressive disorder, dysthymic disorder, a recent history of cocaine and alcohol abuse, panic disorder with agoraphobia, and a history of bulimia nervosa. On Axis II she had borderline, dependent, and self-defeating PDs. She had been in psychotherapy twice weekly with a very supportive therapist for several years prior to hospitalization with whom she continued after discharge. She had a series of three hospitalizations over 3 years, each precipitated by suicidal episodes and intense guilt over wishes to become more independent and to resist familial pressure to make her marriage work and remain a dutiful daughter. A breakthrough came during her third hospitalization, one result of which was a decision to end the marriage, which had remained unconsummated. Following this, her regressive episodes ceased and she resumed her college career path, steering clear of intimate relationships for a period of several years until she established her independent adult identity more. She continued to see her therapist, gradually cutting down to once weekly, then every other week by about 7 years for several years longer. She obtained a good position in her chosen career and began to date, eventually marrying and having a child. By the 14th year of follow-up, she was recovered from all of her Axis I disorders and was functioning at a healthy adult level by global assessment of functioning (GAF) (>71) and in other social roles as well.

This case was selected because it demonstrates two points: how long it can take until someone with treatment-refractory disorders develops a steady rate of change in defensive functioning and how long it takes to develop healthy-neurotic functioning. Over the 13.25 years of follow-up, her defenses were assessed at 17 points in time from 7 dynamic and 10 RAP interviews. Given the length of follow-up, we explored the question of determining the time at which her long-term trends in defensive functioning became evident or stabilized. To do this, we present four figures, each of which displays the linear trends for immature, neurotic, and high adaptive-level defenses using observations up to four increasing lengths of follow-up: 3, 5, 7, and the total 13.25 years. For ease of visual comparison across all four figures, the linear trends of the first three figures are extrapolated out to 14 years.

Figure 6.7 examines the change in defenses over the first 3 years of follow-up, prior to her decision to end her marriage. That this was a highly turbulent period is demonstrated by the increasing levels of immature defenses and accompanying wide variation. Neurotic levels actually decreased, while, unexpectedly, high adaptive-level defenses increased. The intercepts reflect the modeled level of defenses at intake, along with the actual change rates, the change in percentage of overall functioning per year. These are displayed below the graphic presentations for each tripartite defense level. Figure 6.8 displays the trends based on the first 5 years of data, including the early period of stabilization after deciding to end her marriage. By 5 years, different trends have emerged. Immature defenses decreased by 3% per year, high adaptive defenses increased at a slightly slower rate, and neurotic defenses increased very slowly (0.25% per year). Figure 6.9 indicates that the trends are similar at 7 years with the trends for high adaptive and immature defenses in the same direction but at slightly steeper rates than at 5 years. However, the direction of change for the

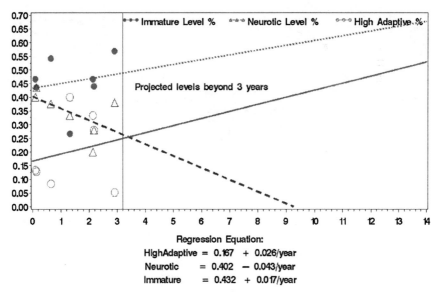

Fig. 6.7 After 3 years, the patient appears somewhat unstable and regressed, with immature defenses increasing and neurotic level defenses decreasing. However, high adaptive-level defenses increase

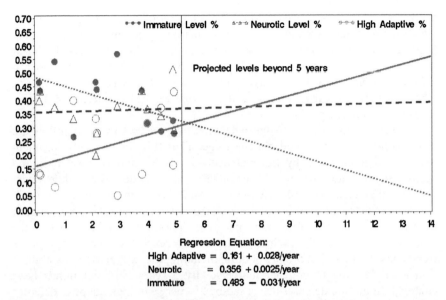

**Fig. 6.8** After 5 years of follow-up, immature defenses decrease, predicted to reach normative levels by 12 years, while neurotic and high adaptive defenses increase

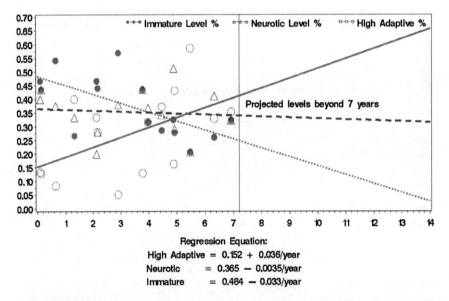

**Fig. 6.9** After 7 years, immature defenses decrease at a rate established by 5 years, while neurotic defenses decrease slightly. High adaptive-level defenses increase still slightly faster than at 5 years

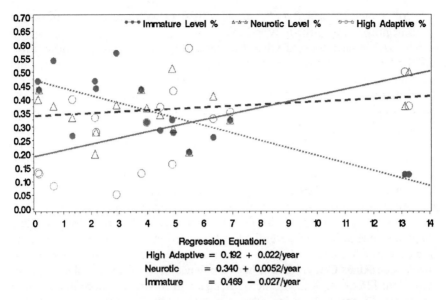

**Fig. 6.10** By over 13 years, immature, neurotic, and high adaptive-level defenses have reached normative levels, having continued on trajectories established by 5 years

neurotic-level defenses shifted toward decreasing, again at a slow rate (–0.35% per year). Finally, Fig. 6.10 displays the data using all 13.25 years. Over this long time frame, immature defenses have decreased to less than 15% of total defensive functioning, while neurotic defenses have increased to almost 40% and mature defense to almost 50% of total defensive functioning. Her ODF – not shown – was scored at 4.38 and 4.53 in her first two interviews – consistent with severe BPD – yet were scored at 6.00 and 5.68 in her last two interviews, indicating that she had achieved a healthy neurotic level of functioning. A simple linear regression model using all observations over the 13 + years estimated that her initial ODF was 4.41, significantly increasing 1.65 points by the end of follow-up to an estimated final $ODF$ of 6.06 $(df = 1.15, F = 20.01, p = 0.0004)$. Variability was much higher during the first half of the follow-up, intake to 6.5 years, than in the second half of the follow-up, intake to 6.5–13.25 years (ODF range 3.79 vs. 1.62 points).

The graphical presentations indicate clearly that as time progressed, the subject's variability tended to decrease leading to relatively stable trends by about 5 years. Graphically this is evident by the similarities of the trend lines at 5, 7, and 13.25 years. Her ODF also clearly was increasing by this time and continued to increase relatively linearly by the end of the 13.25 years. These data are consistent with our first hypothesis. Also, she developed solid healthy functioning in other areas of her life, including work and close relationships, consistent with our third hypothesis. Finally, she did develop rather consistent rates of change between 3 and 5 years, consistent with expectations of individuals as noted in the fourth hypothesis.

The patient deviates somewhat, however, from our second hypothesis. During the first 3 years, the patient had unstable trends for both immature- and neurotic-level defenses, with only the high adaptive-level defenses showing a trend that would be upheld across the four time periods. Thus at 3 years, the patient began improving first in the one area, which we hypothesized would be the last to show improvement. By 5 years, the improvement pattern was largely in line with our second hypothesis, although improvement was greater in high adaptive than in neurotic levels, which is not typical. These trends remained more or less throughout the remainder of follow-up. Our explanation is post hoc but several things are evidently different in this patient's treatment than in our other cases. First, she was well into an ongoing intensive outpatient treatment prior to her first hospitalization. Second, during the first 3 years, she had three hospitalizations of several months duration, each of which included intensive psychotherapy (four sessions per week) with the same therapist at the Austen Riggs Center. Third, her turbulence decreased when she made her important life decision to end her marriage and to strike a more independent position as an adult. We believe that we captured this patient with two distinct trends going on in parallel. The first trend reflects the common experience of the borderline patient in repeated crises related to anaclitic close relationships, which took between 3 and 5 years to stabilize. The second is the self-reflective process, which she was already engaged in and intensified periodically during her residential stays. Thus we feel she was developing insight and some related healthy defenses all along, necessary for her to make her life-altering decision. Had she begun treatment only at intake into the study, it is possible that she might have taken a more typical course, perhaps not showing significant changes in high adaptive-level defenses until some time after her immature defenses began to decrease, but this cannot be known for sure.

## Case D. A woman treated for recurrent depression with 18 months of psychotherapy

This case is that of a 38-year-old woman with one child and a partner of many years, who sought treatment for an episode of recurrent major depression on top of dysthymic disorder. She had some depressive and self-defeating personality traits but did not meet full criteria for a PD. Although she had her first depressive episode in her late teens during university, she had remained largely free of episodes until the previous year during which she experienced a number of serious stressful events in her work and family life, including several serious illnesses of relatives. Everyone who knew her saw her as competent and noncomplaining. Although she handled the recent stressors well from an external point of view, the problems left her with a feeling that she was holding too much in and a sense that disaster was around the corner. Several months into the episode, she saw her general practitioner who prescribed an antidepressant, which helped somewhat, but after several months without greater improvement, she sought psychotherapy.

At intake, she was still moderately depressed with an HRSD-17 score of 21 and a BDI-II score of 19, both indicating moderately severe depression. She received 18 months of dynamic psychotherapy with an experienced clinician initially once but eventually twice weekly. Both patient and clinician described the therapy as very helpful; however, the therapist communicated that this was really a case requiring longer-term treatment. Termination occurred at a time when the patient was beginning to address deeper characterological issues, and thus was experienced as premature by both patient and therapist. Over the course of the therapy, she slowly remitted, attaining recovery from the index episode by month 12 of treatment. Over the last 6 months of treatment and subsequent 24 months of follow-up (30 months total), she had four of eight HRSD-17 scores above 6, indicating a mixed period of recovery interspersed with mild symptoms. Although there were no recurrences of a depressive episode meeting full criteria, this indicates that some vulnerability to depression remained. Figure 6.11 shows the changes in the HRSD-17 score over this time period.

This case demonstrates that characterological issues may lead to some regression in defensive functioning even while the patient may improve

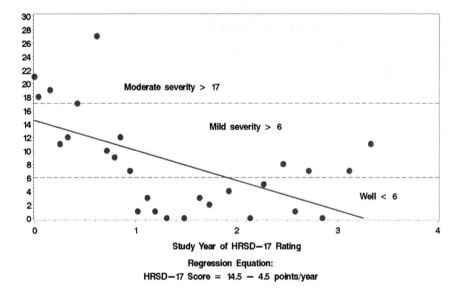

**Fig. 6.11** The Hamilton Rating Scale for Depression –17 (HRSD-17) decreases in severity, indicating the patient is fully recovered (<6) after almost 2 years. However, half the observations from 2.5 years onward are in the mild range, suggesting residual symptoms remain

symptomatically and in other areas of coping. If therapy terminates before the deeper work is done, some vulnerability in defensive functioning may remain, which may be associated with residual symptoms.

### Defenses

The significant characterological issues in this case are reflected in how defenses changed over the course of therapy. Overall defensive functioning changed very slowly but nonsignificantly up to session 83, the last one rated, 2 months from termination. Combining ratings of all three data types (dynamic and RAP interviews and therapy sessions), a linear regression model indicated that her initial ODF (intercept) was 5.29 with a rate of change (slope) of 0.026 points per year, statistically nonsignificant, estimating a final ODF of 5.33 at about 16 months. This indicates that she began and ended about in the midpoint of the range of neurotic functioning. Figure 6.12, which breaks down the change in ODF by interview type, displays three different patterns of change. According to the dynamic interviews, her ODF remains about the same, whereas the RAP interview, which reflects interpersonal interactions, indicates an increase of 0.243 points per year. However, the psychotherapy sessions displayed an interesting pattern: ODF initially displayed a lot of variability, which became more stable by the end of the 18 months of treatment, albeit at a lower level (*ODF* rate of change = −0.194 points per year). In therapy, as the patient stabilized, there

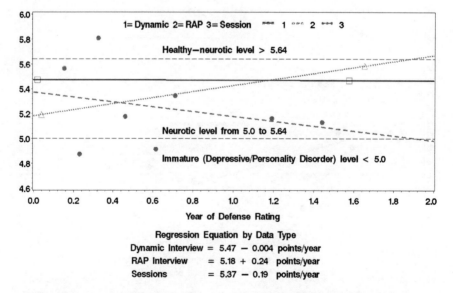

Regression Equation by Data Type
Dynamic Interview = 5.47 − 0.004 points/year
RAP Interview     = 5.18 + 0.24 points/year
Sessions          = 5.37 − 0.19 points/year

**Fig. 6.12** Over the 18 months of treatment, overall defensive functioning (ODF) remains the same in the dynamic interviews, but improves in interpersonal vignettes (RAP interviews), while showing some stabilization and regression in the therapy sessions

was a mild degree of regression in functioning, consistent with an intensive process of dynamic exploration wherein the patient allows neurotic issues and related defenses to emerge for exploration of affective meaning and development of insight. Had therapy proceeded into a longer-term therapy, once hitting a plateau, ODF would have been expected to rise as treatment worked through the underlying characterological issues. Further examination of the details can help support whether this interpretation is correct, that real change is occurring, but the process was not brought to completion in the 18-month time frame.

The above differences in ODF across the three interview types correlate with the degree of structure in each. Beck and Perry [33] found that RAP interviews are more structured than dynamic interviews, while sessions are the least structured. They hypothesized that less-structured interviews would be associated with a diminution in the level of defensive functioning, which is true in this case.

We examined variability comparing the range of ODF in the first half to that in the second half of the period over which defenses were rated (0.93 vs. 0.45 points). This indicated that the variability was decreasing, one indicator of improvement, even though ODF did not yet break significantly higher.

Figure 6.13 examines three groups of defenses. Her immature defenses, which include the depressive defenses, decreased nearly significantly ($p = 0.07$), while her use of repression increased markedly but nonsignificantly ($p = .14$). This indicates that as she traded off her lower-level defenses, she increasingly explored material that had heretofore been more deeply repressed.

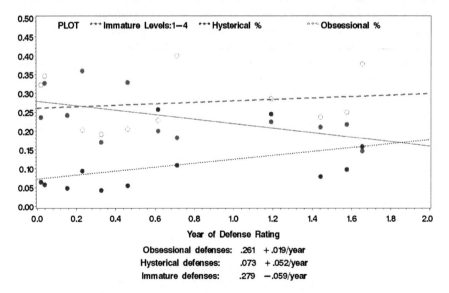

Obsessional defenses: .261 + .019/year
Hysterical defenses: .073 + .052/year
Immature defenses: .279 − .059/year

**Fig. 6.13** During 18 months of therapy, immature defenses decrease while both hysterical and obsessional levels rise, indicating increasing reliance on neurotic mechanisms

The increase in repression indicates that the material is closer to consciousness and within the reach of some exploration. At the same time, there was a slight increase in obsessional defenses as she attempted to understand what she is conflicted about, but was still not able to tolerate the associated affects fully. The mature defenses did not change significantly yet, again indicative that at the time of termination, she was only midway through the process of getting to healthy-neurotic. Were the patient to have continued and completed the work of a longer-term therapy, we would predict that the immature defenses would continue to fall, and in particular the depressive defenses would fall below 7%, the cutoff for individuals without depression. Furthermore, the subject would trade off her hysterical and obsessional defenses for an increase in mature-level defenses.

## Coping

We also assessed coping mechanisms in this case. As briefly described in the introduction, Haan's [6] distinction between defense mechanisms that respond to intrapsychic conflict and coping mechanisms that deal with adaptation to external reality led the way for Lazarus and Folkman's [7] complete separation of coping mechanisms from defenses. Coping mechanisms were thus conceptualized as largely conscious processes that individuals employ in response to stressors or problems encountered in their environment. A recent review of empirical methods for studying coping [8] concluded that coping has a hierarchical structure in which specific instances of coping action patterns (CAPs) can be classified into 12 categories, and these 12 categories can be further grouped into three broader families of coping that are grouped together based on shared objectives. The competence family seeks to coordinate actions in the environment, the relatedness family seeks to coordinate self-reliance and social resources, and the autonomy family seeks to coordinate individual preferences and available options. Each family consists of two more-adaptive coping mechanisms and two less-adaptive coping mechanisms (adaptive processes are listed first). Competence processes include problem-solving, information seeking, helplessness, and escape; relatedness processes include self-reliance, support seeking, delegation, and isolation; autonomy processes include accommodation, negotiation, submission, and opposition. Thus, much like defenses, coping mechanisms are organized into a hierarchy, and it is expected that more-adaptive forms of coping would be related to better psychological and social functioning.

   In the present case example, we used the hierarchical structure of coping to create a manual for coding verbatim text from patient interviews and psychotherapy sessions (Perry et al., ms in preparation). Coping was divided into positive CAPs (more-adaptive coping) negative CAPs (less-adaptive coping). Furthermore, a general score of overall coping functioning (OCF) was constructed as the overall proportion of adaptive coping used by the patient in each transcript (range 0–1.0). Figure 6.14 displays the OCF scores for the interviews

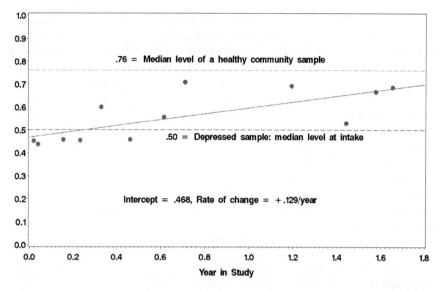

**Fig. 6.14** Overall coping functioning (OCF, the proportion of coping mechanisms that are positive) rises over the 18 months of therapy, but remains shy of normative levels

and sessions. At intake, the subject's score was less than 0.50, which is the mean for subjects with acute depression, indicating that coping is divided equally between positive and negative categories. Simple linear regression found this rate of change (0.129 per year) to be significant ($p = .007$). By the end of treatment, OCF was estimated to have increased to 0.687, indicating that two-thirds of her coping was positive, although this is still below the mean of 0.75 for a community sample of nonill women who were mothers (data still being rated by the authors). Thus she improved measurably but may not have fully reached healthy norms.

We were interested in the relationship between coping and defenses as markers of change of functioning over psychotherapy. The median number of defenses was 58.5, while the median number of CAPs was 24, indicating a ratio of 2.4 defenses to every CAP. Furthermore, across the 12 interviews, the numbers scored for each were highly correlated (Spearman correlation or $r_s = 0.73$, $n = 12$, $p = 0.007$). Not surprisingly, as ODF did not change overall, there was little correlation with OCF across the sessions ($r_s = .16$, n.s.), whereas there was a significant correlation between the immature defense score and OCF ($r_s = -0.72$, $p = 0.008$), as the immature defenses decreased OCF improved. The trade off was largely to neurotic not to mature defenses, with the former correlating at a trend level with OCF ($r_s = 0.51$, $p = 0.09$). Examining some of the individual defenses noted in Fig. 6.13, the increase in repression was correlated with OCF ($r_s = 0.62$, $p = 0.03$), suggesting that as warded off issues became more evident, even though still somewhat repressed, her overall coping improved. Similarly the levels of intellectualization and isolation correlated with OCF ($r_s = 0.58$, $p = 0.05$ and $r_s = 0.48$, $p = 0.12$, respectively). As we posited earlier that her defensive functioning returned to a neurotic level of functioning, as therapy progressed and depression lifted, this suggests that some of her improvement in OCF may have been a return to previous levels of coping available to her as well. One test of this would be the durability of change in both defensive and coping functioning over ensuing years of follow-up. Only time can sort out the state changes from the more resilient trait improvements. In any case, in this subject, the immature defenses were improving and were highly correlated with improved coping. Unfortunately, the termination before changes were seen in high adaptive-level defenses precluded determining whether such changes would have heralded a lift of OCF into healthy normative levels. Overall then, we have evidence of both some convergence and discrimination of defensive and coping functioning.

## Discussion

The four cases presented are relevant to all or most of the hypotheses about how defenses change. Each case was selected to represent a different type of disorder or therapeutic approach, resulting in too few cases to test the validity of the hypotheses. Nonetheless, we can reasonably discuss whether the data from each case support the hypotheses or not, offering very preliminary evidence of validity. Of course, full validation would require larger samples and different treatment conditions and designs, especially for the fourth hypothesis. Table 6.3 presents the findings from each case for each of the hypotheses discussed.

*Hypothesis 1* stated that as patients improve, ODF rises. Cases A–C clearly demonstrated this, while case D demonstrated more limited changes in defensive functioning that resulted in only a small rise in the overall level (ODF). Case A was assessed at only three points in time over a year and showed a move from depressive-immature to a neurotic level by termination, maintained at 1-year follow-up. Although meaningful, it is not clear whether this was a state change, back to the status quo prior to the depressive episode, or whether it represented a move to a new, higher level of defensive functioning. Cases B and C are different in that each patient clearly moved to and remained at a significantly higher ODF over time, consistent with true trait changes. Alongside the rise in ODF was the reduction of variability in defensive functioning as patients improved. Although this is harder to estimate in case A with only three ratings, clearly Cases B–D all showed that over time the range from lowest to highest ODF diminished by half or more. This supports the subhypothesis that as defenses improve, they become more resilient, as indicated by less deviation from their usual level of functioning. Stress does not result in as wide swings in defensive functioning as was evident prior to and during the earlier phases of treatment.

**Table 6.3** Confirmation or disconfirmation of hypotheses by case

| Defensive functioning hypotheses | Case A 20 sessions[a] 1 year[b] | Case B 79 sessions[a] 2 + years[b] | Case C Hundreds[a] 13 + years[b] | Case D 83 sessions[a] 1.5 years[b] |
|---|---|---|---|---|
| 1a. Improvement: general level of ODF rises | Yes ODF + 0.41 Initial = 4.97, final = 5.38 | Yes ODF + 1.09 Initial = 3.55, final = 4.64 | Yes ODF + 1.65 Initial = 4.41, final = 6.06 | ± ODF + 0.04 Initial = 5.29, final = 5.33 |
| 1b. Improvement: variability in defensive functioning decreases | Insufficient data | Yes Decreased Each year | Yes Decreased Early vs. late | Yes Decreased Early vs. late |
| 2. Improvement follows the hierarchy in stages | Yes | Yes | Yes | Yes |
| High Adaptive: | Slight increase | Little change | Steady increase | Little change |
| Neurotic: | Increase | Increase | Increase[c] | Increase |
| Immature: | Decrease | Decrease | Decrease[d] | Decrease |
| 3. Individuals and classes of individuals have unique rates of change, in a given condition: natural history or specific treatment | Recurrent depression : ODF returned to neurotic in months | BPD & NPD meaningful improvement over 2 + years | BPD, SDPD & 8 Axis I disorders: normalized by 13 years | Recurrent depression: ODF stabilized by 16 months |
| 4. Improvement in defensive functioning correlates with improvement in symptoms, functioning | Yes, less depression, improved social role functioning | Yes, markedly improved role functioning: school, work, and relationships | Yes, reached healthy norms in most areas of functioning | Partial: fewer immature defenses and improved depression and coping |

[a] Number of individual therapy sessions during period of study.
[b] Period of study in years, including therapy and any posttherapy follow-up.
[c] Initial 3 years of regression characterized by decrease before increasing through year 13.
[d] Initial 3 years of regression characterized by increase before decreasing through year 13.
BPD, borderline personality disorder; NPD, narcissistic personality disorder; SDPD, self-defeating personality disorder.

*Hypothesis 2* stated that improvement occurs stepwise up the hierarchy, first trading off lower-level defenses, e.g., action or borderline, for defenses somewhat higher on the hierarchy. After this is well under way, then midlevel defenses, such as higher-level immature, e.g., narcissistic defenses, or neurotic defenses diminish as mature defenses increase. Thus the whole hierarchy does not shift at once, but in temporal phases affecting lower defense levels first, followed by mid level, then high level. All four cases demonstrated this in part, and three in full. Each case demonstrated substantial decreases in immature defenses with simultaneous increases in mid level, but not high adaptive-level defenses. Case C was atypical in that high adaptive-level defenses began to increase from intake onward. However, that case was also atypical in that the subject's therapy had been ongoing for several years prior to intake into a naturalistic study, and thus may have been in a later phase of treatment with her therapist than the other three cases in which the total therapy was observed. Cases A and C developed some or a sizable proportion of mature defenses, in the case of the latter as a result of a very long period of treatment and follow-up. Cases B and D improved shy of developing mature defenses, because the treatment in both cases appeared to terminate before completing the therapeutic tasks as reported by both therapists. This relates to the fourth hypothesis as well, regarding the role of patient factors that moderate change. Thus all four cases support the idea that defenses change in stages, but treatment to a healthy level of functioning was not carried out in all cases, which would have provided a more complete picture across the hierarchy.

*Hypothesis 3* posited that different patients or classes of patients and different treatment conditions should be associated with different rates of change in defensive functioning. Four cases can illuminate only some factors that might plausibly be related to the rate of change, or the amount of change over a given time period. Although common experience alone would support this, it remains to define and validate these moderators (i.e., patient characteristics) and mediators (e.g., type of treatment, frequency of sessions, therapeutic alliance, length of treatment, or follow-up).

Case A was characterized by a discrete short-duration depressive episode and good pre-episode personality functioning. The rise of ODF to neurotic levels was accomplished over 20 weeks, concurrent with cessation of depression. However, depressive defenses were still somewhat above healthy norms, and high adaptive-level defenses were just beginning to rise, suggesting that the rise in ODF was at least somewhat state-dependent, and further change after termination would occur at a slower rate. This was in line with the findings of Hoglend and Perry [31], who found that their depressed patients returned to a neurotic level (mean ODF = 5.11) after 6 months. Case D exemplified this more clearly. Her depression was of longer duration and there were more characterological issues, which a longer but not open-ended therapy – limited to 18 months – tried to address. This process included a period of regression in the therapy as deeply repressed issues emerged. When therapy stopped at 18 months per protocol, both patient and therapist felt still "in the middle" of the treatment. As a result, lower-level defenses decreased, neurotic-level defenses increased, but high adaptive defenses did not emerge yet. Thus the patterns of change in depression and defenses were not the same, with the characterological work producing a countertrend in defensive functioning, in the therapy itself, whereas defenses in relationship vignettes (the RAP) did appear to improve.

Both cases B and C had BPD and entered their respective studies in a regressed state. The rate of change was slow but after a period of time became quite steady, after only a year in case B. A rate of change which help-up remarkably until year 13-plus. Notably, over most of this time, she remained with the same therapist. Thus we can see differences between these two cases with PDs – both had BPD – and the two cases with discrete depressive episodes. In the latter, the early years showed unstable defensive functioning, which included periods of regression, before stable rates of change developed. In the two depressive cases, return of functioning was quicker in the presence of mild characterological issues. In case D with more characterological issues, there was improvement in the immature defenses while some regression to more neurotic levels as the deeper work proceeded. In this case, regression was much more limited in depth than in the cases with PDs.

*Hypothesis 4* posited that improvement in defensive functioning should be associated with improvement in symptoms and other aspects of functioning. All four cases followed this pattern. What remains to be determined is whether attaining healthy-neurotic levels of defensive functioning (e.g., *ODF* > 5.64) confers protection from major psychiatric conditions, such as recurrence of major depression, and disruption of generally high levels of functioning, in the face of difficult environmental stressors, such as death of a loved one and loss of a job. Future studies should examine whether individuals who have developed healthy functioning are more likely to remain so if their defensive functioning has also risen to healthy-neurotic levels.

## Some Future Directions

These four cases suggest several further related hypotheses, which include potential interactions between moderators and mediators of defensive change.

A. Episodic disorders, such as major depression, may be associated with rates of change related to the phase of the disorder. The rate of change during the depressive phase through remission may be faster than the subsequent rate of change once remission has occurred while treatment or follow-up continues.

B. Treatment length may paradoxically affect the rate of change over certain periods of time. Short-term treatments (e.g., 20 sessions or less) may be associated with a faster rate of change than is found in longer-term treatments. The faster rate of change may be due to the experience of state effects associated with starting treatment, which wash out in longer-term treatments as characterological work gradually progresses. However, further change may not occur or may occur at a slower pace (viz., point A above).

C. Some patient factors may attenuate the rate of change in both treatment and naturalistic conditions. Likely candidates include having a PD, especially BPD, high levels of Axis I comorbidity, a longer duration of illness, early age of onset, and greater number of prior episodes. As these are validated, they will have implications for the duration, and perhaps the frequency (intensity) of treatment, noted next.

D. The optimal duration of any treatment, which has a goal of improving defensive functioning, will be a function of the patient factors moderating the rate of change. For instance, case B improved markedly but clearly required additional treatment beyond the two plus years in the index therapy, truncated when the therapist had to terminate. Case C required a very long-term treatment (about 10 years, although intensity diminished over time).

E. Related to points C and D is the hypothesis that for more disturbed patients, the beginning of therapy will be followed by a period of induction. In this early phase, the patient and the therapist form an alliance and deal with repeated crises and disruptions to the work of therapy, before engaging in the more steady, fundamental characterological work. During this induction phase, there may appear to be no consistent change in defensive functioning, i.e., a negligible rate of change. Case B, who was highly motivated by the painful regressive experience in the preceding failed therapy, finished the induction phase by the second year, while case C, who was far more dysfunctional, required between 3 and 5 years to achieve a steady rate of change. Following the induction phase, when the patient is thoroughly engaged in the fundamental therapeutic tasks, the patient will develop a faster, more or less linear rate of change over a long time frame, assuming that therapy continues. Of course, each patient under optimal circumstances will still reach a ceiling – healthy-neurotic functioning – at which point the rate of change diminishes toward zero.

F. Any effective treatment should increase the rate of change in defensive functioning when compared to natural history. A related idea is that sufficient treatment may bring the patient to the point where, after termination, the rate of change continues to be positive, even though healthy-neurotic functioning was not attained by termination. This is often called a delayed treatment effect. The patient takes away the ability to continue the work of therapy on his or her own. What remains to be determined is what type of treatment is effective, at what intensity, for which class of patients, after requiring what duration of a treatment induction phase. It is plausible that all treatments including supportive, experiential, interpersonal, cognitive–behavioral, dynamic, and psychoanalysis proper may affect defensive functioning but that the rates of change may differ among them.

## Conclusion

This chapter has examined change in defensive functioning as an outcome in itself as well as in relationship to other outcomes. The issue of how to change defenses is the province of studies of the therapeutic process and has been only touched upon in passing in this chapter. That too is worthy of its own exploration, as we have discussed elsewhere [13, 34]. Ultimately, one could examine defenses in response to the therapist's interventions, with the expectation that a given level of defensive functioning would interact with certain interventions to lead to differences in outcome. This requires that both defenses and interventions intended to affect them be examined together, a step that has begun using several instruments to identify relevant therapeutic interventions [35, 36]. For example, in a study of a four-session brief psychodynamic investigation, in the initial session, a high level of therapist attunement to the level of defensive functioning leads to positive changes in the therapeutic alliance across the following three sessions [37]. A result of studies of this type should be that defenses could be examined at points in treatment as an indicator of the instantaneous effect of the therapeutic process, while they could also be summed, compared across sessions or interviews within or outside of therapy to provide an overall indicator of outcome. Defenses are a robust measure of how personality structure is functioning at any moment in time, which measured over time can reveal whether that structure is changing. Thus we can note the defenses arising in psychotherapy to attune to a patient's functioning, and we can assess defenses over time to measure structural change. This makes the study of defenses one of the most versatile psychodynamic endeavors spanning theory, research, and clinical work. Finally, this chapter described a research agenda that will further bridge process and outcome studies to advance our future understanding of how our treatments work.

**Acknowledgments** This ratings for the individual cases were supported by two grants from the Fund for Psychoanalytic Research (Cases A and D), the National Institute of Mental Health RO1-MH40423 (Case B), and The Erikson Institute of the Austen Riggs Center (Case C).

# References

1. Freud S (1894/1962). The neuro-psychoses of defence. The Complete Works of Sigmund Freud, vol. 2, Standard Edition. London, Hogarth Press, 1962.
2. Freud A (1937/1966). The Ego and the Mechanisms of Defense, Revised Edition. New York, International Universities Press, 1966.
3. Waelder R (1976). The principle of multiple function. In Guttman SA, (ed.), Psychoanalysis: Observation, Theory, Application. New York, International Universities Press. pp. 68–83.
4. Schafer R (1968). Mechanisms of defense. Int J Psychoanal 49: 49–62.
5. Hartmann H, Kris A, Lowenstein RM (1964). Essays on Ego Psychology: Selected Problems in Psychoanalytic Theory. New York, International Universities Press, Inc.
6. Haan N (1963). Proposed model of ego functioning: coping and defense mechanisms in relationship to IQ change. Psychol Monogr 77: 1–23.
7. Lazarus R, Folkman S (1984). Stress, Appraisal and Coping. New York, Springer.
8. Skinner EA, Edge K, Altman J, Sherwood H (2003). Searching for the structure of coping: a review and critique of category systems for classifying ways of coping. Psychol Bull 12: 216–269.
9. Perry JC, Ianni F (1998). Observer-rated measures of defense mechanisms. J Pers 66: 993–1024.

10. Kernberg OF (1967). Borderline personality organization. J Am Psychoanal Assoc 15: 641–685.
11. American Psychiatric Association (1994). Diagnostic and Statistical Manual of Mental Disorders, 4th Edition. Washington, D.C., American Psychiatric Press, pp. 751–757.
12. Perry JC (1993). The study of defense mechanisms and their effects. In Miller N, Luborsky L, Barber J, Docherty J, (eds.), Psychodynamic Treatment Research: A Handbook for Clinical Practice. New York, Basic Books, pp. 276–308.
13. Perry JC, Bond M (2005). Defensive functioning [in personality disorders]. In The American Psychiatric Publishing Textbook of Personality Disorders. Oldham J, Skodol AE, Bender D, (eds.), Washington, D.C., American Psychiatric Press Inc., Chapter 33, pp. 589–609.
14. Vaillant GE (1993). The Wisdom of the Ego. Cambridge, Massachusetts, Harvard University Press.
15. Freud S (1926/1959). Inhibitions, symptoms and anxiety. The Complete Works of Sigmund Freud, vol. 20, Standard Edition. London, Hogarth Press, 1959.
16. Perry JC (2001). A pilot study of defenses in psychotherapy of personality disorders entering psychotherapy. J Nerv Ment Dis 189: 651–660.
17. Perry JC, Cooper SH (1987). Empirical studies of psychological defenses, In Michels R, Cavenar JO Jr., (eds.), Psychiatry, vol. 1. Philadelphia, J.B., Lippincott, Chapter 30, pp. 1–19.
18. Vaillant GE (1976). Natural history of male psychological health: the relation of choice of ego mechanisms of defense to adult adjustment. Arch Gen Psychiatry 33, 535–545.
19. Bader M, Perry JC (2001). Mécanismes de défense et épisodes relationnels lors de deux psychothérapies brèves mère-enfant. (Eng trans. Defense mechanisms and relationship episodes among two brief mother-infant psychotherapies). Psychothérapies 21: 123–131.
20. Kernberg OF (1975). Borderline Conditions and Pathological Narcissism. New York, Jason Aronson.
21. Perry JC, Cooper SH (1986). A Preliminary report on defenses and conflicts associated with borderline personality disorder. J Am Psychoanal Assoc 34: 863–893.
22. Perry JD, Perry JC (2004). Conflicts, defenses and the stability of narcissistic personality features. Psychiatry: Interpersonal and Biological Processes 67: 310–330.
23. Bond M, Gardner ST, Christian J, Sigal JJ (1983). Empirical study of self-rated defense styles. Arch Gen Psychiatry 40: 333–338.
24. Perry JC, Cooper SH (1989). An empirical study of defense mechanisms: I. Clinical interview and life vignette ratings. Arch Gen Psychiatry 46: 444–452.
25. Skodol A, Perry JC (1993). Should an axis for defense mechanisms be included in DSM-IV? Compr Psychiatry 34: 108–119.
26. Perry JC (1990). Defense Mechanism Rating Scales (DMRS), 5th Edition. Cambridge, Massachusetts, published by author.
27. Perry JC, Hoglend P (1998). Convergent and discriminant validity of overall defensive functioning. J Nerv Ment Dis 186: 529–535.
28. Blais MA, Conboy CA, Wilcox N, Norman DK (1996). An empirical study of the DSM-IV Defensive Functioning Scale in personality disordered patients. Compr Psychiatry 37: 435–440.
29. Hilsenroth MJ, Callahan KL, Eudell EM (2003). Further reliability, convergent and discriminant validity of overall defensive functioning. J Nerv Ment Dis 191: 730–37.
30. Perry JC, Henry M (2004). Studying defense mechanisms in psychotherapy using the Defense Mechanism Rating Scales. In Hentschel U, Smith G., Draguns J, Ehlers W, (eds.), Defense Mechanisms: Theoretical, Research and Clinical Perspectives. Elsevier, Amsterdam, Chapter 9, pp. 165–192.
31. Hoglend P, Perry JC (1998). Defensive functioning predicts improvement in major depressive episodes. J Nerv Ment Dis 186(4): 1–7.
32. Waldron S, Helm F and the APS Research Group (2004). Psychodynamic features of two cognitive-behavioral and one psychodynamic treatments compared using the Analytic Process Scales. Can J Psychoanal 12(2): 346–368.

33. Beck S, Perry JC. An empirical assessment of interview structure in five types of psychiatric and psychotherapeutic interviews. Psychiatry: Journal of Biological and Interpersonal Processes (in press).
34. Perry JC (2007). Cluster C personality disorders: Avoidant, obsessive-compulsive, and dependent. In: Gabbard G.O., (ed.), Glen Gabbard's Treatment of Psychiatric Disorders, 4th Edition. American Psychiatric Press, Inc., Washington, D.C., 2007, Chapter 55, pp 835–854.
35. Milbrath C, Bond M, Cooper S, Znoj HJ, Horowitz MJ, Perry JC (1999). Sequential consequences of therapists' interventions. J Psychother Res Pract 8: 40–54.
36. Trijsburg RW, Semeniuk TT, Perry JC (2004). An empirical study of the differences in interventions between dynamic psychotherapy and cognitive-behavioral therapy for recurrent major depression. Can J Psychoanal 12: 325–345.
37. Despland J-N, Despars J, de Roten Y, Stiglar M, Perry JC (2001). Contribution of patient defense mechanisms and therapist interventions to the development of early therapeutic alliance in a Brief Psychodynamic Investigation J Psychother Pract Res 10: 155–164.

# Part II
# Empirical Measures of Psychotherapy Process

# Chapter 7
# Process Measures for Psychodynamic Psychotherapy

Caleb J. Siefert, Jared A. Defife, and Matthew R. Baity

**Abstract** Research focusing on psychodynamic psychotherapy has grown considerably in the past three decades [1]. Recently, there has been growing interest in studying the process of psychotherapy. The present chapter provides a brief review of some measures that are useful for research into psychodynamic psychotherapy. We review ten measures designed to assess the process occurring in psychotherapy. For each measure, we provide a general description of the measure's purpose, scales, and methods, and provide some examples of how the measure has been used by researchers in the past. This chapter is not intended to be comprehensive. Instead, we provide a sample of several different types of measures and measurement methods, all of which are likely to be of interest to investigators who wish to empirically study psychodynamic psychotherapy.

**Keywords** Psychodynamic psychotherapy · Process research · Process measures · Psychotherapy research · Psychotherapy process

## Process Measures

### Why Study Process?

Historically, the empirical study of psychotherapy has relied on randomized controlled clinical trials as the gold standard for evaluating the efficacy of psychotherapy. Recently, however, emphasis has shifted away from demonstrating that psychotherapy is effective and focused on uncovering those specific factors that account for its effectiveness. Researchers are now focusing on specific therapeutic factors, interventions, and patient–therapist interactions, which lead to improved outcomes in psychotherapy [2, 3]. This type of research has been referred to as process research.

C.J. Siefert
Massachusetts General Hospital and Harvard Medical School, Boston, MA
e-mail: csiefert@partners.org

R.A. Levy, J.S. Ablon (eds.), *Handbook of Evidence-Based Psychodynamic Psychotherapy*,    157
DOI: 10.1007/978-1-59745-444-5_7, © Humana Press 2009

There are a number of situations in which process measures are useful. For example, process research is seen as an important compliment to randomized controlled trials (RCT) in determining what aspects of a treatment contribute to patient outcome [4–6]. Randomized controlled trial research frequently utilizes process measures to demonstrate therapists' adherence to a particular form of treatment. However, process measures utilized to measure adherence to a specific form of psychotherapy tend to be limited in focus, assessing only those core features associated with the specific form of treatment being utilized [7]. While effective for assessing adherence to a particular treatment, such measures may be inappropriate or ineffective for studying the processes of other forms of psychotherapy (i.e., psychodynamic psychotherapy), naturalistic treatments, or for comparing process across different types of treatment [e.g., comparing the process occurring in psychodynamic treatment with the process occurring in cognitive–behavioral treatments (CBTs)].

In contrast to adherence-focused measures, a number of more general process measures that can be utilized to study psychotherapy process across *multiple* forms of treatment have been developed. In this chapter, we review a number of process measures designed to assess a wide variety of therapeutic interventions, as well as patient–therapist interactions. Though all of the measures reviewed below are appropriate for psychodynamic psychotherapy, they differ in a number of aspects. Measures differ with regard to interventions rated, methods for making ratings, training required, and the amount of time and effort required. There is no single optimal measure of psychodynamic psychotherapy process. Thus, the selection of a particular measure must be made with the goals of the researcher in mind.

### The Psychotherapy Process Q-Sort

The Psychotherapy Process Q-sort (PQS) [8] was developed by Enrico Jones and colleagues; it quantifies therapeutic process in descriptive theory-neutral terms and is particularly useful in comparing process across various forms of psychotherapy. It has previously been used to study several psychotherapies, including psychodynamic, cognitive–behavioral, interpersonal, humanistic, gestalt, and rational-emotive therapy [9–11].

The PQS contains 100 items that describe therapist actions and interventions (e.g., therapist focuses on patient's feelings of guilt), patient responses (e.g., patient does not feel understood by the therapist), session content (e.g., there is a discussion of scheduling of hours or fees), as well as therapist attitudes (e.g., therapist is distant, aloof) and patient attitudes (e.g., patient is anxious or tense). Raters rate the PQS after reviewing one *entire* psychotherapy session. As with most Q-sorts [12], items are typically printed on small cards and sorted into piles.

The PQS is scored by having external raters sort items into piles based on the items' relevance for describing the session being rated. The manual suggests that raters first sort each item into three separate piles: uncharacteristic, neutral/

irrelevant, and characteristic. Each of these piles is then further broken down into three more piles (resulting in a total of nine piles), which range from pile 1 (extremely uncharacteristic) to pile 9 (extremely characteristic). Items in the middle, pile 5, are considered neutral or unimportant for describing the session. It is important to note that items placed in pile 1 (uncharacteristic) *are not unimportant or irrelevant*, but rather are rated so because their absence is meaningful and important for describing the session. The PQS manual [8] provides item descriptions and examples for when particular items should be rated as extremely characteristic or extremely uncharacteristic. To ensure variance in the ratings, a normal distribution is enforced, which also forces raters to make multiple decisions about the placement of items, and the number of items placed in each of the nine piles differs [13]. Only five items are placed in piles 1 and 9, and the number of items per pile increases as one heads toward the middle (18 items are placed in pile 5).

Using the PQS, researchers can examine how well the process of a particular psychotherapy session adheres to a particular form of psychotherapy [e.g., psychoanalytic, cognitive–behavioral (CB), and interpersonal] by comparing it to session prototypes. Session prototypes for different types of psychotherapy were created by asking expert clinicians to rate the PQS items representing the ideal processes for their form of psychotherapy (e.g., psychodynamic and interpersonal). Expert's ratings were then subjected to Q-type factor analysis and factor scores were used to create prototypes for psychotherapy sessions of specific orientations [2, 3]. To determine the degree to which an individual session adheres to the principles of a particular theoretical orientation, the process ratings for that session can be correlated with these ideal prototypes. This allows researchers to calculate the degree of adherence to a particular therapeutic approach. Additionally, and unlike typical adherence measures, the PQS can assess the various degrees to which multiple therapeutic approaches (e.g., psychodynamic, interpersonal, and CB) are present and utilized within an individual session or series for rated sessions [4].

Reliability for the PQS has been satisfactory across several studies [2–4]. Interrater reliability for all 100 PQS items has been acceptable, with coefficient $\alpha$ between multiple raters reported as ranging from 0.83 to 0.89 [4, 13]. Reliability analyses for individual items have also obtained acceptable reliability ($\alpha$ ranging from 0.50 to 0.95) [4, 11]. The validity of the PQS has been shown through several studies demonstrating its discriminate and predictive power. The discriminant validity of the PQS has been repeatedly demonstrated by its ability to accurately differentiate various forms of psychotherapy from one another. For example, Jones and Pulos [11] used the PQS to compare the process in CBT with psychodynamic therapies, and found that though both treatments reduced symptoms, they utilized strikingly different interventions to do so. The PQS has also been used to predict patients' outcomes. For example, Ablon and Jones [13] used the PQS to study psychotherapy sessions from the National Institute of Mental Health Treatment of Depression Collaborative Research Program and found that across CBT and interpersonal psychotherapy, patient in-session characteristics were related to outcome [13]. The PQS can also be used to examine what specific aspects of treatment relate to patient outcome. This is done by examining the correlations between outcome variables and specific PQS items. For example, in a study on the naturalistic treatment of panic disorder, Ablon, et al. found that though clinicians had described themselves as psychodynamic, their sessions had incorporated a good deal of CBT process. Nonetheless, specific therapeutic interventions not necessarily associated with CBT (e.g., focus on identifying and expressing emotion and feelings) were most strongly related to improved patient outcomes [4].

## Summary

Strengths of the PQS include descriptive items, the wide number of interventions, attitudes, and interactions assessed, use of a Q-sort methodology, the inclusion of multiple psychotherapy prototypes, and its usefulness for multiple research purposes. The PQS provides detailed descriptive information on the unique aspects of a psychotherapy session regardless of therapists' theoretical orientation or therapeutic approach. Psychotherapy Process Q-sort items are also written in a descriptive form designed to require minimal inference on the part of the rater. Thus, raters with differing theoretical orientations can use the measure. It contains 100 items and, while time-intensive, allows for the *detailed* assessment of numerous interventions, attitudes, and patient and therapist interactions. It also includes various interventions from multiple therapeutic orientations (e.g., psychodynamic, CBT, and interpersonal). As such, it is appropriate for rating many different forms of psychotherapy. Its use of a Q-sort methodology and fixed distribution reduces rater biases (e.g., halo effects) and assures that raters make multiple decisions about each item. In addition, prototypes have been developed for a wide variety of psychotherapy approaches, and items are written in a theory-neutral language making the PQS a highly effective measure for comparative psychotherapy process research. The research utility of the PQS is quite broad. It can be used for a number of research purposes, including macro analyses, such as assessing therapists' adherence to a particular therapeutic approach, and micro analyses, such as determining what specific interventions are related to outcome. Researchers interested in comparing various types of treatments, treatments across different treatment providers, adherence to a particular therapeutic approach, or identifying the specific treatment aspects related to patient outcome are likely to find the PQS a highly useful and informative measure.

Despite these strengths, there are also a handful of drawbacks associated with the PQS. The PQS does require fairly intensive training, and it can take some time for raters to become familiar and proficient with all 100 items. Rating the PQS requires some expertise and familiarity with conducting psychotherapy. As such, its authors strongly recommend that raters hold at least masters-level degrees in a therapy-related field. Psychotherapy Process Q-sort ratings also involve a substantial investment of time and energy. Rating a single session requires the rater to review the entire session and then sort all 100 items. As such, the rating process typically takes between 90 and 120 min.

## The Comparative Psychotherapy Process Scale

The Comparative Psychotherapy Process Scale (CPPS) was developed by Mark Hilsenroth and colleagues [14] and is a brief measure of psychotherapy process, tapping the degree to which a therapist uses global techniques of psychodynamic–interpersonal (PI) and/or cognitive-behavioral (CB) psychotherapy. It was developed from empirical literature reviews focusing on the distinctive features of short-term PI and CB psychotherapy [15, 16]. Its items are descriptive and written to reflect between-treatment differences that are core features of CB and PI psychotherapies. Further, as its authors note, unlike measures designed to assess adherence to a manualized treatment, the focus on global and distinctive features of CB and PI psychotherapies makes the CPPS particularly useful for assessing naturalistic (nonmanual-based) forms of psychotherapy [14].

The CPPS contains two subscales (PI and CB), each of which are composed of 10 items. Items are rated on a scale of 0 (not at all characteristic) to 6 (extremely characteristic). Raters rate each item for how characteristic the item is for that particular psychotherapy session after they have watched a videotape of the entire therapy session. Psychodynamic–interpersonal and CB subscale scores on the 10 items on the subscale are summed and then divided by 10 producing an average score that can be interpreted on the 0–6 scale. Each item of the CPPS is written as a statement designed to represent a specific type of intervention (e.g., the therapist allows the patient to initiate the discussion of significant issues, events, and experiences). In addition to subscale scores, item scores represent how characteristic a specific PI or CB intervention is of the rated session.

The psychometric properties of the CPPS have been evaluated across several studies and have recently been summarized by Hilsenroth and colleagues [14]. The internal consistency of both subscales has been reported in the excellent range ($\alpha$ ranging from 0.92 to 0.94). Interrater reliability among external raters using the CPPS has also been found to be reasonably strong. For example, examination of external raters ratings of the CPPS has yielded interclass correlation coefficients (ICC) [17] in the good (0.60–0.74) to excellent ($\geq$0.75) range for the CPPS items across multiple studies [14, 18]. Further, ICCs for the PI and CB subscales have also been reported in the excellent range across studies [14, 18].

Hilsenroth and colleagues [14] have also recently summarized much of the validity data for the CPPS. The CPPS subscales have been shown to be related to similar measures of therapeutic process. Both CPPS subscales and items have been shown to distinguish between psychodynamic and other forms of psychotherapy. Similarly, when experts were asked to rate the CPPS for an imagined "ideal" CB or PI therapy session (CB experts rated an ideal CB session; PI experts rated an ideal PI session), significant differences emerged among the PI and CB subscales. Further, there was excellent internal agreement for the items on each scale. Ratings made by the actual therapist (using a version of the CPPS intended to be rated by the therapist) and supervisor (using the external rater form) have been shown to be highly correlated. Similarly, patients in psychodynamic psychotherapy, when asked to complete a patient version of the CPPS, rated the PI subscale significantly higher than the CB scale.

## Summary

The CPPS has a number of strengths, including the broad research utility of the measure, excellent psychometric properties, the brevity of the measure, and multiple versions. The CPPS can be used to broadly classify a given psychotherapy session, assess the degree to which a therapist made use of PI and/or CB techniques, examine the effects of specific PI or CB interventions [18], and compare the use of various techniques within CB or PI psychotherapies [14]. A particular benefit of the CPPS is its brevity. The measure contains only 20 items, thus requiring a very modest investment of time and energy to rate. Items are clear and distinct, which enhances the speed with which raters can become familiar and reliable with rating the CPPS. Multiple versions (therapist, patient, and external rater) of the CPPS exist, allowing researchers to examine how patient, therapist, and external-rater perspectives of psychotherapy each contribute to the prediction of patient outcome. The psychometric properties of the CPPS are well-documented [14]. Finally, as its authors have noted, it may be particularly well suited for studying and categorizing psychotherapy sessions as they occur in naturalistic treatment settings. As such, the CPPS may be particularly appealing for researchers who are looking for a brief measure for studying real-world treatments.

Since the CPPS was developed based on an empirical review of the core techniques from PI and CB psychotherapies, it focuses on interventions associated with these approaches. As such, it may be less well suited for studying other forms of psychotherapy or may fail to code for other interventions not associated with these approaches. Its items are written to capture the use of more global and distinctive PI and CB techniques. Though this may be optimal for distinguishing PI from CB treatments, it may limit researchers' ability to identify specific microprocesses that are associated with outcome.

## Coding System of Therapeutic Focus

The Coding System of Therapeutic Focus (CSTF) was developed by Goldfried et al. (Goldfried MR, Newman, CF, Hayes, AM, 1989. The coding system of therapeutic focus. Unpublished Manuscript). It was initially designed to assess psychotherapy process by using a theoretically neutral language to examine therapists' verbal interventions and focus in psychotherapy. It was intended to provide a "common metric" for conducting comparative analysis of psychotherapy process across different types of CB and PI psychotherapy [19].

The CSTF attempts to capture the focus of interventions rather than how they are made. It codes 39 areas of therapists' focus that fall within five separate categories: components of client's functioning (e.g., emotions, thoughts, and actions), intrapersonal (connecting client's thoughts and feelings) and interpersonal (e.g., connecting client's actions to another person's actions) links made by the therapist, the time frame of the focus (e.g., focus on the past or the future), people in the client's life on which the focus has been placed (e.g., parent and spouse), and general interventions (e.g., providing support or information) [19]. Each of these dimensions is further broken down into specific coding categories [20]. The unit of analysis for the CSTF is the therapist turn (everything said by the therapist after a patient's utterance). Each turn is coded separately and each category receives a code of present or absent for each turn. Patient's statements are not coded. They can, however, be used to provide contextual information for coding the therapists' turn.

The CSTF is intended to be rated by external raters [19, 20]. To code the CSTF, raters review typed transcripts of psychotherapy sessions. Early studies [21, 22] produced mixed interrater reliability ratings for the various CSTF categories when coded by individual raters. Thus, many subsequent studies using the CSTF have utilized a consensus rating method recommended by Stiles [23]. Utilizing this approach, moderate to good interrater reliabilities have been consistently achieved. For example, Goldfried and colleagues [20] reported good interrater reliability across rating categories, with the vast majority of categories achieving ICCs of 0.60 or higher (ICCs ranging from 0.54 to 0.98). Highly similar interrater reliabilities have been reported in subsequent studies [19, 24]. It should be noted that acceptable interrater reliability ratings for the CSTF have been obtained with highly trained coders. In previous studies, raters have typically been advanced graduate students who have received a relatively high degree of training (48–90 h of training) [19, 20, 24].

There are several studies verifying the discriminant and predictive validity of the CSTF [19–23]. For example, the CSTF has consistently found theoretically predicted differences among both naturalistic [19] and manual-based PI and CB psychotherapies [20]. For example, studies using the CSTF have found that PI therapists than CB therapists were more likely to focus on emotion, intrapersonal patterns, expectations of other's reactions, and more likely to emphasize the therapeutic relationship and client's relationships with their parents [20–22]. Additionally, the CSTF has been useful in predicting therapeutic outcomes on the basis of therapist interventions speaking to the measure's predictive validity [24, 25].

## Summary

The CTSF has a number of strengths including an already rich research tradition, excellent validity data, and unique coding approach enhancing its utility for studying therapeutic process across multiple forms of CB and PI therapy. It has been applied to highly controlled clinical settings [22] as well as to naturalistic settings [19]. Its strong research base allows future findings to be interpreted within the broader context of previous studies. The measure has been proven to be effective for studying various forms of CB and PI interventions, and like the PQS, codes for numerous therapeutic foci, making it an excellent measure for researchers interested in conducting comparative psychotherapy research.

Despite the many strengths of the CTSF, there are also some drawbacks. Previous research establishing the psychometric properties of the measure has provided raters with a rather large amount of training from experts who were involved in the measure's development. Further, most previous research has utilized teams of raters to achieve acceptable reliability ratings. Some investigators may not have the resources required to assemble teams of raters. The CTSF also does not code for patient's response or involvement in the session. As such, this measure cannot be used alone if a researcher wishes to study patient's reactions to treatment interventions. Finally, as some of the measure's creators have noted [26], the CSTF incorporates several variables and rates all of them for each therapist turn. As such, coding with the CSTF is quite labor-intensive. Although this may provide for a more fine-grained analysis of therapeutic process, some researchers may find the CSTF too burdensome. In response to this issue, Samoilov et al. [26] have developed the Therapeutic Focus on Action and Insight (TFAI), which provides a "more feasible alternative for coding psychotherapy process." The TFAI is discussed in further detail below.

## The Interpretive and Supportive Technique Scale

Ogrodniczuk and Piper [27] developed the Interpretive and Supportive Technique Scale (ISTS). The ISTS is a brief measure assessing therapist use and adherence to various interpretive and supportive techniques. It was developed based on a manual for supportive–expressive treatment and from a review of the relevant theoretical and clinical literature [28]. Unlike other process measures assessing supportive and interpretive interventions, the ISTS does not adhere to any one theoretical or technical approach and was developed for use across a range of psychodynamic psychotherapies.

The ISTS is composed of 14 items that are rated for *emphasis* on a 0 (no emphasis)–4 (major emphasis) scale. Seven items focus on interpretive interventions (e.g., makes links between the patient's relationship with the therapist and the patient's relationships with others) and seven items focus on interventions that are more supportive in nature (e.g., provide guidance similar to the role of a family doctor; praise the patient). The ISTS produces a full-scale score derived from all 14 items, as well as scores for 2 subscales. The interpretive subscale is calculated by summing the seven items targeting interpretive interventions, while the supportive subscale is calculated by summing the seven items focusing on supportive interventions. Scores for each scale range from 0 to 28. In addition, its authors have developed and tested a formula for assessing adherence on a bidirectional continuum. The supportive subscale score is subtracted from the interpretive subscale score. Then 28 points are added to the difference. Scores below 28 suggest a more supportive treatment, scores above 28 suggest a more interpretive treatment, scores closer to the middle may represent a treatment in which supportive and interpretive elements are present.

The items of the ISTS were written in a descriptive rather than evaluative fashion and were written at a level designed to minimize the amount of clinical expertise required to rate them. As such, it may be rated by nonclinician external raters with a Bachelors degree or higher. External raters rate the ISTS after reviewing an entire therapy session. A single session is coded at a time, raters code the session after watching the entire session, and the ISTS authors suggest that it requires roughly 1 h to score a session. Ogrodniczuk and Piper [27] provided the initial investigations into the psychometric properties of the ISTS. They found that the full scale of the ISTS has demonstrated excellent internal consistency ($\alpha$ reported as ranging from 0.86 to 0.95). Similarly, the interpretive and supportive subscales have achieved $\alpha$ coefficients ranging from 0.86 to 0.92 and 0.81 to 0.94, respectively [27, 29]. With regard to interrater reliability, ICC scores range from 0.93 to 0.97 for the full scale, 0.84 to 0.88 for the interpretive subscale, and 0.69 to 0.93 for the supportive subscale [27, 29]. The average ICC score across the individual items of the ISTS has been reported as ranging from 0.54 to 0.74 [27]

Ogrodniczuk and Piper [27] also examined the validity of the ISTS. The ISTS was shown to be related to similar measures of therapist technique in predictable ways. For example, in study 2, therapy sessions were rated using the ISTS and the Therapist Intervention Rating System (TIRS) [30]. As expected, ratings for the ISTS interpretive scale were strongly related to therapists' use of interpretations as assessed by the TIRS, and ratings of supportive interventions were associated with noninterpretive interventions assessed by the TIRS. Similarly, external rater ratings of the ISTS were strongly related to therapist's perceptions of their use of technique. The ISTS has also accurately differentiated between manual-based supportive and interpretive treatments. For example, therapy sessions that followed a manual-based interpretive treatment were rated significantly higher on the interpretive scale than sessions that followed a manual-based supportive treatment. A factor analysis of the ISTS revealed a single factor. Factor loadings were positive for all seven supportive items and negative for all seven items on the interpretive scale. These results support the measure's developmental rationale and bidirectional focus that locates interpretive interventions at one end and supportive interventions at the other.

Summary

Strengths of the ISTS include its brevity, initial psychometric data, and ease of ratings. The ISTS possesses a number of strengths including strong psychometric properties, early data speaking to the measure's validity, its brevity, and its multiple uses as a research instrument. As its authors note, the interrater reliability for the ISTS is among the highest reported for process measures, which is impressive given these ratings were obtained with undergraduate raters with a limited amount of training. This speaks to the measure's clarity and ease of use. Of course, further examination of the ISTS psychometric properties is needed to fully evaluate the measure. The ISTS may be particularly useful to researchers who wish to assess how therapists' emphasis on supportive or interpretive techniques within various psychodynamic treatments are related to outcome. The ISTS requires less time and energy to rate than many other process measures. Additionally, the clarity of the items and the measure's focus on emphasis (as opposed to effectiveness) of interventions allows it to be rated by individuals with minimal clinical experience.

Of course, as with most brief process measures, there is a trade off for the measure's brevity. First, the measure assesses a limited number of interventions, assesses more global interventions (as opposed to specific interventions), and does not include items for rating interventions associated with CBT-type treatments (though many of these may be properly coded as supportive). Of course, many of the measure's strengths, such as the speed with which raters can become proficient and reliable with the measure, is likely to be a function of the measure's focus on a smaller set of global interventions. Nonetheless, this may limit the measure's utility for researchers who wish to examine a broad range of techniques. The authors have been fairly clear in terms of their intention for developing a measure for use with psychodynamic psychotherapies. As such, the measure may be less than optimal for assessing CBT or conducting comparative research among different types of treatment (e.g., comparing sessions of psychodynamic psychotherapy to CBT). Despite these limitations, the ISTS represents an excellent young measure. Its relative ease to learn and rate may be appealing to new investigators or to investigators limited in terms of time and resources. Future research with the ISTS will be useful in ultimately determining the measure's utility as a research instrument. Finally, Ogrodniczuk and Piper's [27] initial examination of the psychometric properties of the ISTS serves as an excellent model for future investigators interested in developing and testing their own process measures.

**Vanderbilt Psychotherapy Process Scale**

The Vanderbilt Psychotherapy Process Scale (VPPS) [31, 32]) was one of the first measures designed to objectively assess the process of a psychotherapy session. Its authors set out to identify the key characteristics of the therapeutic interaction and relationship in order to predict which factors lead to a "good" hour. Not only were the developers of the VPPS among the first to examine the "active ingredients" of psychotherapy, they also pioneered a research methodology to investigate therapy process in an empirical manner [32]). Current versions of the VPPS [31, 32] have been developed through empirical studies and advancement of the original measure.

The current version of the VPPS contains 80 items rated on a 1 (not at all)–5 (great deal) scale. Three of the 80 items are designed to assess the global impression of the therapeutic relationship, productivity of the hour, and patient's emotional involvement. All items are unidimensional and are written in descriptive language [31]. Some items describe the behavior of the therapist (e.g., showed warmth and friendliness toward the patient) and some the behavior of the patients (e.g., actively participated in the interaction). In addition, ratings are made about the demeanor and feelings of the patient and the therapist. The VPPS contains eight subscales: Patient Participation; Patient Hostility; Patient Exploration; Patient Dependency; Patient Psychic Distress; Therapist Warmth and Friendliness; Negative Therapist Attitude; and Therapist Exploration [31].

Internal consistency for the VPPS has been reported in the good to excellent range ($\alpha$ reported as ranging from 0.81 to 0.96), and interrater reliability has been reported in the good to excellent range (ICCs ranging from 0.79 to 0.94) [31, 33, 34]. Similar internal consistency and interrater reliability ratings have been achieved by independent investigators in subsequent studies [35]. Although much of the research on this measure has been done in segments of taped sessions, full sessions can also be used. Adequate interrater reliability and internal consistency data exist for both procedures [32, 35]. A VPPS rating manual has also been developed to help with scoring dilemmas and to make the VPPS more attractive to outside researchers.

The validity of the VPPS has been established through studies demonstrating its ability to differentiate different types of psychotherapy. The original version of the VPPS detected differences among psychoanalytic clinicians, experientially informed clinicians, and nonclinical college advisors [36]. The predictive validity of the VPPS has also been shown through its ability, particularly the patient participation and patient hostility subscales, to predict patient-rated outcomes across multiple types of treatment [31, 36]. Similar results were reported by other research labs, which found that the external rater's ratings for the VPPS predicted therapist's rated outcome in psychodynamically informed treatment [37]. In addition to the externally rated VPPS [31], therapist-rated (VPPS-T) and patient-rated (VPPS-P) versions of the VPPS have recently been developed from data derived at a university outpatient sample [32]. Therapist and patient versions contain 45 items (42 items + 3 global assessment items) and have been shown to have adequate psychometric properties [32].

Summary

The VPPS is one of the earliest measures of therapeutic process, and it continues to be a useful measure for assessing process. Its strengths include nontheoretical items that are easy to understand, and the development of multiple versions to be rated by patients, therapists, and external raters. Previous research has shown the VPPS to have a consistent relationship with outcome based on who is providing the ratings. The fact that this finding has been generally replicated in several different data sets is promising evidence for the continued use of this measure. The inclusion of patient, therapist, and external rater forms allows for the assessment of multiple perspectives within the same study. At 45 items, these versions of the VPPS are also relatively low burden and require minimal training to complete.

**Psychodynamic Intervention Rating Scale**

The Psychodynamic Intervention Rating Scale (PIRS) was developed by Cooper and Bond (Cooper S, Bond M, 1992. Psychodynamic Intervention Rating Scale. Unpublished Manuscript) [38] and is designed to assess therapist's use of interpretative and supportive interventions in psychodynamic psychotherapy. It focuses on therapists' utterances (what the therapist actually said). It covers a smaller range of general interventions and defines them in a manner that allows them to be easily categorized. It was developed after reviewing many previous measures of psychotherapy process. Its authors sought to fill a gap in the literature by creating a categorical measure that allowed researchers of psychodynamic psychotherapy to categorize therapist interventions.

The PIRS is a categorical rating system that codes therapist statements into 10 different therapist interventions within two broad categories: supportive and interpretive. The two interpretive interventions assessed are defense interpretations and transference interpretations. The eight supportive interventions assessed are clarification, reflection, direct questioning, acknowledgements, supportive statements, work-enhancing statements, contractual arrangement, and associations [37–39]. The manual for the PIRS defines each intervention clearly and provides examples that help raters differentiate the various interventions from one another [37].

Raters rate every therapist statement, in a given therapy session, by placing it into a category. Each category then receives a session score calculated by dividing the raw count for a category by the total number of interventions made [40]. Additionally, interpretative interventions are rated for depth on a 1–5 scale, with higher scores indicating greater completeness or depth [41–43].

The interrater reliability of the PIRS has been demonstrated in several studies. Milbrath and colleagues [39] reported $\kappa$ coefficients ranging from 0.83 to 0.99 across PIRS categories. Similar $\kappa$ coefficients have been obtained by independent researchers as well [40]. Hersoug and her colleagues [44] have reported mean ICCs ranging from 0.78 to 0.79 for the interpretive interventions and ranging from 0.97 and 0.98 for supportive interventions.

The PIRS has been previously utilized to study both macroprocesses (e.g., the impact of therapist techniques across sessions on patient outcome) and microprocesses (e.g., the immediate in session impact of specific therapist interventions). For example, Milbrath and colleagues used the PIRS to examine both micro and macroprocesses in 20 randomly selected psychotherapy sessions for bereavement. Regarding microprocesses, they found that patient's elaboration of their emotions was followed by therapist's interpretations of defense, which then tended to be followed by greater emotional elaboration. They also found that therapist supportive interventions led patients to disclose more facts, rather than emotions. Regarding macroprocesses, they found that the use of both interpretive and supportive interventions was linked to symptom reduction [39]. The PIRS has also been used to link specific types of interventions with theoretically predictable outcomes. For example, Hersoug and colleagues [44] found that therapists' use of interpretive, but not supportive, techniques was linked to a reduction in the use of maladaptive defenses.

Summary

The PIRS is unique in that it is a categorical rating system specifically designed for the study of psychodynamic psychotherapy interventions. The scale was not intended to be a comparative measure and does not include items tapping interventions associated with other therapeutic approaches (e.g., CBT). However, its focus on core psychodynamic interventions may allow it to be used for comparing differing forms of psychodynamic psychotherapy (e.g., relational and interpersonal). The PIRS builds on previous measures by differentiating two forms of interpretations (transference and defense). In fact, much of the previous research conducted with this measure has sought to investigate the impact of different types of interpretations [40–44]. However, the transference interpretation category is very broadly defined and incorporates all statements made by the therapist referring to the therapeutic relationship. Further, the valence (positive or negative) of transference interpretations is not assessed [44]. Thus, some researchers are specifically interested in studying various types of transference interpretations or differentiating here and now therapist comments (e.g., sounds like you feel angry at me right now) from more interpretive comments (e.g., I think the anger you are experiencing toward me right now is related to the anger you as a child when your father was cold and unsupportive). The PIRS has been used to study both the immediate [39] and/or the aggregate impact of therapeutic interventions [44]. Early investigations with the PIRS have revealed fairly strong psychometric properties for the measure, with good to excellent interrater reliability achieved in multiple studies across multiple labs.

There are also some difficulties associated with using the PIRS. The measure places therapists' turns into one intervention category, which can be problematic at times as multiple interventions may be made in one turn. Additionally, it is not always easy to place an intervention into a single category. Further, some statistical analyses are limited by the use of a categorical rating format. In many studies, the use of interpretive and supportive interventions is expressed as a proportional score (the number of interpretive interventions divided by the total number of interventions). Across therapist differences and even within treatment differences in the number of interventions made will affect the proportional scores obtained.

## Recently Developed Measures of Therapeutic Process

### The Analytic Process Scales

Scharf and colleagues developed the Analytic Process Scales (APS; Scharf RD, Waldron S, Firestein SK, Goldberger M, Burton AM, 2004. The analytic process scales (APS) coding manual. Unpublished Manuscript). The APS is a recently developed measure designed to assess the degree of "analytic process" occurring in psychotherapy. It focuses on "well-defined features, observable at the clinical surface" (Scharf RD, Waldron S, Firestein SK, Goldberger M, Burton AM, 2004. The analytic process scales (APS) coding manual. Unpublished Manuscript). It was developed by a team of highly experienced psychoanalysts and may be of interest particularly to researchers who wish to study psychodynamic psychotherapy or psychoanalysis proper. Though the measure focuses on interventions and interactions associated with a psychodynamic process, its authors have attempted to create the measure in a manner that allows it to assess psychodynamic process across various forms of psychotherapy (e.g., psychodynamic; CBT).

The APS is composed of 36 total variables: 14 patient variables for rating the patient's communications, 4 rater variables for rating the desirability or appropriateness of particular interventions based on the patient's communications, and 18 therapist variables for rating therapist's interventions. Five patient variables tap the content of the patient's communication (e.g., to what degree does the patient speak about romantic or sexual matters?), three tap the quality of patient's productions (e.g., to what degree is the patient identifiably responding to the therapist's intervention in a potentially useful manner?), and six tap patient features (e.g., how clearly does the patient convey experiences permitting the rater to delineate his/her conflicts?). The four rater variables assess rater's suggestions for appropriate interventions, given the patient's communication (e.g., to what degree would it be desirable to encourage elaboration of this segment?). Four therapist variables tap the types of specific interventions made (e.g., to what degree does the therapist clarify in this segment?), seven variables focus on the aims of intervention (e.g., to what degree does the therapist focus on patient's conflicts?), four variables focus on the characteristics of the therapist's interventions (e.g., therapist's intervention appears to be hostile), and three variables focus on the intervention's quality (e.g., to what degree is this a good intervention?). All of the APS variables are rated on a five-point Likert scale ranging from 0 (none) to 4 (strong), with the midpoint being 2 (moderate). In an effort to improve reliability across different raters, the APS manual contains examples of fictionalized case illustrations serving as vignettes for scoring each variable at the 0, 2, and 4 levels.

Like previous measures, the APS is designed to be rated by external raters who review transcripts or tape-recorded psychotherapy sessions. The unit of analysis for the APS is both "psychotherapeutically meaningful segments" (Scharf RD, Waldron S, Firestein SK, Goldberger M, Burton AM, 2004. The analytic process scales (APS) coding manual. Unpublished Manuscript) and the entire session. Analytic Process Scale raters first rate three types of meaningful segments that occur in psychotherapy: patient segments, therapist segments, and joint segments. Patient and therapist segments refer to a period of time that begins and ends with a significant change from the speaker or large-scale changes in the psychological theme. A joint segment refers to moments in the session "when the contributions of patient and therapist are so interwoven that separating them would produce fragments with insufficient psychological meaning" (Scharf RD, Waldron S, Firestein SK, Goldberger M, Burton AM, 2004. The analytic process scales (APS) coding manual. Unpublished Manuscript). The 14 patient variables and 4 rater variables are used to assess patient segments, while 18 APS variables are applied to rate therapist segments. All 36 variables are used to rate therapist and patient contributions within joint segments, respectively.

After rating all individual segments, raters are asked to provide ratings for the entire session (referred to as whole-session scores). The authors suggest that whole-session scores should be made as if one is characterizing the session to a colleague. Thus whole-session scores should not simply be an attempt by the rater to aggregate or average segment ratings for the hour, but instead should attempt to capture the most meaningful and pivotal features of the session. As an alternative to rating both segments and the whole session, raters can simply be asked to make whole-session scores for a psychotherapy session.

Initial investigations into the reliability of the APS [45–47] suggest that the APS has adequate interrater reliability. Median alpha coefficients for the therapist variables have been reported as ranging from 0.57 to 0.71, and the median alpha coefficients for the patient variables range from 0.73 to 0.82 [45, 46]. Both highly experienced clinicians and less-experienced clinicians (e.g., psychology interns) have been able to reliably rate psychotherapy sessions using the APS [46]. Using the methods described in the APS manual, raters have also been able to reliably cut psychotherapy sessions into meaningful segments ($\kappa = 0.86$) [46]. Though these properties are promising, as proponents of the APS note [46], further research is required to evaluate the APS's properties.

Research with the APS is still in the early stages. For example, Waldron and colleagues [47] used the APS to rate psychotherapy sessions from two CBT therapists and one therapist practicing short-term psychodynamic psychotherapy (STPP) and found significantly more psychodynamic process in the STPP sessions as compared to the CBT sessions. Additionally, these authors found that the quality of the therapist's communication, as assessed by the APS, was related to patient productivity (higher quality was related to higher productivity).

Summary

The APS is a promising new measure of treatment process designed to assess the presence of analytic process within psychotherapy. It is the only measure reviewed that was developed entirely by experienced psychoanalysts (Scharf RD, Waldron S, Firestein SK, Goldberger M, Burton AM, 2004. The analytic process scales (APS) coding manual. Unpublished Manuscript). The clinical techniques assessed by the APS are strongly associated with psychodynamic treatments (e.g., clarification and interpretation). Though appealing to investigators studying psychodynamic treatments, it may also limit the measures useful in assessing other forms of psychotherapy or conducting research that makes comparisons across multiple forms of treatment. Though its authors claim that the measure can be used in psychodynamic and CBT psychotherapies and have provided some evidence for this [44, 45], the APS assesses interventions strongly associated with psychodynamic psychotherapy (e.g., clarification and interpretation) and makes no effort to tap interventions associated with other forms of treatment. Thus, it may not be optimal for comparative process research. Conversely, it may be capable of examining analytic process within other types of therapy. A unique feature of the APS is variables that attempt to assess process across sessions. Its authors suggest that the smallest number of successive session's raters need to review prior to making formal ratings with the APS is 3 or 4. For the rated session, scores can be assigned to segments of a session, the entire session, or both. When segments are rated, each variable is rated for every session segment. Although offering the potential benefit of understanding the process of a single session within a broader psychotherapy, review of multiple sessions requires a larger time commitment from raters than many other measures and is also more labor-intensive. Moreover, the option of whole-session scores may relieve some of this burden. Early investigations into the psychometrics of the measure as well as its research utility have involved a small number of cases. Investigations into the validity of the measure, while promising, are still in the early stages and need to be further investigated. It is important to note that the APS is a very new process measure. Early studies [45–47] have been promising with regard to the usefulness of the measure.

**Achievements of Therapeutic Objectives Scale**

The Achievements of Therapeutic Objectives Scale (ATOS; McCullough L, Larsen AE, Schache E, Andrews S, Kuhn N, 2003. Achievement of Therapeutic Objectives Scale: ATOS scale. Unpublished Manuscript) was developed by McCullough and colleagues in an effort to create a measure that was not focused on the therapist intervention, but instead attempts to identify therapeutic objectives and assess how the patient is adaptively responding to treatment (McCullough L, Larsen AE, Schache E, Andrews S, Kuhn N, 2003. Achievement of Therapeutic Objectives Scale: ATOS scale. Unpublished Manuscript). Unlike the previous measures discussed, the ATOS was designed to measure patient behaviors indicating assimilation of the therapeutic interventions [6]. Stated differently, the measure attempts to capture the "mini-outcomes" occurring within psychotherapy sessions. Though the measure was created for use in research focusing on short-term dynamic psychotherapy (STDP), the authors have attempted to write items in theory-neutral language that focuses on common factors across treatments. This focus on the achievement of treatment-specific objectives (as opposed to a theoretically defined idea of optimal outcome) allows the measures to be used across many types of psychotherapy. In fact, the manual contains examples of how items are scored for both CBT and STDP treatments and a model for how the ATOS can be applied to additional treatments. In this chapter, we discuss the ATOS as it applies to STDP.

The ATOS contains seven subscales tapping STDP objectives: recognition of defensive behavior (Insight), desire to change maladaptive behaviors/defenses (Motivation), physical experience of conflicted feelings (Exposure), the capacity to express feelings adaptively (New Learning), regulation of negative emotions (i.e., anxiety, guilt, shame, or pain) in session (Degree of Inhibition), improvement in sense of self, and improvement in relations with others. Raters also select the predominant affect focus for each 10-min segment. To score the ATOS, external raters review videotapes (audiotapes or transcripts may also be used, but the authors *strongly* suggest the use of videotape). Consistent with its focus on microoutcomes, raters rate 10-min segments of the session at a time. For each 10-min segment, each objective is rated on a 0 (least adaptive)–100 (most adaptive) scale. Specific anchors for the 0–100 scale are provided in the manual for each objective. The manual notes that objectives should not be rated unless there is "clear and unambiguous behavioral data" from which to make the rating. Raters are asked to jot down a descriptive behavioral example (e.g., quoting the patient or highlighting a nonverbal behavior, such as crying) as a rationale for their rating. When there is no such data for an objective, a rating of "No Data" is given. The authors have suggested that it takes *at least* 8–12 h of training to become reliable on the measure, but more strongly suggest that 20–30 h are optimal [6].

The reliability of the ATOS has been systematically examined in a series of five studies across three research labs used to enhance the reliability of the measure [6]. The first four scales of the current version of the ATOS have produced moderate to excellent interrater reliability for individual raters (ICCs ranging from 0.66 to 0.84) from McCullough's lab, and fair to moderate interrater reliability for group ratings (ICCs ranging from 0.43 to 0.77 across groups). Ratings of segment's affect focus using the ATOS achieved perfect reliability across two studies in McCullough's lab ($\kappa = 1.00$). In a subsequent follow-up study, using raters from an alternative lab in Italy, the first four ATOS scales demonstrated moderate interrated reliability (ICCs ranging from 0.61 to 0.78) for individual raters, and agreement for a segment's affect focus was excellent ($\kappa = 0.74$).

## Summary

The ATOS is a promising new measure that has been under development and investigated by McCullough and her colleagues for over 10 years. It is highly unique in its focus of the immediate assimilations by the patient of the objectives of psychotherapy within a session. Its use of segments allows researchers to examine how therapist techniques, patient–therapist interactions, and the content of patient utterances impact patient's subsequent behavior in relation to the objectives of therapy within the same session.

A clear strength of the ATOS is consistency with which McCullough and her colleagues have used empirical data to improve the measure. For example, the decision to code 10-min segments as opposed to 50-min sessions was decided on the basis of an early study, demonstrating "too much variation within the 50-min period" [6]. Similarly, McCullough and her colleagues are currently conducting research to systematically establish the number of hours required to become proficient with the measure.

The ATOS does demand a small time commitment in terms of training. However, it also boasts a web-based interactive training program that has been previously demonstrated as reasonably effective for training new raters [6]. Due to the relative newness of the measure, there are very few studies that have utilized the measure thus far. Additionally, more information regarding the validity of the measure is needed before the research utility of the ATOS can be fully appreciated [6]. For now, it remains an exciting and promising new measure for examining microprocesses within psychotherapy sessions.

## Therapeutic Focus on Action and Insight

The TFAI [26] is a recently developed measure of therapeutic process. It was developed to be a shorter and less labor-intensive measure based on the CSTF (Goldfried MR, Newman CF, Hayes AM, 1989. The coding system of therapeutic focus. Unpublished Manuscript). The TFAI was developed from an exploratory factor analysis of CSTF-coded archival data for PI and CB sessions of "high clinical impact" [26].

The TFAI contains 12 coding categories tapping the two factors: Construction of Meaning and Facilitating Action. It also differs from the CSTF in that it is designed to be used with audiotapes and written in a language that would allow less-experienced raters (e.g., undergraduate students) to reliably code the measure. The initial investigation into the TFAI's reliability produced excellent interrater reliability across two undergraduate raters (ICCs of 0.94 for the Construction of Meaning factor and 0.88 for the Facilitating Action factor). Therapeutic Focus on Action and Insight ratings also had high correlations with the CSTF and differentiated CB from PI psychotherapy.

Summary

Though this measure is new and still in the early phase of investigation, it does possess some notable strengths. The initial investigation into the measure's psychometric properties is promising. Further, these properties were achieved with the use of audiotapes and undergraduate student raters. Although much less laborious than the CSTF, it maintains a similar focus and approach. Thus, future findings using the TFAI may be compared to previous findings from research involving the CSTF. Surprisingly, we were unable to find additional subsequent studies that have utilized the TFAI. This is unfortunate, given many of the measure's strengths identified in its initial development. As such, the reliability, validity, and research utility of the TFAI need to be further examined by future researchers before its usefulness can be determined.

## Conclusion

The empirical study of psychodynamic psychotherapy represents one of the most exciting advances within the field of psychology. Although empirical research may never be able to perfectly capture the full spectrum of what occurs in psychotherapy, there is little doubt that it will continue to lend itself to the refinement of theory and practice. Further, as paradigms, technology, methods, and measures improve, we no doubt will continue to experience a growth in our understanding of the changes that occur as a result of psychotherapy, as well as the mechanisms that bring those changes about. The advances in methods and measures used to study psychotherapy process represent one such advance that will no doubt advance our knowledge.

Though the study of psychodynamic process is in and of itself interesting, it is essential that process be studied in relation to various outcomes. Traditional clinical research has focused on the reduction of symptoms as the primary method for assessing treatment response [48]. There is little question that effective treatment involves the reduction of symptoms. However, a growing number of theorists, clinicians, and researchers have suggested that the benefits of psychodynamic psychotherapies are likely to go beyond symptom reduction. Further, since the focus and goals of psychodynamic treatments may differ substantially from other forms of treatment, research into treatment outcomes may need to include measures specifically tailored to tap constructs closely related to the goals of psychodynamic psychotherapy in addition to traditional symptom measures [48, 49]. The inclusion of outcome measures suitable for studying change processes in psychodynamic psychotherapy was unfortunately beyond the scope of this chapter. Fortunately, reviews of such measures have previously been written [48–51].

In this chapter, we have attempted to provide researchers, particularly those who may be new to psychotherapy research, with an introduction to some of the exciting measures and methods developed for the study of the process of psychotherapy. We regret is that we are limited with regard to the number of measures we could include in this chapter, as well as the amount of information we could include pertaining to each measure's history, development, use in previous research, and potential use for future research. Some process measures were not included because substantial reviews of their use and psychometric properties already exist [30, 52, 53]. Nonetheless, we hope the chapter provides new researchers with an introduction to a wide variety of measures designed to assess what actually happens between therapist and patient in psychotherapy. Further, we hope that investigators will incorporate measures of therapeutic process into their future research. Such research will no doubt contribute to the growing understanding of the various factors within psychotherapies that account for their effectiveness.

# References

1. Fonagy P, Kächele HH, Krause R, Jones E, Perron R. IPA: An open door Review of Outcome Studies in Psychoanalysis. London: University College London (1999).
2. Ablon JS, Jones EE. How expert clinicians' prototypes of an ideal treatment correlate with outcome in psychodynamic and cognitive–behavioral therapy. Psychother Res 1998;8:71–83.
3. Ablon JS, Jones EE. Validity of controlled clinical trials of psychotherapy: Findings from the NIMH treatment of depression collaborative research program. Am J Psychiatry 2002;159:775–783.
4. Ablon JS, Levy RA, Katzenstein T. Beyond brand names of psychotherapy: Identifying empirically supported change processes. Psychotherapy: Theory, Research, Practice, Training 2006;43:216–231.
5. Garfield SL. Some comments on empirically supported treatments. J Consult Clin Psychol 1998;66:121–125.
6. McCullough L, Kuhn N, Andrews S, Valen J, Hatch D, Osimo F. The reliability of the achievement of therapeutic objectives scale. (ATOS): A research and teaching tool for psychotherapy. J Brief Therapy 2004; 2, 2–18.
7. Waltz J, Addis ME, Koerner K, Jacobson N. Testing the integrity of a psychotherapy protocol: Assessment of adherence and competence. J Consult Clin Psychol 1993;61:620–630.
8. Jones EE. Therapeutic action: A guide to psychoanalytic therapy. Northvale, NJ: Jason Aronson, 2000:316–361.
9. Coombs MM, Coleman D, Jones EE. Working with feelings: The importance of emotion in both cognitive–behavioral and interpersonal therapy in the NIMH treatment of depression collaborative research program. Psychotherapy: Theory, Research, Practice, Training 2002;39:233–244.
10. Jones EE, Cumming JD, Horowitz MJ. Another look at the nonspecific hypothesis of therapeutic effectiveness. J Consult Clin Psychol 1988;56:48–55.
11. Jones EE, Pulos SM. Comparing the process in psychodynamic and cognitive – behavioral therapies. J Consult Clin Psychol 1993;61:306–316.
12. Block J. The Q-sort method in personality assessment and psychiatric research. Springfield, IL: Charles C Thomas, 1961.
13. Ablon JS, Jones EE. Psychotherapy process in the NIMH Collaborative Research Program. J Consult Clin Psychol 1999;67:64–75.

14. Hilsenroth MJ, Blagys MD, Ackerman SJ, Bonge DR, Blais MA. Measuring psychodynamic-interpersonal and cognitive–behavioral techniques: Development of the comparative psychotherapy process scale. Psychotherapy: Theory, Research, Practice, Training 2005;42:340–356.
15. Blagys MD, Hilsenroth MJ. Distinctive features of short-term psychodynamic-interpersonal psychotherapy: A review of the comparative psychotherapy process literature. Clin Psychol Sci Pract 2000;7:167–188.
16. Blagys MD, Hilsenroth, MJ. Distinctive features of short-term cognitive–behavioral psychotherapy: A review of the comparative psychotherapy process literature. Clin Psychol Rev 2002;22:671–706.
17. Shrout PE, Fleiss JL. Intraclass correlations: Uses in assessing rater reliability. Psychol Bull 1979;86:420–428.
18. Siefert CJ, Hilsenroth MJ, Weinberger J, Blagys MD, Ackerman SJ. The Relationship of patient defensive functioning and alliance with therapist technique during short-term psychodynamic psychotherapy. Clin Psychol Psychother 2006;13:20–33.
19. Goldfried MR, Raue PJ, Castonguay LG. The therapeutic focus in significant sessions of master therapists: A comparison of cognitive–behavioral and psychodynamic interpersonal interventions. J Consult Clin Psychol 1998;66:803–810.
20. Goldfried MR, Castonguay LG, Hayes, AM, Drozd, JF, Shapiro, DA. A comparative analysis of the therapeutic focus in cognitive–behavioral and psychodynamic-interpersonal sessions. J Consult Clin Psychol 1997;65:740–748.
21. Goldsamt LA, Goldfried MR, Hayes AM, Kerr S. Beck, Meichenbaum, and Strupp: A comparison of three therapies on the dimension of therapist feedback. Psychotherapy, 1992;29:167–176.
22. Kerr S, Goldfried MR, Hayes AM, Castonguay LG, Goldsamt L. Interpersonal and intrapersonal focus in cognitive – behavioral and psychodynamic – interpersonal therapies: A preliminary analysis of the Sheffield Project. Psychother Res 1992;2:266–276.
23. Stiles WB, Development of a taxonomy of verbal response modes. In Greenberg LS & Pinsof WM (eds.) The Psychotherapy Process: A Research Handbook, New York: Guilford Press, 1986: 161–199.
24. Castonguay LG, Goldfried MR, Wiser S, Raue PJ, Hayes AM. Predicting the effect of cognitive therapy for depression: A study of unique and common factors. J Consult Clin Psychol 1996;64:497–504.
25. Hayes AM, Castonguay LG, Goldfried MR. Effectiveness of targeting the vulnerability factors of depression in cognitive therapy. J Consult Clin Psychol 1996;64:623–627.
26. Samoilov A, Goldfried MR, Shapiro DA. Coding system of therapeutic focus on action and insight. J Consult Clin Psychol 2000;68:513–514.
27. Ogrodniczuk JS, Piper WE. Measuring therapist technique in psychodynamic psychotherapies. J Psychother Pract Res 1999;8:142–154.
28. Piper WE, Joyce AS, McCallum M, Azim HF, Ogrodniczuk JS. Interpretive and supportive psychotherapies: Matching therapy and patient personality. Washington, DC: American Psychological Association, 2002.
29. Piper WE, McCallum M, Joyce AS, Rosie JS, Ogrodniczuk JS. Patient personality and time-limited group psychotherapy for complicated grief. Int J Group Psychother 2001;51:525–552.
30. Piper WE, Debbane EG, de Carufel FL et al. A system for differentiating therapist interpretations and other interventions. Bull Menninger Clin 1987;51:532–550.
31. O'Malley SS, Suh CS, Strupp, HH. The Vanderbilt Psychotherapy Process Scale: A report on the scale development and a process-outcome study. J Consult Clin Psychol 1983;51:581–586.
32. Smith SR, Hilsenroth MJ, Baity MR, Knowles ES. Assessment of patient and therapist perspectives on process: A revision of the Vanderbilt psychotherapy process scale. Am J Psychother 2003;57:195–205.

33. Suh CS, O'Malley SS, Strupp HH. The Vanderbilt Psychotherapy Process Scale (VPPS). J Cogn Psychother 1989;3:123–154.
34. Piper WE, Ogrodniczuk JS, Joyce AS, McCallum M, Rosie JS, O'Kelly JG, Steinberg PI. Prediction of dropping out in time-limited interpretive individual psychotherapy. Psychotherapy 1999;36:114–122.
35. Smith MF, Tobin SS, Toseland RW. Therapeutic processes in professional vs. peer counseling, adult daughter or daughter-in-law caregivers of frail elderly. Soc Work 1992;37:345–351.
36. Gomes-Schwartz B. Effective ingredients in psychotherapy: Prediction of outcome from process variables. J Consult Clin Psychol, 1978;46:1023–1035.
37. Windholz MJ, Silberschatz G. Vanderbilt Psychotherapy Process Scale: A replication with adult outpatients. J Consult Clin Psychol 1988;56:56–60.
38. Bond M, Bannon E, Grenier, M. Differential effects of interventions on the therapeutic alliance with patients with personality disorders. J Psychother Pract Res 1998;7:301–318.
39. Milbrath C, Bond M, Cooper S, Znoj H, Horowitz MJ, Perry JC. Sequential consequences of therapist interventions. J Psychother Pract Res 1999;8:40–54.
40. Despland JN, de Roten Y, Despars J, Stigler M, Perry JC. Contribution of patient defense mechanisms and therapists interventions to the development of early therapeutic alliance in brief psychodynamic psychotherapy. J Psychother Pract Res 2001;10:155–164.
41. Banon E, Evan-Grenier M, Bond M. Early transference interventions with male patients in psychotherapy. J Psychother Pract Res 2001;10:79–92.
42. Hersoug AG, Bogwald KP, Hoglend P. Are patient and therapist characteristics associated with the use of defence interpretation in brief dynamic psychotherapy? Clin Psychol Psychother 2003;10:209–219.
43. Hersoug AG, Hoglend P, Bogwald KP. Is there an optimal adjustment of interpretation to patient's level of functioning. Am J Psychother 2004;58:349–361.
44. Hersoug AG, Bogwald KP, Hoglend P. Changes of defensive functioning: Does interpretation contribute to change. Clin Psychol Psychother 2005;12:288–296.
45. Waldron S, Helm FL. Psychodynamic features of two cognitive–behavioural and one psychodynamic treatment compared using the analytic process scales. Can J Psychoanal 2004;12:346–368.
46. Waldron S, Scharf R, Crouse J, Firestein SK, Burton A, Hurst D. Saying the right thing at the right time: A view through the lens of the analytic process scales (APS). Psychoanalytic Q 2004;74:1079–1125.
47. Waldron S, Scharf R, Hurst D, Firestein SK, Burton A. What happens in psychoanalysis: A view through the lens of the Analytic Process Scales (APS). Int J Psychoanal 2004;85:443–466.
48. Blatt SJ, Auerbach JS. Psychodynamic measures of therapeutic change. Psychoanal Inq 2003; 23:268–307.
49. Wallerstein RS. Assessment of structural change in psychoanalytic therapy and research. J Am Psychoanal Assoc 1988;36:241–261.
50. Crits-Christoph P, Gladis M, Connoley MB. Outcome Measurement in Patient's Receiving Psychosocial Treatments. In IsHak WW, Burt T, Sederer LI. (eds.) Outcome measurement in psychiatry: A critical review. Washington, DC: American Psychiatric Publishing, 2002:121–138.
51. McCullough L. Standard and Individualized Psychotherapy Outcome Measures: A Core Battery. In Miller N, Luborsky L, Barber JP, Docherty JP, (eds.) Psychodynamic treatment research: A handbook for clinical practice. New York: Basic Books, 1993:469–496.
52. Hill CE, Nutt EA, Jackson S. Trends in psychotherapy process research: Samples, measures, researchers, and classic publications. J Couns Psychol 1994;41:364–377.
53. Hill CE. An overview of four measures developed to test the hill process model: Therapists intentions, therapist response modes, client reactions, and clients behaviors. J Couns Dev 1992;70:728–739.

# Chapter 8
# Countertransference and Personality Pathology: Development and Clinical Application of the Countertransference Questionnaire

Ephi J. Betan and Drew Westen

*Mario, an accountant in his early 30s, came to therapy angry and ready to challenge the parameters of treatment (i.e., time, fees, and interventions). He displayed barely concealed disdain toward his therapist and therapy despite a desperate plea for help. He was isolated, new to the city with few attachments to tether him to the world. He was in conflict with his supervisor and coworkers after only a few months at his new job. He was intensely suspicious – of authority figures, of peers, of family, of strangers, of everyone with whom he came in contact. He was terrified of his internal experience of ever-impending annihilation of self. Seeking help was necessary to contain his terror, yet stimulated his expectation of intrusion and damage.*

*From the start, he criticized his therapist's therapeutic style, choice of words, and efforts to explore his reactions. Most times the therapist ventured to speak, her words triggered the patient's angry outbursts. He demanded the therapist repeat verbatim the words he wanted to hear, and it seemed he could not tolerate anything but perfect and absolute mirroring. Paraphrasing, using synonyms, pointing out the controlling quality of his demands brought an onslaught of criticism of the therapist's personhood with accusations that the therapist was inhuman, disingenuous, and even nonhuman. The patient's efforts to dehumanize and annihilate the therapist intensified during periods of consistent attendance. Normally, however, the patient arrived 30 min late if he arrived at all.*

*Interpretations of Mario's need to control the interaction and fears of differ-ence, along with attempts to articulate the therapist's understanding of the links between Mario's early experiences and presentation in the treatment, sometimes seemed to quiet his anger and promote collaboration. However, at other times, he experienced these interventions as the therapist's withdrawal and abandonment, intensifying his anxiety and rage.*

*In the face of ongoing interpersonal assaults, it became increasingly difficult for the therapist to think her own thoughts. She felt stilted and stifled, as well as angry in response to what she experienced as Mario's effort to control her. At each*

---

E.J. Betan
Clinical Psychology Program at Argosy University/Atlanta,
e-mail: ebetan@argosy.edu

R.A. Levy, J.S. Ablon (eds.), *Handbook of Evidence-Based Psychodynamic Psychotherapy*,     179
DOI: 10.1007/978-1-59745-444-5_8, © Humana Press 2009

*appointment, waiting to see if Mario would arrive, the therapist hoped he would miss, dreaded that he would attend, and worried about his well-being.*

## Countertransference

Freud first introduced the concept of *countertransference* in 1910 [1], in his address to the Nuremberg Psychoanalytic Congress, noting that the patient's influence on the analyst's unconscious feelings can interfere with analytic treatment. His view of countertransference was similar to that of transference in that he considered the analyst's reactions reflected neurotic distortions from the past. Freud elaborated relatively little on countertransference, maintaining that the analyst must begin with a self analysis, and "anyone who cannot succeed in this self analysis...[is] unable to treat neurotics by analysis" (p. 145). This early, narrow view of countertransference as an impediment to treatment rendered the analyst's responses as shameful and inappropriate, if not pathological, and stymied open discussions.

Over time, however, writers broadened the concept of countertransference, recognizing that the analyst's reactions to the patient may have diagnostic and therapeutic relevance and facilitate treatment [2–6]. Paula Heimann was among the earliest to refer to countertransference as all of the feelings an analyst experiences toward a patient, generally labeled as the totalistic approach. She suggested that "the analyst's immediate emotional response to his patient is a significant pointer to the patient's unconscious processes and guides him towards fuller understanding" (p. 83). In this, she held that the analyst's countertransference is a product of the analytic relationship, and it is "the patient's *creation,* it is part of the patient's personality" (p. 83). Winnicott also highlighted useful aspects of countertransference and differentiated an "objective countertransference," suggesting that at times, a therapist's response may be a natural reaction to the patient's personality or extreme behaviors.

In introducing the concept of *projective identification,* Klein [7] opened the door for viewing the analyst's responses as a reflection of the patient's efforts to evoke feelings in the therapist that either the patient cannot tolerate [8] or correspond with the patient's internal object relations [9, 10]. In a similar way, Racker [4] distinguished between *concordant* and *complementary* identifications by the analyst, whereby the analyst experiences the central emotions a patient is feeling or the analyst identifies with the internal objects of the patient, respectively. From a contemporary Freudian perspective, Sandler [11] introduced the notion of *role responsiveness,* in which the analyst acts in a manner congruent with an internalized relationship paradigm the patient unconsciously seeks to recreate. Earlier, Sandler et al. [5] noted that countertransference could be best understood as the analyst's specific emotional reactions aroused by specific patient qualities. Wachtel [12, 13] proposed the similar concept of *cyclical psychodynamics,* by which patients, driven by their fears, wishes, expectations, and behaviors, often create self-fulfilling prophecies in interpersonal relations.

Despite growing appreciation of countertransference as a clinically meaningful experience that could shed light on the dynamics of the patient and the treatment, empirical studies of countertransference are limited [14–18]. Recent research using largely nonclinical samples provides indirect support for countertransference as a response to what the patient evokes, demonstrating that depressed people tend to engage in interpersonal behaviors that elicit rejection and criticism from significant others that matches their own self-criticism [19–24] and that people who are rejection-sensitive tend (through needy, angry, and otherwise distancing behavior) to elicit rejection and hence to confirm and reinforce their internal working models of relationships [25]. Swann and colleagues [26] have demonstrated that some of these processes occur in clinical settings as well.

In research specific to countertransference, a series of analogue studies have defined countertransference as the therapist's reactions to a patient that are based solely on the therapist's unresolved conflict and as a result, have operationalized countertransference in terms of a therapist's avoidant behaviors (i.e., disapproval, silence, ignoring, mislabeling, and changing the topic) [27–32]. These studies focus on negative countertransference and are limited to what countertransference tells us about the therapists. Furthermore, the studies do not investigate the specific internal emotional responses or thoughts associated with countertransference reactions.

This chapter reports on the factor structure and reliability of the Countertransference Questionnaire [33] designed to assess the range of cognitive, affective, and behavioral responses therapists have to their patients. To our best knowledge, this is the only broad measure of countertransference with ecological validity in its application to directly studying clinicians' countertransference reactions in treating patients. Although Najavits and colleagues [34] developed the Ratings of Emotional Attitudes to Clients by Treaters scale (REACT), a clinically subtle measure of countertransference, it is restricted primarily to the study of therapist responses to patients in treatment for substance abuse.

The Countertransference Questionnaire is an empirically valid and reliable measure of countertransference responses that can be applied to a range of diagnostic and clinical populations [33]. We were especially interested in studying the relationship between patients' personality pathology and countertransference reactions in order to test clinically derived hypotheses that have never been put to empirical investigation. In addition, to illustrate the potential clinical and empirical uses of the instrument, we will report on prototypes of the "average expectable" countertransference responses to patients with a personality disorder. Delineating the specific content and domains of countertransference may help therapists understand and anticipate their reactions toward patients, as well as further clarify how countertransference influences clinical work and can have diagnostic value.

## Our Data Source: A Practice Research Network Approach

Using a practice network approach, we solicited data from randomly selected, experienced (at least 3 years of post-licensure or post-residency experience and at least 10 hours per week of direct patient care) psychiatrists and psychologists from the membership registers of the American Psychiatric and American Psychological Associations. Each participant provided data on a randomly selected patient from his or her caseload. With this approach, clinically experienced observers, skilled in clinical inference and diagnosis, use standardized instruments to provide data on a large, representative sample of patients seeking treatment. Although this approach avoids problems traditionally associated with extensive clinical inference [35–40], the most important objection is the possibility of bias in clinical judgment [41]. However, recent research suggests that clinicians can in fact make highly reliable and valid judgments if their observations and inferences are quantified using psychometric instruments [42–47].

Our clinician sample included 78% psychologists and 22% psychiatrists, and 58.6% were male. The majority saw patients in private practice (80.1%) but also worked in other settings, including hospital (31.5%), forensic (8.3%), clinic (7.7%), or school (5%) settings. As might be expected, psychiatrists were more likely to have primary or secondary employment in hospital settings. Clinicians identified their theoretical orientations most commonly as psychodynamic (40.3%), eclectic (30.4%), and cognitive–behavioral (20.4%).

Clinicians could participate either by pen-and-paper or on an interactive website (www.psychsystems.net). Web vs. paper participants did not differ on any variable studied here (e.g., countertransference factor scores; eight $t$-tests). Clinicians received a modest honorarium ($85) for a procedure that took 3–4 h to complete, with a response rate of approximately 10%. Psychologists responded at a substantially higher rate than psychiatrists to the solicitation, allowing us to assess for biases imposed by differential training or response rates. Despite a roughly 3:1 difference in response rate, we found no differences between patients described by psychologists and psychiatrists significant at $p < 0.01$ on any variable of interest (age, sex, race, socioeconomic status, education level, treatment length, or countertransference factor scores; 14 $t$-tests).

In addition to the Countertransference Questionnaire, described in detail below, participating clinicians completed a number of measures in standardized sequence. For the present study, we used The Clinical Data Form (CDF) [28, 29] to assess demographic, diagnostic, and etiological variables, including the clinicians' basic demographic data (sex, years of experience, discipline, theoretical orientation, and employment site) and the patient's data (age, sex, race, education level, socioeconomic status, and Axis I diagnoses). Clinicians also completed ratings of the patient's adaptive functioning, developmental history, and family history. To assess Axis II disorders, clinicians rated each criterion of each of the DSM-IV Axis II diagnoses, randomly ordered, as present or absent.

To obtain a cross section of psychotherapy patients seen in clinical practice and to increase external validity, we asked clinicians to select the last patient they saw during the prior week who met study criteria. The criteria included a nonpsychotic patient at least 18 years old in treatment for a minimum of eight sessions (to maximize the likelihood that they would know the patient well enough to provide a reasonably accurate description of the patient). Each clinician described only one patient in order to minimize rater-dependent biases. Clinicians provided no identifying information about the patient (such as name, initials, or social security numbers), and we instructed them to use only information already available to them from their contacts with the patient so that data collection would not compromise patient's confidentiality or interfere in any way with ongoing clinical work.

In accord with our efforts to obtain a sample stratified by sex, patients were half male and half female, with an average age of 40.5 years (SD 13.4). The sample was 93% Caucasian. Most were middle class (56.4%), with 2.8% rated as poor, 24.3% as working class, and 16.6% as upper class. The mean GAF score was 58.0 (SD 12.9). Length of treatment averaged 19 months (SD 30.0) with a median of 13 months, indicating that the clinicians knew the patients very well. The most common diagnoses reported by clinicians were major depressive disorder (49%), dysthymic disorder (37.7%), generalized anxiety disorder (25.6%), and adjustment disorder (24.7%).

## The Countertransference Questionnaire: Development and Factor Structure

The Countertransference Questionnaire (Zittel C, Westen D, 2003, The countertransference questionnaire. Unpublished manual) (download at http://www.psychsystems.net/lab) is a normed, psychometrically valid clinical-report instrument that assesses countertransference patterns in psychotherapy for both clinical and research purposes. The 79 items measure a wide range of thoughts, feelings, and behaviors expressed by therapists toward their patients. We generated the items based on a review of the clinical, theoretical, and empirical literature on countertransference and related variables, and several experienced clinicians reviewed the initial item set for comprehensiveness and clarity. To ensure that clinicians of any theoretical orientation could use the instrument, we wrote the items in everyday language, without jargon. Items assess a range of responses, from relatively specific feelings (e.g., "I feel bored in sessions with him/her") to complex constructs such as "projective identification" (e.g., "More than with most patients, I feel like I've been pulled into things that I didn't realize until after the session was over").

### Factor Structure

Based on results of a principal components analysis using Kaiser's criteria and the screen plot, we ran factor analyses with 7, 8, and 9 factors to maximize interpretability using several estimation procedures. We used the most coherent solution, the eight-factor Promax (oblique) solution using maximum likelihood estimation. This solution accounted for 69% of the variance and included factors well marked by at least five items each, suggesting a stable factor structure unlikely to be substantially affected by sample size [48]. To create the factor-based scores, we included items loading $\geq 0.50$ for factors 1 and 2, $>0.40$ for factor 3, and $\geq 0.375$ for factors 4–8 to maximize reliability (coefficient $\alpha$). Intercorrelations among the eight factors ranged from $-0.16$ to $0.58$, with a median of $0.30$.

It should be noted that we ruled out theoretical bias as an alternative explanation for the conceptual coherence and clinical relevance of the factor structure. Eliminating the clinicians who espoused a psychodynamic orientation (40% of the sample), we conducted a second factor analysis (remaining $N = 108$) using the same rotation and estimation procedures. The results reproduced the same factor structure, except that the factors appeared in a slightly different order. This outcome suggests that the coherence of the factor structure is not bound to psychodynamic theoretical beliefs of participating clinicians.

## A Portrait of Countertransference: Eight Dimensions

The factor analysis generated eight distinct factors (33, p. 893). The items and highest factor loadings are provided following brief descriptions of each factor. As typically occurs in factor analytic studies, a substantial number of items [25] that did not load strongly on any single factor are not listed here. Whether we delete or rework those items in the future will depend on (a) replication of the factor structure in a second sample using confirmatory factor analysis, and (b) whether those items prove useful in composite portraits of different disorders (see below).

**Factor 1, Overwhelmed/Disorganized** (coefficient alpha = .90), involves a desire to avoid or flee the patient and strong negative feelings including dread, repulsion, fand resentment.

| | |
|---|---|
| I feel resentful working with him/her | .72 |
| I wish I had never taken him/her on as a patient | .71 |
| When checking phone messages, I feel anxiety or dread that there will be one from him/her | .69 |
| S/he frightens me | .67 |
| I feel used or manipulated by him/her | .62 |
| I return his/her phone calls less promptly than I do with my other patients | .61 |
| I call him/her between sessions more than my other patients | .60 |
| I think or fantasize about ending the treatment | .59 |
| I feel mistreated or abused by him/her | .55 |
| I feel pushed to set very firm limits with him/her | .54 |
| I feel angry at him/her | .52 |
| I feel repulsed by him/her | .50 |

**Factor 2, Helpless/Inadequate** (coefficient alpha = .88), was marked by items capturing feelings of inadequacy, incompetence, hopelessness, and anxiety.

| | |
|---|---|
| I feel I am failing to help him/her or I worry that I won't be able to help him/her | .84 |
| I feel incompetent or inadequate working with him/her | .80 |
| I feel hopeless working with him/her | .78 |
| I think s/he might do better with another therapist or in a different kind of therapy | .67 |
| I feel overwhelmed by his/her needs | .62 |
| I feel less successful helping him/her than other patients | .62 |
| I feel anxious working with him/her | .61 |
| I feel confused in sessions with him/her | .52 |

**Factor 3, Positive (coefficient alpha = .86),** characterizes the experience of a positive working alliance and close connection with the patient.

| | |
|---|---|
| I look forward to sessions with him/her | .69 |
| S/he is one of my favorite patients | .67 |
| I like him/her very much | .67 |
| I find it exciting working with him/her | .58 |
| I am very hopeful about the gains s/he is making or will likely make in treatment | .52 |
| I have trouble relating to the feelings s/he expresses | −.48 |
| If s/he were not my patient, I could imagine being friends with him/her | .44 |
| I feel like I understand him/her | .43 |
| I feel pleased or satisfied after sessions with him/her | .43 |

**Factor 4, Special/Overinvolved** (coefficient alpha = .75), indicates a sense of the patient as special relative to other patients, and "soft signs" of problems maintaining boundaries, including self-disclosure, ending sessions on time, and feeling guilty, responsible, or overly concerned about the patient.

| | |
|---|---|
| I disclose my feelings with him/her more than with other patients | .64 |
| I self-disclose more about my personal life with him/her than with my other patients | .64 |
| I do things, or go the extra mile, for him/her in way that I don't do for other patients | .52 |
| I feel guilty when s/he is distress or deteriorates, as if I must be somehow responsible | .39 |
| I end sessions overtime with him/her more than with my other patients | .39 |

**Factor 5, Sexualized** (coefficient alpha = .77), describes sexual feelings towards the patient or experiences of sexual tension.

| | |
|---|---|
| I find myself being flirtatious with him/her | .99 |
| I feel sexually attracted to him/her | .89 |
| I feel sexual tension in the room | .78 |
| I tell him/her I love him/her | .62 |

**Factor 6, Disengaged** (coefficient alpha = .83), depicts feeling distracted, withdrawn, annoyed, or bored in sessions.

| | |
|---|---|
| I feel bored in sessions with him/her | .82 |
| My mind often wanders to things other than what s/he is talking about | .72 |
| I don't feel fully engage in sessions with him/her | .53 |
| I lose my temper with him/her | .46 |
| I watch the clock with him/her more than with my other patients | .46 |
| I feel annoyed in sessions with him/her | .42 |

**Factor 7, Parental/Protective** (coefficient alpha = .80), captures a wish to protect and nurture the patient in a parental way, above and beyond normal positive feelings toward the patient.

| | |
|---|---|
| I feel like I want to protect him/her | .69 |
| I feel nurturant toward him/her | .68 |
| I have warm, almost parental feelings toward him/her | .67 |
| I wish I could give him/her what others never could | .53 |
| I feel angry at people in his/her life | .45 |

**Factor 8, Criticized/Mistreated** (coefficient alpha = .83), describes feeling unappreciated, dismissed, or devalued by the patient.

| | |
|---|---|
| I feel unappreciated by him/her | .75 |
| I feel criticized by him/her | .63 |
| I feel dismissed or devalued | .60 |
| I feel am "walking on eggshells" around him/her, afraid that if I say the wrong thing she/he will explode, fall apart, or walk out | .56 |
| I have to stop myself from saying or doing something aggressive or critical | .44 |

The factor structure offers a complex portrait of countertransference processes that highlight the nuances of therapists' reactions toward their patients. The dimensions are distinct and go beyond the cursory divisions between "positive" and "negative" countertransference. For example, we identified distinct experiences of negative countertransference – i.e., feeling overwhelmed and disorganized, helpless and inadequate, disengaged, or mistreated with a patient. Similarly, the sexualized, special/overinvolved, and parental/protective factors all suggest affiliation or closeness, but with distinct clinical roots and implications for treatment.

The complexity of countertransference responses captured by the measure corresponds with clinical observation. Certainly, the feelings of dread and fear associated with the overwhelmed/disorganized factor are consistent with clinical descriptions of countertransference reactions to patients with borderline disorders [49] in addition to research on disorganized and unresolved attachment patterns [50, 51]. Narcissistic pathology has been connected repeatedly with feelings of incompetence (factor 2), helplessness (factor 2), and boredom (factor 6) in clinicians [52–54].

Although the clinical literature is rich in cogent descriptions of therapist reactions, empirical investigation of countertransference as it occurs in clinical practice avoids the subjectivity of clinical observation that is generally based on a single author's clinical experience with a limited number of cases. The Countertransference Questionnaire, used with a practice network approach, allowed us to pool the experience of dozens of clinicians and thereby identify common patterns of countertransference reactions that are not readily apparent to an individual observer or from even an in-depth review of the clinical literature. Delineating the specific domains of countertransference may aid therapists in increasing awareness of and management of the myriad reactions we have toward patients.

## Countertransference and Personality Pathology

As noted earlier, the broad view of countertransference affirms that our reactions to patients are meaningful to understanding the patient and the treatment. The majority of discussions of countertransference in practice focus on treatment of difficult populations, for example, those with a trauma history [55], substance abuse, or personality disorder. These are patients who typically arouse intense, and we would suggest common, reactions on the part of the clinician. Persons carrying the same personality disorder diagnosis have similar modes of emotional, cognitive, and interpersonal functioning (indeed, DSM diagnoses are based on these dimensions); therefore, it is expected that they would evidence similar relational patterns and thereby evoke consistent reactions from therapists.

To study the relationship between countertransference and personality pathology, we examined the associations between the eight countertransference factors and the DSM-IV personality disorder clusters. We used the clusters for the initial analyses because of the extensive comorbidity of the Axis II disorders; we followed up with partial correlation analyses for specific disorders based on the initial cluster-level analyses. We described our hypotheses, analyses, and results in detail in an earlier publication [33]; here, we report only the significant results.

First, as we hypothesized, Cluster A (odd/eccentric) showed a significant association with Criticized/Mistreated countertransference. Contrary to our predictions, however, Cluster A was not correlated with the Disengaged factor. Patients with paranoid, schizoid, and schizotypal disorders are often characterized as disinterested in or uncomfortable with other people. These social deficits inhibit establishing a comfortable relationship, and the patients are often described as aloof, cold, or withdrawn. In turn, we had expected that a clinician would disengage, i.e., feel bored, distracted, and annoyed. However, we found, instead, that clinicians working with patients with paranoid, schizotypal, and schizoid disorders feel unappreciated, criticized, dismissed, and devalued by these patients. Our research has highlighted an important nuance in counter-transference reactions toward patients displaying interpersonal detachment and mistrust. Therapists value intimate connections with their patients, both as a key mechanism of therapeutic action and as an affirmation of their identity and efficacy as clinicians. It makes sense that in working with patients who disavow their needs for or recoil from others, therapists endorse feeling mis-treated and rejected. These patients essentially disavow key aspects of thera-pists' talent, skills, and functioning. With this knowledge, therapists can be more attuned to ways in which they experience attacks to their self-esteem and personhood when working with patients with Cluster A disorders.

The data supported the hypothesis that Cluster C (anxious) disorders would be associated with the Parental/Protective factor, indicating desire to protect and take care of the patient. These countertransference feelings are likely related to patients with Avoidant and Dependent disorders. These patients are similar in that they tend to be acutely sensitive in their relationships, be preoccupied with rejection, and suffer intense anxiety. Their early experience may be marked by unmet needs, criticism, and unpredictable attachment by their parents. They struggle to establish healthy self-concept and relationships. Clinicians endorse feeling drawn to basically reparent, to provide patients what they did not receive, and to heal attachments in the face of the patients' passivity in or avoidance of relationships. The therapists' pull to assume caretaking capacities for and to feel so strongly on behalf of their patients provides diagnostic insight into the patients' dynamics that tend to make others respon-sible for their self-concept. Important here is that the Parental/Protective factor involves countertransference feelings and does not indicate any actions on the part of the therapist, unlike the countertransference experiences associated with Cluster B disorders. To the extent this suggests that clinicians are less likely to act out and more likely to experience their countertransference at an emotional level, it may indicate less disturbed dynamics on the part of both the patient and the therapeutic interaction; however, this warrants empirical investigation.

The Cluster B (dramatic–erratic) disorders were associated, as we predicted, with the Overwhelmed/Disorganized, Helpless/Inadequate, and Sexualized factors, but not the Special/Overinvolved factor. Essentially, what we found is that patients with antisocial, borderline, histrionic, narcissistic disorders arouse intense feelings; this is not especially surprising given the interpersonal demands and serious distortions in self and other representations associated with these disorders. Our work provides empirical confirmation of the complex nature of these intense feelings. The Overwhelmed/Disorganized factor captures a multi-faceted constellation of negative feelings, which involve dreading contact with the patient, feeling angry with and resentful of the patient, and actively avoiding the patient (returning phone calls less promptly and setting firm limits). Thera-pists also feel unable to help their patients with Cluster B personality disorders; their sense of inadequacy and helplessness leave them feeling overwhelmed, anxious, and confused by their patients. Interestingly, therapists also experience sexual attraction with these patients despite their acute feelings of helplessness and dread. In addition, we found support for our hypothesis that borderline personality disorder is associated with the Special/Overinvolved factor, which captures problems maintaining boundaries, including self-disclosure, ending sessions on time, and feeling guilty, responsible, or overly concerned about the patient. Loving and erotic feelings may serve as a way to avoid the increasing hostility and anxiety that the therapists experience with their patients who present severe disturbances in self and interpersonal functioning. As Gabbard [56] summarizes, "... the therapist's loving feelings are frequently in the service of disavowing negative feelings involving aggression, contempt, sadism, and hate" (p. 314). This may be a key to therapists' vulnerability to boundary crossings with Borderline and Histrionic patients in particular [57, 58] and warrants further empirical investigation.

Although we did not predict it, the Cluster B disorders showed an association with the Disengaged factor, and in follow-up analyses, we confirmed our hypothesis that narcissistic personality disorder would account for this correlation. In fact, we found that the other Cluster B disorders showed no significant associations with therapist disengagement. Our work to create a prototype of countertransference responses to narcissistic patients echoes this finding, as discussed below.

## Typical Countertransference Responses to Narcissistic Patients

Our research enabled us to create a composite description of countertransference reactions that clinicians experience in working with patients who met the DSM-IV criteria for narcissistic personality disorder. In doing so, we reported the items that were most descriptive and least descriptive of countertransference responses to patients with this disorder as detailed in Table 8.1 and 8.2. Our earlier publication [33] details the analyses.

We found that patients with narcissistic personality disorder tend to arouse a range of angry feelings in clinicians, including feeling annoyed, frustrated, resentful, or enraged, as well as concerns about acting on these feelings. Clinicians experience their narcissistic patients as devaluing, critical, unappreciative, or manipulative of the therapist, as well as brittle and apt to erupt in anger. Not surprisingly, these clinicians also report feeling bored, distracted, disengaged, avoidant, and hopeless, with a desire to terminate treatment. Interestingly, feelings of inadequacy or incompetence were not among the most descriptive items of countertransference with narcissistic patients. Clinicians were least likely to endorse feeling compassion, positive anticipation of sessions, or hope for the patient's prognosis.

Kernberg [54] characterizes narcissistic patients as displaying intense self-absorption and superficial modes of relating to others. In addition to grandiose fantasies and excessive need for admiration and recognition from others, Kernberg

**Table 8.1** Countertransference reactions to patients meeting DSM-IV criteria for narcissistic personality disorder ($N$ = 13): standardized countertransference items most descriptive of therapist response

| Item | Mean |
|---|---|
| I feel annoyed in sessions with him/her | 1.63 |
| I feel used or manipulated by him/her | 1.42 |
| I lose my temper with him/her | 1.38 |
| I feel mistreated or abused by him/her | 1.29 |
| I feel resentful working with him/her | 1.24 |
| I talk about him/her with my spouse or significant other more than my other patients | 1.17 |
| I feel I am "walking on eggshells" around him/her, afraid that if I say the wrong thing she/he will explode, fall apart, or walk out | 1.10 |
| When checking my phone messages, I feel anxiety or dread that there will be one from him/her | 1.07 |
| I feel unappreciated by him/her | 1.04 |
| At times I dislike him/her | 1.04 |
| I have to stop myself from saying or doing something aggressive or critical | 1.04 |
| My mind often wanders to things other than what s/he is talking about | 0.99 |
| I feel criticized by him/her | 0.98 |
| I feel angry at him/her | 0.98 |
| I watch the clock with him/her more than with my other patients | 0.97 |
| I get enraged at him/her | 0.97 |
| I dread sessions with him/her | 0.93 |
| I feel dismissed or devalued | 0.91 |
| I feel like I'm being mean or cruel to him/her | 0.91 |
| I feel hopeless working with him/her | 0.88 |
| I feel sexual tension in the room | 0.88 |
| I think or fantasize about ending the treatment | 0.87 |
| I feel bored in sessions with him/her | 0.86 |
| I wish I had never taken him/her on as a patient | 0.85 |
| I feel interchangeable – that I could be anyone to him/her | 0.84 |
| I don't feel fully engaged in sessions with him/her | 0.83 |
| I return his/her phone calls less promptly than I do with my other patients | 0.82 |
| I feel like my hands have been tied or that I have been put in an impossible bind | 0.80 |
| I feel envious of or competitive with him/her | 0.78 |
| I feel frustrated in sessions with him/her | 0.76 |

Note: Means are in standard deviation units, and describe the number of standard deviations the average narcissistic patient in the sample is above the sample mean on each item.

describes narcissistic patients as having "serious deficiencies in their capacity to love and to be concerned about others" (p. 15). Kernberg [54] attributes therapists' difficult countertransference reactions to the narcissistic patient's "consistent efforts to deny the existence of the psychotherapist as an independent person" (p. 232).

Returning to our clinical example, Mario's therapist is beset by feelings similar to those captured in our prototype of countertransference responses to narcissistic patients. Frustrated with and resentful of Mario's inability to

**Table 8.2** Countertransference reactions to patients meeting DSM-IV criteria for narcissistic personality disorder ($N = 13$): standardized countertransference items least descriptive of therapist response

| Item | Mean |
| --- | --- |
| I like him/her very much | −0.32 |
| I feel compassion for him/her | −0.42 |
| I am very hopeful about the gains s/he is making or will likely make in treatment | −0.47 |
| I look forward to sessions with him/her | −0.47 |
| S/he is one of my favorite patients | −0.52 |

Note: Means are in standard deviation units, and describe the number of standard deviations the average narcissistic patient in the sample is above the sample mean on each item.

acknowledge the therapist as a separate being, the therapist found herself withdrawing: she consciously wished Mario would leave treatment, lamenting that she ever took him on as a patient and feeling relieved when he would miss a session. In the moments she could not think her own thoughts, she had disengaged from the patient and the treatment. In the moments she could not bring herself to repeat Mario's words, she had rejected his mirroring transference needs, unable to tolerate becoming merely an "impersonal function" [59] that parrots the patient's words to confirm his sense of himself. Bleiberg [60] describes similar experiences in working with children who present narcissistic disturbances, conveying his feelings of dread, irritation, helplessness, and boredom. He also describes wanting to show his patients who was "really in charge." Alternating between dread and anger in ways similar to the experiences captured in our empirical portrait, the therapist found herself embroiled in a power struggle – a struggle to preserve her identity and existence in relation to Mario, who could not recognize the other for fear of losing himself. Hanna Segal [61] wrote, "In narcissism, life-giving relationships and healthy self-love are equally attacked" (p. 75). In the countertransference response to the patient's destruction of self and other, the therapist is bound to experience anger, dread, and avoidance.

Gabbard [62] distinguished between oblivious and hypervigilant narcissism, referring to predominant interpersonal styles of narcissistic patients. Oblivious narcissism (overt) refers to patients who are unconcerned with their impact on others, so invested in their own omnipotence to the exclusion of actual relationships [59]. They are more likely to exhibit the grandiosity and exhibitionism characteristic of the DSM-IV diagnosis of narcissistic personality disorder. They are akin to "thick-skinned" narcissists. Hypervigilant narcissists (covert) are "thin-skinned," acutely aware of others, inhibited, and vulnerable to experiencing shame. Their grandiosity emerges in inhibited fantasy as opposed to manifesting overtly in uninhibited behaviors. Our composite description captures countertransference experiences with the oblivious narcissist more so than the hypervigilant narcissist. This is not surprising given that the clinicians reported on their experiences working with patients who met DSM-IV criteria for narcissistic personality disorder. The hypervigilant narcissism has received far less attention and is not represented in the DSM-IV. However, this is an important clinical distinction that would likely evoke distinct countertransference patterns.

Mario displayed tendencies toward both the oblivious and hypervigilant narcissistic styles. He was acutely vulnerable to experiencing shame and also profoundly careless in his relationships, driven by his desire to feel affirmed and special in the eyes of others. As the analytic space collapsed in the face of his pressures to control how his therapist related to him, Mario attacked, as Segal anticipated, the possibility of reciprocity and mutual respect in his relationship with his therapist. The therapist was confronted with blatant and veiled attacks on her personhood, her sense of efficacy and agency, and her desire to connect.

In order to "use" her countertransference, the therapist must get close to her feelings about Mario. Perhaps seemingly simple at the surface, but in reality, facing countertransference feelings can be profoundly threatening because the therapist must face terribly discomforting feelings of hate, rage, and annihilation. Mario's therapist needed to find space to think her thoughts, to reflect on her feelings of dread and anger, and to recognize how feeling devalued and criticized impacted her way of being with Mario. She needed, too, to turn her attention to considering how her experience of feeling controlled and invisible might provide hints to understanding Mario's internal experience of himself and his relationships. These reflections on her countertransference reactions could be a means to empathic connection with Mario's early experience.

We pick up here Fonagy's concept of reflective functioning with hopes of usefully extending his ideas to the treatment relationship. Reflective functioning [63] refers to the capacity to mentalize, to step back from immediate experience and think about others' and one's own beliefs, feelings, and desires that may motivate behaviors. Fonagy and colleagues have discussed and researched this capacity to think about mental states mainly as a child's developmental achievement that depends on the caregiver's capacity to consider his/her mental state and that of the child. They link the parents' mentalization capacities to the creation of secure attachment in the children, writing and establishing empirically that, "We believe that the parent's capacity to adopt the intentional stance toward a not yet intentional infant, to think about the infant in terms of thoughts, feelings and desires in the infant's mind and in their own mind in relation to the infant and his or her mental state, is the key mediator of the transmission of attachment. . . ." (p. 431). They further posit that the capacity to think about the mental world of another and one's self enables one to establish a coherent and meaningful sense of self and relationship to others.

Fonagy and his colleagues propose that those with limited capacity to mentalize are apt to turn to action and projective identification to establish a sense of coherence. In this regard, the other (the parent, but we could usefully extend this to the therapist) becomes the recipient of aspects of the self that feel alien and create a sense of incoherence of self. This indicates the child's (or patient's) attempt to create a meaningful, coherent sense of self by ridding oneself of the feelings that are incongruent. Many patients with narcissistic dynamics struggle with a fragile hold on their sense of self. In turn, their grandiosity and entitlement serve to make others feel inferior and impotent in order to stave off the anxieties of fragmentation. However, in taking on these feelings, the parent (therapist) is apt to lose "touch with the [child's] mental world" (p. 441), as well as her own mental world, I would conjecture.

Thrown off balance by the power of the patient's interpersonal provocations, Mario's therapist felt she could not think her own thoughts; at moments, she lost touch with her own mental world. Fonagy's work on reflective functioning provides cues to the management of intense countertransference feelings. Regulating strong emotions and making them meaningful depends on this capacity to step back from the immediate experience and think about "plausible interpretations of behaviors in terms of … underlying mental states" (p. 430). Reflection involves thinking about one's experience in a way that contextualizes the feelings and behaviors in interpersonal and/or developmental terms, for example.

One benefit of our empirical portrait of countertransference responses to patients presenting with narcissism is that it helps contextualize the experience. First, the therapist, beset by anger, hopelessness, and feeling devalued, could turn to the profile to anchor her countertransference experiences. Second, the results suggest a very specific constellation of countertransference feelings that are typical in working with narcissistic patients; given this, the character dynamics and internal representations of self and other become more apparent. This allows a therapist to begin to conceptualize the transference–countertransference dynamics. With a stronger hold on her own mental world, anchored in thinking about the patient diagnostically, Mario's therapist could begin to consider the objects represented in the transference–countertransference interplay of feelings and enactments. She could begin to consider who is inadequate, powerless, and abandoned. Who devalued, controlled, and abandoned? With this restored capacity to reflect, the therapist would now have the potential to direct the treatment rather than to respond unwittingly to Mario's pressures. She could choose how to respond based on her understanding of Mario's key dynamics and vulnerabilities. She might, for example, highlight to Mario his need to devalue the therapist; provide the mirroring function of a self-object without yet expecting Mario to recognize her subjectivity; or drawing on the concept of projective identification, contain and help metabolize what Mario disavows and/or reflect back the confused, helpless, angry/rageful, and exploited feelings he carries. The key in this sits with the therapist's openness to her experiences, assuming her reactions to be meaningful and motivated by, in part, the interpersonal context of the therapy relationship and the patient's internal world.

## Discussion

By virtue of reflecting the collective experience of clinicians in practice, the Countertransference Questionnaire normalizes feelings, desires, and behaviors that can otherwise be disconcerting or even shameful to the therapist who holds herself to an ideal of unwavering empathy, positive regard, and beneficence (e.g., wanting to get rid of the patient, feeling enraged with the patient, and sexual fantasies about the patient). In this vein, this measure can serve as a tool in training programs. The knowledge that others also have strong reactions toward patients can diminish the pull toward denial and, consequently, our potential for unwittingly acting out that which we disavow. In a related vein, the measure can help therapists organize and make sense of what can be subtle, even inchoate, responses to patients. The items and the factors anchor emotions, thoughts, and behavior in clear, easy to understand language that is nonetheless descriptive of complex dynamics. A key contribution of our measure is to provide a framework in which to conceptualize those countertransference reactions that disrupt the treatment alliance and the therapist's engagement with and empathy for the patient. Since a lack of awareness of countertransference responses can interfere with the care a patient receives, and, conversely, awareness can facilitate ensuring the welfare of the treatment, this represents an important area for all clinicians. It is vital to treatment for the therapist to learn to attend to his own reactions, which are often unconscious, as a means of understanding the patient [64].

Our findings suggest that countertransference reactions occur in coherent and predictable patterns in the treatment of personality pathology. This supports the broad view of countertransference reactions as useful in the diagnostic understanding of the patient's repetitive interpersonal patterns associated with psychological disturbance. Indeed, the results lend support to the idea that patients with personality disorder elicit "average expectable countertransference" [33] responses that likely resemble responses by other significant people in the patient's life, similar to Winnicott's concept of "objective countertransference" and Wachtel's work on cyclical psychodynamics.

A contemporary postmodern view of psychotherapy, or a two-person psychology, would discount the concept of objective countertransference because, from a postmodern perspective, it is never possible to tease out the therapist's subjectivity in understanding the therapist's feelings about or reactions to the patient. We do not discount that the clinician's history and the interaction between the clinician's and patient's dynamics can elicit very personal reactions that speak to the clinician's internal world and conflicts. However, as Geltner [65] has also pointed out, being aware of the idiosyncratic or personal ways we respond to patients is not mutually exclusive from recognizing the patterns in which countertransference responses are systematically related to patient's enduring personality styles. Jones [66],[1] in his psychotherapy process research, observed that patient and therapist engaged in repetitive, reciprocal patterns of interaction that were distinct for each dyad. He developed a two-person conceptualization of therapeutic action that took into account how "the unconscious psychological processes of each influence the other" (p. 467). His concept takes into account that both the patient's intrapsychic conflicts and the therapist's response to these conflicts manifest in the therapeutic interaction. Jones suggested that self-awareness, and thereby change, in the patient occurs only as

---

[1] We thank Raymond Levy for pointing out the connection between Jones' and our work.

the therapist attempts to understand the patient through the relationship they establish. His research lends support to a connection between patient change and interpretation of these repetitive patterns of interaction; in turn, he found that unacknowledged and uninterpreted countertransference experiences can result in therapeutic stalemate. We advocate a both/and approach to conceptualizing countertransference – that is, understanding countertransference as both a manifestation of the therapist's intrapsychic conflict or unresolved issues and an indication of the influence of the patient's conflicts and ways of being and relating on the therapist. The concept of overdetermination captures the complexity of human motivation and interaction.

In our future work, we hope to identify additional countertransference constellations to help clinicians anticipate potential countertransference challenges inherent in working with multiple forms of personality disturbance. We hope, too, to turn our attention to countertransference patterns associated with other clinical populations that exhibit disturbances in object relations and self-experience, such as survivors of childhood sexual abuse or patients with eating disorders. An important addition to our research on empirical prototypes of countertransference reactions involves also understanding the contribution of the therapist, as well as the interaction between therapist and patient variables. Such research would help refine our understanding of our concept of average expectable countertransference responses and may contribute to enhancing our understanding of the variables that impact patient–therapist match. Finally, given the centrality of the therapist's contributions in contemporary, two-person conceptualizations of psychotherapy, it would be relevant to use the Countertransference Questionnaire in a study of psychotherapy outcome.[2]

# References

1. Freud S. The Future Prospects of Psychoanalytic Therapy. In: Wolstein B, (eds.) Essential papers on countertransference. New York: NY: New York University Press 1988:16–24.
2. Heimann P. On counter-transference. Int J Psychoanal 1950; 31:81–84.
3. Kernberg O. Notes on countertransferences. J Am Psychoanal Assoc 1965; 13(1):38–56.
4. Racker H. The meanings and uses of countertransference. Psychoanal Q 1957; 26:303–57.
5. Sandler J, Holder A, Dare C. Basic psychoanalytic concepts: IV. Countertransference. Br J Psychiatry 1970; 117(536):83–88.
6. Winnicott DW. Hate in the counter-transference. Int J Psychoanal 1949; 30:69–74.
7. Klein M. Notes on some schizoid mechanisms. Int J Psychoanal 1946; 27:99–110.
8. Bion W. Learning from experience. London: Heinemann, 1962.
9. Gabbard GO. A contemporary psychoanalytic model of countertransference. J Clin Psychol 2001; 57(8; 8):983–981.
10. Ogden TH. Projective identification and psychotherapeutic technique. New York: Jason Aronson, 1982.
11. Sandler J. Countertransference and role-responsiveness. Int Rev Psychoanal 1976; 3(1):43–47.

[2] Leon Hoffman was very helpful in suggesting these last two ideas for future research.

12. Wachtel P. Psychoanalysis and behavior therapy. New York: Basic Books , 1977.
13. Wachtel PL. Resistance as a problem for practice and theory. J Psychothe Integr 1999; 9(1):103–117.
14. Brody F, Farber B. The effects of therapist experience and patient diagnosis on counter-transference. Psychotherapy 1996; 33:372–380.
15. Colson DB, Allen JG, Coyne L and Dexter N. An anatomy of countertransference: Staff reactions to difficult psychiatric hospital patients.Hosp Community Psychiatry 1986; 37(9):923–928.
16. Holmqvist R, Armelius B. The patient's contribution to the therapist's countertransference feelings. J Nerv Ment Dis 1996; 184(11):660–666.
17. McIntyre SM, Schwartz RC. Therapists' differential countertransference reactions toward clients with major depression or borderline personality disorder. J Clin Psychol 1998; 54:923–931.
18. Dubé JÉ, Normandin L. The mental activities of trainee therapists of children and adolescents: The impact of personal psychotherapy on the listening process. Psychotherapy: Theory, Research, Practice, Training 1999; 36(3):216–228.
19. Coyne JC. Depression and the response of others. J Abnorm Psychol 1976; 85:186–193.
20. Gotlib IH, Beatty ME. Negative responses to depression: The role of attributional style. Cogn Ther Res 1985; 9(1):91–103.
21. Gurtman MB. Depressive affect and disclosures as factors in interpersonal rejection. Cogn Ther Res 1987; 11:87–99.
22. Hokanson JE, Sacco WP, Blumberg SR, Landrum GC. Interpersonal behavior of depressive individuals in a mixed-motive game. J Abnorm Psychol 1980; 89:320–332.
23. Pettit JW, Joiner, TE. Negative Feedback-Seeking. In: Pettit JW, Joiner, TE (eds.). Chronic depression: Interpersonal sources, therapeutic solutions. Washington, DC: American Psychological Association, 2006: 41–53.
24. Swann WB. The trouble with change: Self-verification and allegiance to the self. Psychol Sci 1997; 8(3):177–180.
25. Downey G, Freitas AL, Michaelis B, Khouri H. The self-fulfilling prophecy in close relationships: Rejection sensitivity and rejection by romantic partners. J Pers Soc Psychol 1998; 75(2):545–560.
26. Giesler R, Josephs RA, Swann WB. Self-verification in clinical depression: The desire for negative evaluation. J Abnorm Psychol 1996; 105(3):358–368.
27. Hayes JA, Gelso CJ. Effects of therapist-trainees' anxiety and empathy on counter-transference behavior. J Clin Psychol 1991; 47(2):284–290.
28. Hayes JA, Gelso CJ. Male counselors' discomfort with gay and HIV-infected clients. J Couns Psychol 1993; 40(1):86–93.
29. Rosenberger EW, Hayes JA. Origins, consequences, and management of countertransference: A case study. J Couns Psychol 2002; 49:221–232.
30. Sharkin BS, Gelso CJ. The influence of counselor trainee anger-proneness and anger discomfort on reactions to an angry client. J Couns Dev 1993; 71(5):483–487.
31. Yulis S, Kiesler DJ. Countertransference response as a function of therapist anxiety and content of patient talk. J Consult Clin Psychol 1968; 32:413–419.
32. Robbins SB, Jolkovski MP. Managing countertransference feelings: An interactional model using awareness of feeling and theoretical framework. J Couns Psychol 1987; 34:276–282.
33. Betan E, Heim AK, Conklin CZ, Westen D. Countertransference phenomena and personality pathology in clinical practice: An empirical investigation. Am J Psychiatry 2005; 162:890–898.
34. Najavits LM, Griffin ML, Luborsky L, Frank A, Weiss RD, Liese BL, Thompson H, Nakayama E, Siqueland L, Daley D, Onken LS. Therapists' emotional reactions to substance abusers: A new questionnaire and initial findings. Psychotherapy: Theory, Research, Practice, Training 1995; 32(4):669–677.

35. Westen D, Harnden-Fischer J. Personality profiles in eating disorders: Rethinking the distinction between Axis I and Axis II. Am J Psychiatry 2001; 165:547–562.
36. Morey LC. Personality disorders in DSM-III and DSM-III-R: Convergence, coverage, and internal consistency. Am J Psychiatry 1988; 145:573–577.
37. Shedler J, Westen D: Dimensions of personality pathology: An alternative to the five factor model. Am J Psychiatry 2004; 161: 1743–1754..
38. Westen D, Shedler J. Revising and assessing axis II, part I: Developing a clinically and empirically valid assessment method. Am J Psychiatry 1999; 156:258–272.
39. Westen D, Shedler J. Revising and assessing axis II, part II: Toward an empirically based and clinically useful classification of personality disorders. Am J Psychiatry 1999; 156:273–285.
40. Wilkinson-Ryan T, Westen D. Identity disturbance in borderline personality disorder: An empirical investigation. Am J Psychiatry 2000; 157:528–541.
41. Garb HN. Clinical Judgment. In: Garb HN, (ed.) Studying the clinician: Judgment research and psychological assessment. Am Psychol Assoc 1998:173–206.
42. Achenbach TM. As others see us: Clinical and research implications of cross-informant correlations for psychopathology. Curr Dir Psychol Sci, 2006; 15:94–98.
43. Hilsenroth MJ, Ackerman, SJ, Blagys, MD, et al. Reliability and validity of DSM-IV axis V. Am J Psych 2000; 157:1858–1863.
44. Nakash-Eisikovits O, Dieberger A, Western D. A multidimensional meta-analysis of pharmacotherapy for bulimia nervosa: Summarizing the range of outcomes in controlled clinical trials. Harv Rev Psychiatry 2002; 10:193.
45. Westen D, Rosenthal R. Quantifying construct validity: Two simple measures. J Pers Soc Psychol 2003; 84:608–618.
46. Westen D, Muderrisoglu S. Reliability and validity of personality disorder assessment using a systematic clinical interview: Evaluating an alternative to structured interviews. J Pers Disord 2003; 17:350–368.
47. Westen D, Muderrisoglu S, Fowler C, Shedler J, Koren D. Affect regulation and affective experience: Individual differences, group differences, and measurement using a Q-sort procedure. J Consult Clin Psychol 1997; 65:429–439.
48. Fabregar LR, Wegener DT, MacCallum RC, Strahan EJ. Evaluating the use of exploratory factor analysis in psychological research. Psychol Methods 1999; 4:272–299.
49. 2003 Not found, but it could be this one: Adler G. Borderline psychopathology and its treatment. New York: Aronson, 1985.
50. Cassidy J, Mohr JJ. Unsolvable fear, trauma, and psychopathology: Theory, research, and clinical considerations related to disorganized attachment across the life span. Clin Psychol Sci Pract 2002; 8:275–298.
51. Main M, Kaplan N, Cassidy J. Security in infancy, childhood, and adulthood: A move to the level of representation. Monogr Soc Res Child Dev 1985; 50(1–2):66–104.
52. Altshul VA. The so-called boring patient. Am J Psychother 1977; 31:533.
53. Blieberg E. Stages in the treatment of narcissistic children and adolescents. Bull Menninger Clin 1987; 51:296–313.
54. Kernberg O. Further contributions to the treatment of narcissistic personalities. Int J Psychoanal 1974; 55:215–240.
55. Walker M. Supervising practitioners working with survivors of childhood abuse: Counter transference; secondary traumatization and terror. Psychodynamic Practice: Individuals, Groups and Organisations 2004; 10(2):173–193.
56. Gabbard GO. Lessons to be learned from the study of sexual boundary violations. Am J Psychother 1996; 50(3):311–322.
57. Gutheil TG. Boundary issues and personality disorders. J Psychiatr Pract 2005; 11(2):88–96.
58. Gabbard GO. Psychiatrists In-Practice Examination (PIPE). J Psychiatr Pract 2006; 12(6):406–408.
59. Kohut H. The psychoanalytic treatment of narcissistic personality disorders: Outline of a systematic approach. Psychoanal Study Child 1968; 23:86–113.

60. Blieberg E. Stages in the treatment of narcissistic children and adolescents. Bull Menninger Clin 1987; 51:296–313.
61. Segal H. Phantasy and Reality. In: Schafer R (eds.) The contemporary Kleinians of London. Madison, CT: International Universities Press, Inc, 1997:75–95.
62. Gabbard GO. Two subtypes of narcissistic personality disorder. Bull Menninger Clin 1989; 53(6):527–532.
63. Fonagy P, Target M, Gergely G. The developmental roots of borderline personality disorder in early attachment relationships: A theory and some evidence. Psychoanal Inq 2003; 23:412–459
64. Ogden T. Primitive edge of experience. Lanham, MD: Jason Aronson 1989
65. Geltner P. The concept of objective countertransference and its role in a two-person psychology. Am J Psychoanal 2006;66(1):25–42.
66. Jones E. Therapeutic action: A new theory. Am J of Psychotherapy 2001;55:460–474

# Part III
# Theory, Technique, and Process in Psychodynamic Psychotherapy

# Chapter 9
# Alliance, Negotiation, and Rupture Resolution

Jeremy D. Safran, J. Christopher Muran, and Bella Proskurov

## Introduction

More than one hundred years have passed since "the talking cure" was introduced as a treatment for psychological problems. Considerable scientific effort over the last 60 years has been spent to determine whether psychotherapy, in general, is effective, and if so, what factors underlie the mechanism of change. With the growing demand of the health care system and the public in general for accountability, there has been a continuous pressure on the mental health field to provide empirical support for the treatments we offer to our patients. This has given rise to the initiatives of the American Psychological Association and American Psychiatric Association to formulate practice guidelines and identify empirically supported interventions and treatments. The focus of these efforts has been on high-quality comparative outcome studies on techniques or brand-name therapies for single categorical disorders, while the therapeutic relationship has been ignored or addressed only vaguely [1]. However, quantitative reviews and meta-analyses of psychotherapy outcome literature consistently reveal that specific techniques account for only 5–15% of the outcome variance [1]. Moreover, technical interventions do not exist in a vacuum; they are applied in a context of patient–therapist relationship. In other words, all techniques and interventions are relational acts [2], and the therapist as a person is a central agent of change [3]. Therefore, empirical investigation of the therapeutic relationship and attempts to discover elements and factors that make this relationship effective are essential and relevant to clinical practice.

Psychotherapy research over the last several decades found the therapeutic alliance to be one of the most important elements of the therapeutic relationship. The therapeutic alliance has been consistently shown to be a robust predictor of positive outcome [4]. Building and maintaining good therapeutic alliance appears to be essential for the success of treatment. At the same time, ruptures in the alliance have been conceptualized as important change events

J. D. Safran
Department of Psychology New School for Social Research,   65 Fifth Avenue, New York, NY 10003, USA,
e-mail: Safranj@newschool.edu

R.A. Levy, J.S. Ablon (eds.), *Handbook of Evidence-Based Psychodynamic Psychotherapy*,       201
DOI: 10.1007/978-1-59745-444-5_9, © Humana Press 2009

and have become a subject of empirical investigation [5]. This emphasis on the importance of repairing alliance ruptures was of course anticipated by Kohut [6] among others.

The literature review that follows will discuss the existing body of literature on the therapeutic alliance, including the history of the concept, measurement of the alliance, empirical research on the relationship between the alliance and the outcome, the concept of the ruptures in the alliance, and the research on the ruptures and their resolution.

## Overview of Psychotherapy Research

Although scientific investigations of psychotherapy effectiveness began as early as the1920 s, increasingly empirically valid and methodologically sound psychotherapy research flourished in the second half of the 20th century. Stimulated by the controversial article of Eysenck, who after a review of 24 studies concluded that psychotherapy was not effective [7], research initially focused on the efficacy of psychotherapy. The advance of meta-analytic techniques allowed researchers to examine multiple empirical studies conducted with thousands of patients having various psychological problems treated by various therapeutic techniques. Multiple comprehensive reviews of outcome research have come to one basic conclusion: psychotherapy, in general, has been shown to be effective [8–11]. Furthermore, psychotherapies have effects beyond those of spontaneous remission and of various no-treatment controls: the average treated person is better off than 80% of untreated control subjects [11]. The effect sizes produced in psychotherapy are as large as or larger than those produced by various medical interventions (e.g., medication). Finally, according to Lambert and Bergin [11], these findings cannot be "explained away by reference to methodological weaknesses in the data reviewed or by reviewing methods" (p. 149).

Psychotherapy outcome research has also examined the effectiveness of various types of psychotherapy in treating the broad spectrum of anxiety and depressive disorders, and interpersonal problems. Numerous reviews of empirical studies comparing a wide range of psychotherapies have found no significant difference between their effectiveness [10, 11]. As Luborsky [12] once quipped, "Everyone has won and all must have prizes." Although a small but consistent advantage for cognitive and behavioral techniques over dynamic and humanistic approaches has been found by some meta-analytic reviews of literature [13–15], it has been argued that these results can be attributed to methodological artifacts [10, 11]. Most recently, Lambert and Barley [10] examined more than 50 meta-analytic reviews of outcome research. They concluded that "while statistically significant differences can sometimes be found favoring the superiority of one treatment over another, these differences are not so large that their practical effects are noteworthy" (p. 19). It should be mentioned, however, that a few specialized techniques have shown superiority with

some specific diagnostic categories (e.g., exposure treatment with specific phobic disorders and response prevention for obsessive–compulsive disorders) [16].

The prevailing explanation of the general finding of the equivalence in outcome among highly diverse therapies is the existence of the "common" or
"nonspecific" factors that are present in all forms of therapy and lead to positive
change [11]. Examples of common factors include therapist's empathy, warmth,
acceptance, patient's trust and feeling of being understood, and the therapeutic
alliance. Although there is substantive evidence that common factors account
for a significant amount of patient's improvement in psychotherapy [10], the
common factor model of change has been critiqued by authors who emphasize
that the specific techniques cannot be separated from the interpersonal nature
of a therapeutic encounter [17, 18]. According to Butler and Strupp [17],
"techniques gain their meaning and, in turn, their effectiveness from the particular interaction of the individuals involved" (p. 33), and psychotherapy is
the "systematic use of a human relationship for therapeutic purposes" (p. 36).
Whether one adheres to the common factor model of change or to the more
complex view of therapeutic process outlined by Butler and Strupp, one thing
is clear: the therapeutic relationship is vital in contributing to the success of
treatment.

Considerable research effort has been devoted to studying numerous variables involved in building a successful therapeutic relationship. One of the most
important factors emerging from both the outcome studies and the psychotherapy process research is the therapeutic alliance.

## Theory and Empirical Research on the Therapeutic Alliance

This section will review the theoretical conceptualization of the therapeutic
alliance (also known as working alliance, helping alliance, or simply alliance),
measuring the alliance and the empirical research on the alliance.

### Conceptualization of the Alliance

The concept of the alliance begins its history in the early psychoanalytic literature. It was Freud who first suggested the necessity of making patient an active
"collaborator" in the analytic process [19]. Freud was primarily concerned with
the transferential unconscious-based aspects of the relationship between patient
and analyst; however, he proposed the existence of the "unobjectionable positive
transference" [20], which should not be analyzed since it provides the patient
with the motivation necessary for reality-based collaboration with an analyst in
order to conquer unconscious fear and rejection of exploring repressed material.
Although Freud considered the resolution of transference neurosis as the main

instrument of change, he also acknowledged the role of analyst's friendliness and affection as "the vehicle of success in psychoanalysis" [21].

Sterba [22], building on Freud's structural model, coined the term "ego alliance" to reflect a "split in the [patient's] ego" between its observant and participant functions. This split allows the patient to use his rational, reality-based elements of the ego to ally with the therapist in order to self-observe and accomplish therapeutic tasks.

Zetzel [23], crediting the term to Bibring, distinguished between the therapeutic alliance and the transference neurosis. She argued that the patient's capacity to build the alliance depends on early developmental experiences, which result in his or her ability to form a stable trusting relationship. Zetzel insisted that if the patient lacks this ability in the beginning of treatment, the therapist needs to respond to the patient's "basic needs and anxieties" [24] and create a supportive relationship before attempting the analysis proper (i.e., interpretation of unconscious conflicts). Essentially, Zetzel was the first who conceptualized the alliance as having a direct impact on the effectiveness of therapy.

Greenson [25] continued to clarify the difference between the transferential aspects of the therapeutic relationship and the real relationship between patient and therapist, including undistorted perceptions, authentic trust, and respect. Greenson distinguished between the working alliance, the ability of patient and therapist to work together on the tasks of analysis, and the therapeutic alliance, which refers to the capacity of the therapeutic dyad to form a personal bond.

The concept of the alliance allowed the practitioners of psychoanalysis to be more flexible in terms of technique and to depart from the traditional classical ideals of abstinence and neutrality [2]. However, psychoanalysts continued to believe that the core mechanism of change was insight, whereas the alliance was a necessary but not sufficient condition for change [18].

From a different theoretical perspective, Rogers [26, 27], although not using the term alliance, posited the quality of the therapeutic relationship as both necessary and sufficient condition for clinical change. He conceptualized the therapeutic relationship as a set of therapist-offered conditions, such as empathy, unconditional positive regard, and congruency. However, Rogers attributed the key responsibility for forging the therapeutic relationship to the therapist and did not address the role of the patient in this process.

During the 1970 s, with the advance of the empirical investigations of the therapeutic process, the concept of the alliance ceased to be the feature of purely psychoanalytic discourse and started to become a more general construct applicable to various types of treatment. Although working from the psychodynamic perspective, Luborsky [28] provided a description of the alliance that fits therapeutic process in general. He proposed that the alliance developed in two phases. Early in treatment (i.e., Type I), the alliance involves the patient's belief that treatment would be helpful and that the therapist is providing a supportive, warm, and caring relationship. This creates condition in which the treatment can be undertaken. Later in treatment (i.e., Type II), the alliance is based on a "sense of working together in a joint struggle against what is impeding the patient"

(p. 94). Thus it involves the patient's faith in the therapeutic process itself, commitment to some of the concepts underlying the therapy (e.g., the source of the problems), and an experience of collaboration with the therapist.

In his seminal contribution, Bordin [29, 30] offered a transtheoretical reformulation of the alliance concept. Building on Greenson's concepts of the real relationship and the alliance and reflecting Rogers' ideas of facilitative conditions, he suggested that the alliance consists of three interdependent components: tasks, goals, and bond. The *tasks* refer to specific activities that patient and therapist will engage in over the course of treatment in order to facilitate the desired change. These activities will differ depending on the modality of treatment (e.g., keeping an automatic thoughts record in cognitive–behavioral therapy (CBT), "two-chairs" exercise in the Gestalt therapy, or free association in the classical psychoanalysis). The *goals* are the desired outcomes, which are the targets of the treatment. The *bond* refers to the affective quality of the patient–therapist relationship and includes feelings of mutual trust and respect, liking, and confidence. According to Bordin [30], the bond "grows out of [patient's and therapist's] experience of association in a shared activity" (p.16). All three components of the alliance influence each other in an ongoing fashion during the course of treatment. That is, the ability to agree on goals and tasks of therapy contributes to patient's feelings of being understood and respected, and the sense of the mutual trust within the therapeutic dyad. In reverse, the positive feelings (i.e., the bond) allow patient and therapist to successfully negotiate the agreement on goals and tasks.

Several authors have highlighted the significance of Bordin's conceptualization of the alliance to psychotherapy theory, research, and practice [2, 31, 32]. First, his transtheoretical conceptualization allowed the concept of alliance to spread to other than psychoanalytic therapeutic traditions. According to Wolfe and Goldfried [33], the alliance became the "quintessential integrative variable" spanning all forms of treatment modalities, including experiential [34], cognitive–behavioral [35–38], couples and family therapy [39, 40], and group therapy [41]. Second, Bordin's formulation offered an alternative to the traditional dichotomy between technical and relational factors in psychotherapy by emphasizing that these two aspects are not separate but interdependent elements of therapy. Finally, building on Bordin's model and emphasizing a relational perspective, Safran and Muran [2, 18, 42] have recently offered a reconceptualization of alliance as *negotiation*. This reconceptualization will be discussed in detail in a separate section of this paper.

## Measuring the Alliance

As Horvath and Bedi [4] have pointed out, much of our knowledge about the alliance derives from the empirical studies that define the alliance by the instruments used to measure it. That is, the measures of the alliance "contribute to the definition of the construct" (p. 39). Currently there are more than 24 different alliance measures in use by psychotherapy researchers [4]. There are several important families of instruments that are used in the majority of empirical studies specifically designed to measure the alliance [4, 43, 44].

The Penn scales were developed by Luborsky and his colleagues (HAcs [28]; HAr [45]; HAq [46]) at the Penn Psychotherapy Project to empirically test Luborsky's [28] psychodynamic conceptualization of the Type I and Type II helping alliances. These instruments assess two dimensions of the alliance: (1) a warm, supportive, accepting relationship and (2) patient's experience of collaboration and participation with the therapist in working toward the goals of the treatment. Luborsky and colleagues created the Penn scales that rate the alliance from patients', therapists', and independent observers' perspective.

The Vanderbilt scales (VPPS [47, 48]; VTAS [49]) were developed by Strupp and his colleagues to measure the process dimensions of the Vanderbilt I project. The original 80-item Vanderbilt Psychotherapy Process Scale (VPPS) was an observer-rated measure of the therapist–patient relationship and the psychotherapy process. It was later refined to contain 44 items that specifically measure the alliance (Vanderbilt Therapeutic Alliance Scale). The alliance components in these measures include Patient's Participation, Patient's Exploration, Patient Motivation, Patient's Acceptance of Responsibilities, Therapist's Warmth and Friendliness, and Negative Collaboration.

The California–Toronto scales include the instruments developed over time by researchers from the University of Toronto and the Langley Porter Psychiatric Institute in San Francisco. The Therapeutic Alliance Rating Scale (TARS) [50, 51] was guided by the psychodynamic conceptualization of the alliance and combined items from other scales (the VPPS, the VTAS, and the HAcs). It focuses mostly on the affective dimensions of the alliance and measures its four components: Patient's Positive Contribution, Patient's Negative Contribution, Therapist's Positive Contribution, and Therapist's Negative Contribution. The most recent meta-analysis of the studies on the alliance and outcome [43] found that the TARS did not significantly correlate with the outcome. The authors advise against using this measure for future studies interested in the association between the alliance and the outcome. The California researchers revised the TARS based on factor-analytic studies and created the California Therapeutic Alliance Rating Scale (CALTARS) [52]. A subsequent revision resulted in creating the California Psychotherapy Alliance Scales (CALPAS) [53]. The current CALPAS assess four aspects of the alliance as conceptualized by Gaston [54], which are as follows: (1) the Patient Working Capacity scale reflects patient's ego strength and his or her capacity to work purposefully in therapy, (2) the working alliance is assessed by the Patient Commitment scale, (3) the therapist's contribution to the alliance is measured by the Therapist Understanding and Involvement scale, and (4) the Working Strategy Consensus scale reflects the collaborative agreement between the patient and the therapist on the treatment goals and tasks. The CALPAS offers versions that are rated by patients, therapists, and independent observers.

The Working Alliance Inventory (WAI) [55] was developed to measure Bordin's [29] transtheoretical model of the alliance as consisting of three components: the bond, the agreement on goals, and the agreement on tasks. To allow measurement of the alliance from different perspectives, Horvath and colleagues developed patient, therapist, and independent observer-rated versions of the WAI. A shortened 12-item version of the WAI was also developed [56]. Subsequent studies [56] suggested that the WAI appears to be measuring one general alliance factor, as well as the three specific alliance factors of task, goal, and bond. However, there is also evidence that patients make relatively little distinction between the task and the goal dimensions of the scale [57], while therapist are able to make more distinctions among these dimensions [58].

Several studies that compared different alliance measures (the CALPAS, the Penn, the VTAS, and the WAI) reported that all instruments demonstrated high internal consistency and good interrater reliability [59, 60]. The recent meta-analysis of the alliance literature [43] reported the overall average reliability of the alliance scales based on various estimation methods to be 0.79 ($n = 93$, SD $= 0.16$). When interrater reliability was used, the average reliability was 0.77 ($n = 33$, SD $= 0.15$), whereas when Cronbach's $\alpha$ was reported, the average alliance scale reliability was 0.87 ($n = 44$, SD $= 0.10$). Horvath and Bedi [4] summarized the existing findings regarding the overlap between different instruments and reported medium to high (ranging from 0.34 to 0.87) intercorrelations between various measures of the alliance. Horvath and Bedi [4] also report that factor-analytic examination of the most popular measures indicates three underlying factors present, to varying degrees, in all measures: "personal bonds, energetic involvement in treatment (collaborative work), and collaboration/agreement on the direction (goal) and substance (tasks) of treatment." However, it does not appear that each scale measures the identical construct. Although each instrument reflects the core dimensions, they also assess some features of the relationship that other measures do not.

## The Empirical Research on the Alliance

Numerous studies examining the relationship between the strength of the alliance and the outcome of treatment have been conducted over the past 20 years. These studies use different instruments to measure the alliance and outcome, address various psychiatric disorders (e.g., depression, personality disorders, and substance abuse), and various treatment modalities (e.g., psychodynamic, behavioral, and cognitive). The advance of the meta-analytical methods allows us to integrate the vast empirical evidence and to identify patterns in the literature. Several meta-analytic reviews of the alliance literature [4, 43, 61] have provided evidence linking the quality of the alliance to the treatment outcome. Horvath and Symonds [61] found an overall effect size of 0.26 between the alliance and the outcome based on 24 studies. Martin and colleagues [43] reviewed 79 studies and reported a slightly smaller effect size of 0.22. Most recently, Horvath and Bedi [4] located 10 additional studies published after Martin and colleagues conducted their review and presented their results based on 89 studies. Across all these studies, the average relation between the alliance and the outcome was 0.21, and the median effect size was 0.25 [4]. Although, as Horvath and Bedi pointed out, the magnitude of this relation may not appear very impressive, "the impact of the alliance across studies is far in excess of the outcome variance that can be accounted for by techniques." [4, pg. 61] In other words, the quality of the patient–therapist relationship is more important than the treatment modality.

Although the earlier analyses of the alliance studies suggested that the client-rated alliance was a better predictor of the outcome than the therapist-rated alliance, and that the therapists' ratings showed poor correlations with the patients' [61], some more recent studies indicate that therapists' assessment of the alliance becomes a better predictor of outcome later in therapy [58]. Some researchers found that ratings of the alliance from the independent observer perspective have significant correlations with outcome, while both patient and therapist ratings were not as predictive [60]. Horvath and Bedi [4] reported that patient- and observer-rated alliance have a similar relation to outcome (regardless of the source of outcome ratings), while therapist-rated alliance and outcome are somewhat less related. Horvath and Bedi [4], along with other researchers [59, 62, 63], pointed out that each rater's view of the alliance reflects a qualitatively different aspect of it and provides unique information about the therapeutic relationship. It is, therefore, important to continue studying the alliance from all perspectives.

One of the issues that has been discussed over the years in alliance literature is the possible role of a "halo effect," which is the exaggerated relations between the alliance and the outcome due to the fact that both the alliance and the outcome are rated by the same participants. Horvath and Bedi [4] concurred with the conclusions of others [43, 61] in finding no difference between the effect sizes based on the "same-source" alliance and outcome ratings and the effect sizes based on studies with different sources of the alliance and outcome assessment.

The relationship between alliance ratings at different points in treatment and the final outcome has been investigated by many researchers. Horvath and Symonds [61] found that the early and late alliance measures predict outcome better than the alliance assessments obtained in the middle phase of treatment or the alliance averaged across treatment. According to Horvath and Bedi [4], subsequent investigations confirmed this trend. There is substantial empirical evidence that establishing a strong alliance early in therapy is paramount to the success of treatment and that the alliance measured between the third and fifth sessions is a consistent predictor of final therapy outcome [4]. Moreover, the strength of the alliance after the first session has been shown to be a good predictor of dropout from treatment [64, 65]. These findings also speak against the suggestion that the relation between alliance and outcome is merely an artifact and a by-product of treatment gains [32].

Several researchers attempted to investigate the development of the alliance over the course of treatment. Gelso and Carter [66] suggested that the alliance in successful treatment follows a curvilinear trajectory: initially established strong alliance deteriorates during the middle phase of treatment due to therapist's increasing challenge to patient's dysfunctional relational schemas and improves again toward the end of treatment. The empirical evidence in support of this hypothesis is mixed. Some studies found that the alliance remains stable across the time [67, 68], while others found evidence for the linear growth [58]. Kivlighan and Shaughnessy [69] examined the development of the alliance across four sessions of counseling and discovered three patterns of alliance development: stable alliance, linear alliance growth, and quadratic alliance growth. A pattern of quadratic alliance development was associated with greater improvement on outcome measures when compared to other patterns of alliance development. Tracey and Ray [70] also found that this quadratic trend differentiated good from poor outcome cases, with the good ones showing the high–low–high trajectory. Although not finding the support for the cyclical model of alliance development for patients and therapists on a group level, Bachelor and Salame [67] indicated that individual therapists' and patients' perceptions of various aspects of the alliance showed variation over one time period or another. They concluded that "single assessments of many facets of the participants' perceptions of the relationship cannot be assumed to be representative of their perceptions throughout the course of therapy" (p. 49). The evidence for the dynamic, labile nature of the alliance comes from the longitudinal case studies of more or less successful therapies [71, 72]. These studies found high–low–high pattern of alliance development in good outcome cases and suggested that the course of the alliance in a successful therapy is characterized by a series of ruptures and repairs.

Stiles and his colleagues [73] examined the patterns of alliance development in 79 patients who underwent short-term CBT or psychodynamic–interpersonal treatment for depression. They found that patients whose pattern of alliance development was characterized by episodes of sharp declines in the strength of the alliance followed by a quick return to previous or higher levels (i.e., rupture–repair sequences) made larger gains in treatment compared to other patients. Similarly, in their study of 30 patients who were treated with cognitive therapy for personality disorders, Strauss and his colleagues [74] discovered that most of the patients who reported rupture–repair episodes also reported symptom reductions of 50% or more on all outcome measures.

## Ruptures in Therapeutic Alliance and their Resolution

Although the concept of ruptures in therapeutic alliance (also called strains, breaches, tears in the alliance) is relatively new, working through impasses or difficulties in therapeutic relationship has long been considered pivotal in the process of therapeutic change [2, 75]. In psychoanalytic theory, working through patient's resistance, which was initially seen as an impediment to the analytic process, eventually was conceptualized as the core mechanism of change by the ego psychological school [2, 30]. According to Kohut [6], empathic failures on the part of a therapist are not only inevitable in the course of the therapeutic process but are, in fact, ascribed a central role in the process of change. Therapist's ability to attend to empathic failures by validation of patient's subjective experience and affective attunement results in patients internalizing these "therapist's self-object functions" and patient's capacity to tolerate disappointments and develop a cohesive sense of self. Alexander and French [76] suggested that change takes place through the corrective emotional experience, which the therapist provides by behaving differently from the patient's parents in a conflict situation and thus disconfirming patient's expectations and beliefs about interpersonal relations. A similar concept was proposed and empirically tested by Weiss, Sampson and their colleagues from the Mount Zion Psychotherapy Research Group [77], who theorized that people's problems result from the pathogenic beliefs about interpersonal relationships. These pathogenic beliefs (e.g., that anger will lead to retaliation or that dependence will lead to abandonment) originated as a result of interactions with significant others in the past. According to Weiss and colleagues [77], the process of disconfirming the patient's pathogenic beliefs constitutes a central mechanism of change, and patients unconsciously submit therapist to "transference tests" in order to disconfirm these beliefs. Their empirical studies showed that the disconfirmation of pathogenic beliefs is related to both immediate (i.e., in session) and ultimate outcome [77].

The concept of the alliance rupture overlaps to a certain degree with constructs such as resistance, empathic failure, and transference test [2, 78, 79]. However, the concept of the alliance rupture "has a certain heuristic value because of its link to current psychotherapy research and because of its transtheoretical status" [78]. It is understood to be a function of both patient and therapist contributions – a conceptualization that further distinguishes it from constructs such as resistance, which tend to emphasize the patient's contribution. Alliance ruptures are conceptualized as a type of therapeutic enactment, i.e., periods of unconscious mutual influence between patient and therapist [18, 80]. Enrico Jones [81] calls these unconscious enactments "repetitive interaction structures," and he and his colleagues have devoted considerable attention to investigating them empirically.

An alliance rupture is broadly defined as a strain or breakdown in the collaborative process between patient and therapist, a deterioration in the quality of relatedness between patient and therapist, a deterioration in the communicative situation, or a failure to develop a collaborative process from the outset [5, 75, 78, 80, 82, 83]. Alliance ruptures vary in intensity and duration from minor tension, which can go unnoticed even by a skilled therapist to major problems in communication that, if unresolved, can lead to premature termination or negative outcome [5, 83]. Ruptures can occur during different phases of treatment and with various frequencies.

Bordin [30] awarded central importance to the dynamics of strains in the alliance during the process of therapeutic change. Safran and his colleagues have discussed at length, from both theoretical and empirical perspectives, the importance of investigating alliance ruptures [2, 5, 78, 82–84]. They suggested that alliance ruptures inevitably occur in the course of treatment and can provide a valuable opportunity for therapeutic change. Safran [82] outlined three factors that make alliance ruptures "important therapeutic junctures." First, negative patient–therapist interactions in which therapists respond to patients' hostile communications with similar hostile communications have been shown to result in poor outcome and treatment failure [85]. Second, ruptures provide the therapist with an opportunity to explore patients' expectations and beliefs that constitute their core dysfunctional interpersonal schema, since they often emerge when therapist unwittingly participates in maladaptive interpersonal cycles. Finally, the exploration and resolution of the ruptures can provide the patient with a corrective emotional experience and can modify their dysfunctional interpersonal schemas.

Ruptures in therapeutic alliance have only recently become a subject of rigorous empirical investigation. Safran and colleagues [5] reviewed the existing research related to the alliance ruptures and outlined several emerging trends. First, it appears that patients often avoid revealing their negative feelings about therapists and therapy process [86–88] while even experienced therapists are unable to detect problems in the relationship with patients [87, 88]. Two studies conducted retrospective analyses of therapeutic impasses from patients' [89] and therapists' [90] perspectives. The first study showed that when misunderstandings occurred in a context of poor therapeutic relationship and patients were not able to assert their negative feelings about being misunderstood, they eventually quit therapy. Moreover, when the misunderstanding occurred in a context of good relationship, patients were willing to openly confront their therapists about their negative feelings, and patients and therapists engaged in a mutual repair process over some period of time, the misunderstandings were resolved, which led to an enhanced relationship with the therapist and to patient's growth. The second study conducted a qualitative analysis of therapists' recollection of ruptures that led to unilateral termination. The study showed that patients did not reveal their dissatisfaction until they prematurely terminated, and therapists reported that they were not aware of any problems in the relationship until patients quit therapy.

Second, even when therapists become aware of ruptures in the alliance, they find it difficult to address them in a way leading to their repair and improvement in the alliance. In fact, they may unwittingly contribute to further deterioration of the relationship and to poor outcome of treatment. Several studies [91–94] found that in poor outcome cases, therapists, confronted with ruptures in the alliance, attempted to address them by increasing adherence to the treatment model in a rigid and unconstructive fashion (i.e., challenging distorted cognitions in the CBT modality or transference interpretations in psychodynamic therapy). Critchfeld and colleagues [31] used the Structural Analysis of Social Behavior, a well-established measure of interpersonal process, to examine the differences in the nature of therapeutic relationship between cases with good outcome, declining outcome (high level of functioning at termination but a low level at 12-month follow-up), and poor outcome (low level of functioning at both termination and follow-up) in CBT for generalized anxiety disorder. They found that patients in the declining and poor outcome groups showed higher level of control toward therapists. Therapists in the poor outcome group responded to this behavior with the increased attempts to control the session, thus engaging in a power struggle and a vicious cycle of negative interpersonal process, as opposed to therapists in the declining outcome group who granted patients more interpersonal distance. These findings are similar to those of the Vanderbilt studies, which also used the SASB to measure the interpersonal process [95, 96]. Strupp and colleagues found that the interpersonal process associated with poor outcome was characterized by negative complementarity (interpersonally disaffiliative communications) and higher evidence of therapists' hostile control. Therapists in the Vanderbilt II study who underwent extensive training in a manualized form of psychodynamic treatment specifically focused on patient–therapist relationship and managing maladaptive interpersonal patterns, however, showed more negative disaffiliative process and became more authoritarian and defensive, despite exhibiting good adherence to the model. In fact, as mentioned before, it appears that, faced with the difficulties in therapeutic relationship, therapists increased rigid adherence to the model, which negatively affected the alliance and the outcome.

Several small-sample qualitative studies attempted to investigate factors that contribute to the resolution of the alliance ruptures. Foreman and Marmar [97] selected six patients who initially displayed poor alliance out of a sample of 52 patients undergoing short-term dynamic psychotherapy of bereavement. Of these patients, three had improved alliance over the course of treatment and had good outcome, while the other three did not improve alliance and had poor outcome. The researchers found that the alliance improved when therapists directly addressed patient's defenses, guilt and expectation of punishment, patient's negative feelings toward the therapist, and linked the problematic feeling in relation to therapist with patient's defenses. When therapists' interventions failed to directly address problems in the relationship, the alliance did not improve.

Lansford [98] specifically studied weakening and repairs in the alliance by looking at six cases in short-term psychotherapy. Independent raters assessed the effectiveness in repairing weakened alliance by observing segments of sessions and were able to predict outcome based on the degree of successful resolution of ruptures. She also found that when patients initiated addressing problems in the relationship and worked with therapists to repair weakened alliance, it resulted in the highest patients' alliance ratings. Lansford emphasized the role of addressing strains in the alliance during the process of change by stating that "if weakenings [in the alliance] were successfully repaired and resolved, then one could say that the person had been able...to change what was most painful or difficult in his or her life" (p. 366).

Safran, Muran, and colleagues [2, 5, 78, 83, 99] have conducted a series of studies investigating the roles of alliance rupture and resolution in treatment process and outcome. Guided initially by the task-analytic paradigm for the psychotherapy research [100, 101], we have developed and refined a model of the rupture resolution process. Following task analysis procedures, we have employed a combination of qualitative and quantitative methods, and oscillated back and forth between theory building and empirical analysis to progressively refine this model [102].

The preliminary model of the rupture resolution was based on psychodynamic and interpersonal theory [99] and included several stages. First, the patient reenacts with the therapist his or her characteristic maladaptive interpersonal pattern (e.g., anticipating abandonment, patient withdraws). The therapist unwittingly responds in a complementary fashion, thus contributing to the dysfunctional interpersonal cycle (e.g., reacting to patient's withdrawal, the therapist becomes bored, unresponsive, or frustrated). In the next stages, the therapist becomes aware of his role in the enactment and begins disembedding from the negative process by metacommunicating to the patient about the current interaction. He or she explores the patient's experience of it in the "here and now" and accepts responsibility for his or her own contribution to the interaction.

This model was refined through a series of small-scale, intensive, qualitative and quantitative studies. The studies involved identifying sessions with ruptures and rupture resolution, exploratory and qualitative analyses of these sessions using various measures of psychotherapy process in order to operationalize different dimensions of the model components, and testing the hypothesized resolution model on different samples (for more detailed discussion of the model development see [78]). The resulting general model of rupture resolution includes four stages of interactions between patient and therapist: (1) attending to the rupture marker, (2) exploring the rupture experience, (3) exploring the avoidance, and (4) emergence of wish or need. Rupture events were categorized into two major types: confrontation ruptures and withdrawal ruptures [99]. A confrontation rupture is characterized by an aggressive and accusatory statement of resentment or dissatisfaction in regard to the therapist or some aspect of the therapy process. A withdrawal rupture is characterized by patient disengaging from the therapist, some aspect of the therapy process or from his or her own internal experience. The resolution process for confrontation and withdrawal ruptures follows different exploratory pathways (stages 2, 3, and 4). The typical progression in the resolution of confrontation ruptures involves moving through feelings of anger to feelings of disappointment and hurt over having been failed by the therapist to contacting underlying vulnerability and the wish to be nurtured. The avoidant operations in this case typically involve fear of being too vulnerable associated with the expectation of rejection by therapist.

The progression in the resolution of withdrawal ruptures involves moving through increasingly clearer articulations of discontent to self-assertion and becoming aware of the wish for agency. The avoidance that emerges usually concerns the fear of one's aggression and the expectation of retaliation by the therapist.

As mentioned above, small quantitative studies were conducted to test the resolution model (see [78]). The results of these studies provided evidence consistent with the presence of the hypothesized components of the model in resolution sessions and demonstrated statistically significant differences between resolution and nonresolution sessions [77]. The clear limitation of these studies is a small number of cases on which the findings are based. Currently, a study that will attempt to verify the model on a large number of cases is in progress.

In the course of the development of the model of rupture resolution described above, Safran and his colleagues [5, 99] created a self-report measure for identifying ruptures in the alliance and rupture resolution events and establishing their relationship to overall outcome. The postsession questionnaire (PSQ) is completed by both patient and therapist after each psychotherapy session. It includes direct questions about the presence of a rupture in the alliance ("Did you experience any problem or tension in your relationship with your therapist/patient during the session?") and their resolution ("To what degree do you feel this problem was resolved by the end of the session?" [rated on a five-point scale]), as well as the Rupture Resolution Questionnaire (RRQ) specifically designed to identify the presence of experiences hypothesized to be associated with the rupture resolution process (RRQ; Safran JD, Muran JC, Winkelman E. Rupture Resolution Questionnaire. In: Unpublished measure. New York, 1996). This measure will be discussed in more detail below. Several studies (see [99] for a review) demonstrated the psychometric properties of the PSQ, including its ability to detect ruptures and rupture resolution, as well as its predictive validity. In a study of 128 cases [103], patient- and therapist-reported resolution (as measured by a direct query) was found to be positively related to depth of in-session exploration and therapeutic alliance, as rated by patient and therapist. Early session patient and therapist reports of rupture resolution negatively predicted patient dropout. These findings were based on medium to large effects ($r = .22–.48$).

The proposed model of the rupture resolution was further investigated through a series of studies that examined the efficacy of brief relational therapy (BRT) [2], a short-term treatment that integrates principles emerging from rupture resolution research with principles of relational Psychoanalysis. A treatment study of 128 personality-disordered patients compared the BRT, short-term psychodynamic treatment of a more traditional nature, and CBT [103]. Although all three treatments were equally effective for patients who completed treatment, the BRT was significantly more superior to the other two modalities based on the dropout rates. Another study attempted to evaluate the efficacy of the BRT with patients who have difficulties in establishing a therapeutic alliance and are at risk for premature termination [104]. Sixty patients were randomly assigned to either the psychodynamic treatment or CBT model. Patients were monitored early in treatment to identify those who were having difficulties in establishing an alliance with their therapists and were at risk for dropout. These patients were offered to be reassigned to a therapist from another treatment condition: either to BRT or to the control for their previous treatment (i.e., patients who were treated in the CBT modality were transferred to the traditional psychodynamic treatment, whereas patients from the traditional psychodynamic treatment were switched to the CBT). Of the 60 patients in the study, 18 met criteria for a switch and were offered an opportunity to be reassigned. Ten patients agreed to be transferred to another treatment modality. Of the five patients assigned to the BRT, three completed treatment with good outcome, one had to leave the city due to a job change after completing midphase (with good outcome), and one dropped out. Of the five patients transferred to the control conditions, all five dropped out. Although the sample size in this study was small, it provided preliminary evidence of the superiority of BRT, a treatment which employs interventions specifically geared to rupture resolution for patients who have difficulties in establishing and maintaining the therapeutic alliance and are, therefore, at risk for poor outcome and dropout.

## Clinical Illustration of the Resolution Process in Confrontation Ruptures

Cindy was a participant in the above-discussed study evaluating the efficacy of the BRT with patients who have difficulties in establishing therapeutic alliance and are at risk for premature termination [104]. She was a 38-year-old divorced woman who was attempting to make it in a career as an actress. She sought short-term therapy to work on what she termed her lack of self-confidence, as well as a tendency toward procrastination and a lack of perseverance. Cindy described the relationships in her life as generally "shaky," and herself as a "negative and angry person." She also reported having difficulty in separating from her family. Cindy reported having been in longer-term therapy on three previous occasions, but was uncertain about whether or not these experiences had been beneficial.

The sessions described below were ones in which Cindy had reported that there had been a problem or tension in her relationship with therapist. The sessions selected were those that had achieved the highest ratings on the resolution question ("To what extent was [this problem] resolved by the end of the session?" rated on a five-point scale), from Cindy in each of the treatment conditions (CBT and BRT). The two senior authors (JDS and JCM) examined videotapes of these sessions and combined their observations to develop consensually based narratives describing the most salient features of each session.

## Before Reassignment (cognitive–behavior therapy, Session 5; Resolution rating: 3)

Cindy is an angry, critical, single woman in her mid-thirties, with a dramatic manner. The therapist (a woman of approximately the same age) is 5 minutes late for the session and Cindy is upset that the therapist is "rattled about being late," because it indicates to her that "you get rattled like I do." The therapist denies being rattled and then attempts to explore Cindy's concerns about her in greater detail. Cindy admits to not having confidence in the therapist or the treatment. Throughout the session, the therapist has somewhat of an edge to her and Cindy seems to be alternately angry and cowed. She admits to attending a weight control clinic at the same time she is in treatment, and the therapist speculates that Cindy may be trying to undermine her treatment. When asked what her motivation for this might be, Cindy compliantly speculates that maybe she does not want to beat her father. The therapist says, "Don't specula-te...what would happen if you took the next step?" Cindy responds, "I feel badly talking about this. I feel I'm making you angry at me. I feel like I'm being difficult." The therapist asks Cindy to think about how she might be able to test their relationship or experiment to see if there is some way that she can become more trusting about the therapy. "Why don't you experiment with putting aside your doubts? What would that be like for you?" Cindy suggests that she could try, but she appears compliant and subdued. The therapist suggests that it is important for them to actually start working and to adopt a problem-solving attitude. When asked what she is experiencing, Cindy replies that she is feeling reprimanded and that she feels like she is being difficult. Consistent with study protocol, Cindy was offered a transfer to a different treatment and therapist.

## After Reassignment (Brief Relational Therapy, Session 6; Resolution rating: 3)

Cindy begins the session with an angry, demanding tirade, "I don't feel this is helping me. There is nothing worthwhile about this." The therapist (a man of approximately the same age) responds, "I guess I'm feeling a little stuck. I understand there hasn't been the kind of progress you want... and I guess... watching the tapes, I'm aware that I've also been acting a little defensive... I guess feeling that you're questioning my competency. And it may be affecting my work a little." Cindy responds, "That's your problem. The bottom line is that I'm stuck. And I resent your implying that it's my fault." The therapist replies, "Well, we need to come up with a way of working together that's more profitable for you." Cindy responds: "That makes me feel there's no plan here. I feel we're directionless. You don't work with dreams. I want to feel you can handle me." The therapist attempts to empathize, "you're really feeling angry about not getting what you want here." This leads to a shift in Cindy's focus. She tells the therapist about a community meeting she participated in between sessions, during which she felt angry, powerless, humiliated and "like a child."

The therapist attempts to explore her feelings, and she vacillates between anger and tears in a somewhat histrionic style. She lists a litany of slights she has experienced in her life and then returns the focus to therapeutic relationship by asking the therapist what he meant earlier when he said he "felt stuck." The therapist replies, "I want to apologize if it felt I was blaming you. I'm just trying to understand what's going on here." Cindy responds, "I think I'm being cooperative." The therapist says, "Did you hear me saying that you're not?" Cindy, "I guess I feel like I get the message that it's not okay to be angry." The therapist acknowledges that he may, at times, communicate this but takes responsibility for his contribution: "When you get angry at me it gets to me sometimes. It's not that you shouldn't get angry...but I let it get to me sometimes."

Cindy softens and suggests that she may in part be "dumping" on him because it feels like a "safe place." "I can act powerful here, but I can't in real life." She becomes tearful, lapses into hysterical crying, and then abruptly stops. The therapist says, "I feel like you're kind of asking me for help, and I'd like to take care of you. I'm just not sure how right now." At first Cindy denies asking for help, but later in the session she spontaneously suggests that maybe she's being overly dramatic, but that she really does want his help and sympathy. This request has an authentic flavor to it (clinical example reprinted with permission from Safran JD, Muran JC, Samstag L, Winston A. Evaluating an alliance focused treatment for potential treatment failures. Psychotherapy 2005;42: 512–531).

This session clearly contains some of the same themes as the session with the previous therapist: Cindy's anger at the therapist, her questions about the therapist's competence, and her concerns about being blamed for being uncooperative and for being angry. In contrast, however, the therapist responds less defensively. He acknowledges responsibility for his own feelings and his contributions to the interaction and attempts to explore the interaction between them. He attempts to empathize with her anger at him and the unmet needs underlying her anger. Cindy gradually moves from an angry, demanding, blaming stance to one in which she accepts some responsibility for her displaced anger and begins to acknowledge her more vulnerable feelings. This transition on the patient's part, from demanding and blaming to acknowledgement of underlying vulnerability, is characteristic of the resolution process in confrontation ruptures.

## Reconceptualizing the Alliance

Building on Bordin's [29, 30] transtheoretical tripartite model of alliance, contemporary relational psychoanalytic thinking [105, 106], and their empirical research on alliance ruptures and their resolution, Safran and Muran [2, 5, 18] have proposed a reconceptualization of the alliance as an "ongoing process of intersubjective negotiation, that is, the negotiation of the respective needs of two independent subjects." As discussed above, three dimensions of the alliance outlined by Bordin (bond, tasks, and goals) are interdependent and influence each other in an ongoing fashion. When disagreements about therapeutic tasks and goals arise, a strong preexisting bond between patient and therapist allows them to constructively negotiate the problem. Moreover, successful resolution of the rupture through negotiation between different perspectives enhances patient's feelings of trust and provides patient with an experience of authentic relatedness [84]. Furthermore, in the process of a constructive negotiation with a therapist, patient develops a capacity to negotiate the needs of the self versus the needs of the others, which, according to Safran and Muran [5], constitutes an "ongoing challenge of human existence" [5, p. 236].

Safran and his colleagues [5, 18] emphasize that negotiation of therapeutic tasks and goals is a ubiquitous phenomenon in psychotherapy occurring both explicitly and implicitly (out of conscious awareness of participants). However, when there is a rupture in the alliance, the process of negotiation itself becomes the most salient feature of the change-producing therapeutic process. Safran and colleagues [5] also point out that this process should not be aimed at superficial agreement and compliance but rather reflect a "genuine confrontation between individuals with conflicting views, needs, or agendas" (p. 236).

As described above, Winkelman, Safran, and Muran (Safran JD, Muran JC, Winkelman E. Rupture Resolution Questionnaire. In: Unpublished measure. New York, 1996) developed a self-report measure, the RRQ, to identify the presence of experiences hypothesized to be associated with the process of rupture resolution. The RRQ can be conceptualized as a measure of alliance as negotiation. Unlike most measures of the alliance described in the previous section, which focus on the agreement between patient and therapist, the RRQ focuses on experiences associated and resulting from the constructive negotiation of conflict between them. Initially, 68 items believed to reflect the patient's experience of constructive negotiation of the therapeutic relationship were generated by a team of psychotherapy researchers. These items were subjected to a content validation procedure involving relevancy ratings first by 10 senior clinicians and then by 60 graduate students in clinical psychology or recently graduated clinicians. Based on the results of the reliability and item analyses, 18 items were retained to construct the RRQ. Patients were asked to fill out the RRQ whenever they had indicated that they experienced a problem or tension in their relationship with their therapists during the session. The items of the RRQ are reprinted below:

Please rate the extent to which each of the following statements reflects your experience during this session

| Not at all | | Somewhat | | | Definitely |
|---|---|---|---|---|---|
| 1. I felt a closer connection with my therapist | 1 | 2 | 3 | 4 | 5 |
| 2. I discovered feelings toward my therapist that I had not been fully aware of | 1 | 2 | 3 | 4 | 5 |
| 3. My therapist and I were able to work through a conflict and connect in a stronger way | 1 | 2 | 3 | 4 | 5 |
| 4. I saw how I was contributing to the difficulties my therapist and I were having | 1 | 2 | 3 | 4 | 5 |
| 5. I acted in a way that felt more authentic or genuine for me | 1 | 2 | 3 | 4 | 5 |
| 6. I recognized and accepted my therapist's limitations | 1 | 2 | 3 | 4 | 5 |
| 7. I felt freer to make mistakes with my therapist | 1 | 2 | 3 | 4 | 5 |
| 8. I became aware of ways in which I avoid creating conflicts and misunderstandings with my therapist | 1 | 2 | 3 | 4 | 5 |
| 9. I saw that I can expose risky feelings and not be rejected/ criticized by my therapist | 1 | 2 | 3 | 4 | 5 |
| 10. I began to get the sense that I don't have to protect my therapist | 1 | 2 | 3 | 4 | 5 |
| 11. I felt more comfortable with expressing vulnerability or anger toward my therapist | 1 | 2 | 3 | 4 | 5 |
| 12. I told my therapist something I had been hesitant to say | 1 | 2 | 3 | 4 | 5 |
| 13. I felt able to disagree with my therapist | 1 | 2 | 3 | 4 | 5 |
| 14. I began to accept a part of myself which I had not fully acknowledged before | 1 | 2 | 3 | 4 | 5 |
| 15. I said something to my therapist which I had felt for a while and it left me with a sense of relief | 1 | 2 | 3 | 4 | 5 |
| 16. I saw that I was doing something to distance myself from my therapist or push him/her away | 1 | 2 | 3 | 4 | 5 |
| 17. I felt more trusting of my therapist | 1 | 2 | 3 | 4 | 5 |
| 18. I was afraid something I said would upset or hurt my therapist but I found out that it did not | 1 | 2 | 3 | 4 | 5 |

The studies of the psychometric properties of the instrument [107, 108] found the RRQ to be a soundly reliable instrument with an adequate internal consistency (Cronbach's $\alpha = 0.87$). Concurrent validity was established by examining the relationship between the RRQ and various measures of psychotherapy process. The RRQ was shown to be positively related to patient and therapist ratings of session helpfulness, depth of therapeutic exploration, and strength of the therapeutic alliance as measured by the WAI. Predictive validity was examined by analyzing the relationships between the RRQ and patient- and therapist-rated measures of the global outcome of treatment. The RRQ was found to be a significant predictor of the improvement in the patient's overall level of functioning (as rated by therapist), a significant predictor of the decrease in severity of patient's interpersonal problems (as rated by therapist), and a significant predictor of the decrease in the severity of symptoms (as rated by patient). The correlation coefficients were in the medium range (0.28–0.41).

In addition, the RRQ was found to make a unique and significant contribution above and beyond the WAI to predict the improvement in interpersonal functioning as rated by therapist. Overall, these results suggest that this measure is a potentially useful instrument for future research on psychotherapy process and outcome.

## Summary and Conclusions

More than 60 years of empirical research on psychotherapy outcome and process strongly supports the following findings: (1) psychotherapy in general is effective; (2) different types of psychotherapy are equally effective in producing therapeutic change; (3) measures of therapeutic relationship correlate more highly with outcome than do specialized therapy techniques; and (4) the quality of the therapeutic alliance appears to be the most robust predictor of the outcome.

The concept of the therapeutic alliance has been refined over the years, with multiple instruments designed to measure it, thereby contributing to the definition of the construct. The recent reconceptualization of the alliance as an ongoing negotiation requires further empirical investigation. The alliance appears to be dynamic, and fluctuations in the alliance (i.e., ruptures and resolutions) appear to be important change-related events in the therapy process. The empirical research on alliance ruptures and resolution is promising. However, the number of studies investigating this issue is limited; most of the studies are qualitative and based on small sample sizes. Nevertheless, the preliminary evidence suggests that the process of recognizing and addressing ruptures in the therapeutic alliance may play an important role in preventing patient dropout and in facilitating good outcome. There is also evidence that even experienced clinicians experience difficulties in recognizing and resolving ruptures in the alliance. Continued research on the mechanism of rupture resolution will clearly have implications for practice, potentially providing clinicians with guidelines on how to effectively deal with problems in the alliance.

## References

1. Norcross JC. Empirically supported therapy relationships. In: Norcross JC, ed. Psychotherapy relationships that work. New York: Oxford University Press; 2002. p. 3–16.
2. Safran JD, Muran JC. Negotiating the therapeutic alliance: A relational treatment guide. New York: Guilford Press; 2000.
3. Lambert MJ, Okiishi JC. The effects of the individual psychotherapist and implications for future research. Clinical Psychology: Science and Practice 1997; 17: 364–366.
4. Horvath AO, Bedi RP. The alliance. In: Norcross JC, ed. Psychotherapy relationships that work. New York: Oxford University Press; 2002.

5. Safran JD, Muran JC, Samstag LW, Stevens C. Repairing alliance ruptures. In: Norcross JC, ed. Psychotherapy relationships that work. New York: Oxford University; 2002.

6. Kohut H. How does analysis cure? Chicago: University of Chicago Press; 1984.

7. Garfield SL, Bergin AE. Introduction and historical overview. In: Bergin AE, Garfield SL, ed. Handbook of psychotherapy and behavior change. 4th edn New York: Wiley; 1994. p. 3–18.

8. Bergin AE, Lambert MJ. The evaluation of therapeutic outcomes. In: Garfield SL, Bergin AE, eds. Handbook of psychotherapy and behavior change. 2nd edn. New York: Wiley; 1978. p. 217–270.

9. Hoglend P. Psychotherapy research: New findings and implications for training and practice. Journal of Psychotherapy Practice and Research 1999; 8: 257–263.

10. Lambert MJ, Barley DE. Research summary on the therapeutic relationship and psychotherapy outcome. In: Norcross JC, ed. Psychotherapy relationships that work. New York: Oxford University Press; 2002. p. 17–32.

11. Lambert MJ, Bergin AE. The effectiveness of psychotherapy. In: Bergin AE, Garfield SL, eds. Handbook of psychotherapy and behavior change. 4th edn New York: Wiley; 1994. p. 143–189.

12. Luborsky L, Singer B, Luborsky L. Comparative studies of psychotherapies: Is it true that "everyone has won and all must have prizes"? Archives of General Psychiatry 1975; 32(8): 995–1008.

13. Dobson KS. A meta-analysis of the efficacy of cognitive therapy for depression. Journal of Consulting and Clinical Psychology 1989; 57: 414–419.

14. Shapiro DA, Shapiro D. Meta-analysis of comparative therapy outcome research: A replication and refinement. Psychological Bulletin 1982; 92: 581–614.

15. Svartberg M, Stiles TC. Therapeutic alliance, therapist competence and client change in short-term anxiety-provoking psychotherapy. Psychotherapy Research 1994; 4: 20–33.

16. Lambert MJ. Implications of outcome research for psychotherapy integration. In: Norcross JC, Goldstein MR, eds. Handbook of psychotherapy integration. New York: Basic; 1992.

17. Butler SF, Strupp HH. Specific and nonspecific factors in psychotherapy: A problematic paradigm for psychotherapy research. Psychotherapy 1986; 23: 30–39.

18. Safran JD. The relational turn, the therapeutic alliance and psychotherapy research: Strange bedfellows or postmodern marriage? Contemporary Psychoanalysis 2003; 39: 449–475.

19. Breuer J, Freud S. The standard edition of the complete psychological works of Sigmund Freud. London: Hogarth Press; 1893–1895/1995.

20. Freud S. An outline of psycho-analysis. Standard Edition ed. London: Hogarth Press; 1940/1964.

21. Freud S. The dynamics of transference. Standard Edition ed. London: Hogarth Press; 1912/1958.

22. Sterba R. The fate of the ego in analytic therapy. International Journal of Psycho-Analysis. 1934; 15: 117–126.

23. Zetzel E. Current concepts of transference. International Journal of Psycho-Analysis 1956; 37: 369–375.

24. Zetzel E. The analytic situation. In: Litman RE, ed. Psychoanalysis in America. New York: International Universities Press; 1966. p. 86–106.

25. Greenson R. The technique and practice of psychoanalysis. New York: International Universities Press; 1967.

26. Rogers CR. Client-centered therapy. Boston: Houghton Mifflin; 1951.

27. Rogers CR. The necessary and sufficient conditions of therapeutic personality change. Journal of Counseling Psychology 1957; 21: 95–103.

28. Luborsky L. Helping alliances in psychotherapy. In: Clanghorn JL, ed. Successful psychotherapy. New York: Brunner/Mazel; 1976.

29. Bordin E. The generalizability of the psychoanalytic concept of the working alliance. Psychotherapy: Theory, Research and Practice 1979; 16: 252–260.
30. Bordin E. Theory and research on the therapeutic working alliance: New directions. In: Hovarth AO, Greenberg LS, ed. The working alliance: Theory, research and practice. New York: John Wiley & Sons; 1994. p. 13–37.
31. Constantino MJ, Castonguay LG, Schut AJ. The working alliance: A flagship for the "scientist-practitioner" model in psychotherapy. In: Tryon GS, ed. Counseling based on process research: Applying what we know. Boston: Allyn and Bacon; 2002.
32. Horvath AO, Luborsky L. The role of the therapeutic alliance in psychotherapy. Journal of Consulting and Clinical Psychology 1993; 61(4): 561–573.
33. Wolfe BE, Goldfried MR. Research on psychotherapy integration: Recommendations and conclusions from an NIMH workshop. Journal of Consulting and Clinical Psychology 1988; 56: 448–451.
34. Watson J, Greenberg LS. Alliance ruptures and repairs in experiential therapy. In Session: Psychotherapy in Practice 1995; 1: 19–32.
35. Arnkoff D. Two Examples of Strains in the Therapeutic Alliance in an Integrative Cognitive Therapy. In Session: Psychotherapy in Practice 1995; 1: 33–46.
36. Goldfried MR, Castonguay LG. Behavior therapy: Redefining strengths and limitations. Behavior Therapy 1993; 24: 505–526.
37. Newman C. The therapeutic relationship and alliance in short-term cognitive therapy. In: Safran JD, Muran JC, eds. The therapeutic alliance in brief psychotherapy. Washington, DC: American Psychological Association Press; 1998. p. 95–122.
38. Raue PJ, Goldfried MR. The therapeutic alliance in cognitive behavioral therapy. In: Horvath AO, ed. The working alliance: Theory, research and practice. New York: John Wiley & Sons; 1994. p. 131–152.
39. Rait DS. The therapeutic alliance in couples and family therapy: Theory in practice. In Session: Psychotherapy in Practice 1995; 1(1): 59–72.
40. Rait D. Perspectives on the therapeutic alliance in brief couple and family therapy. In: Safran JD, Muran JC, eds. The therapeutic alliance in brief psychotherapy. Washington DC: American Psychologic Association Books; 1998. p.171–191.
41. MacKenzie KR. The alliance in time-limited group psychotherapy. In: Safran JD, Muran JC, eds. The therapeutic alliance in brief psychotherapy. Washington, D.C.: American Psychological Association Books; 1988. p. 193–216.
42. Safran JD, Muran, JC. The resolution of ruptures in the therapeutic alliance. Journal of Counseling and Clinical Psychology 1996; 64: 447–458.
43. Martin DJ, Garske JP, Davis MK. Relation of the therapeutic alliance with outcome and other variables: A meta-analytic review. Journal of Counseling and Clinical Psychology 2000; 68(3): 438–450.
44. Horvath AO. Research on the alliance. In: Horvath AO, Greenberg LS, eds. The working alliance: Theory, research, and practice. New York: Wiley; 1994. p. 259–286.
45. Luborsky L, Crits-Cristoph P, Alexander L, Margolis M, Cohen M. Two helping alliance methods for predicting outcomes of psychotherapy: A counting signs vs. a global rating method. Journal of Nervous and Mental Disease 1983; 171: 480–491.
46. Luborsky L, McLellan AT, Woody GE, O'Brien CP, Auerback A. Therapist success and its determinants. Archives of General Psychiatry 1985; 42: 602–611.
47. O'Malley SS, Suh CS, Strupp HH. The Vanderbilt Psychotherapy Process Scale: A report on the scale development and a process-outcome study. Journal of Consulting and Clinical Psychology 1983; 51(4): 581–586.
48. Gomes-Schwartz B. Effective ingredients in psychotherapy: Prediction of outcome from process variables. Journal of Consulting and Clinical Psychology 1978; 46(5): 1023–1035.
49. Hartley DE, Strupp HH. The therapeutic alliance: Its relationship to outcome in brief psychotherapy. In: Masling J, editor. Empirical studies in analytic theories. New Jersey: Erlbaum; 1983. p. 1–37.

50. Marziali E. Three viewpoints on the therapeutic alliance: Similarities, differences, and associations with psychotherapy outcome. The Journal of Nervous and Mental Disease 1984; 172: 417–423.
51. Marziali E, Marmar C, Krupnick J. Therapeutic alliance scales: Development and relationship to psychotherapy outcome. American Journal of Psychiatry 1981; 138(3): 361–364.
52. Marmar CR, Weiss DS, Gaston L. Toward the validation of the California Therapeutic Alliance Rating System. Psychological Assessment 1989; 1(1): 46–52.
53. Gaston L, Marmar C. The California Psychotherapy Alliance Scales. In: Horvath AO, Greenberg LS, eds. The working alliance: Theory, research, and practice. New York: Wiley; 1994. p. 85–108.
54. Gaston L. The concept of the alliance and its role in psychotherapy; theoretical and empirical considerations. Psychotherapy 1990; 27: 143–153.
55. Horvath AO, Greenberg LS. Development and validation of the Working Alliance Inventory. Journal of Consulting and Clinical Psychology 1989; 36(2): 223–233.
56. Tracey TJ, Kokotovic AM. Factor structure of the Working Alliance Inventory. Psychological Assessment 1989; 1(3): 207–210.
57. Hatcher RL, Barends AW. Patient's view of the alliance in psychotherapy: Exploratory factor analysis of three alliance measures. Journal of Consulting and Clinical Psychology 1996; 64: 1326–1336.
58. Kivlighan DM, Shaughnessy P. Analysis of the development of the working alliance using hierarchical linear modeling. Journal of Counseling and Clinical Psychology 1995; 42(3): 338–349.
59. Tichenor V, Hill CE. A comparison of six measures of working alliance. Psychotherapy: Theory, Research, Practice and Training 1989; 26(2): 195–199.
60. Fenton LR, Cecero J, Nich C, Frankforter T, Carroll KM. Perspective is everything: the predictive validity of working alliance instruments. Journal of Psychotherapy Practice and Research 2001; 10(4): 262–268.
61. Horvath AO, Symonds BD. Relation between working alliance and outcome in psychotherapy: A meta-analysis. Journal of Consulting and Clinical Psychology 1991; 38: 139–149.
62. Hatcher RL, Barends A, Hansell J, Gutfreund MJ. Patient's and therapist's shared and unique views of the therapeutic alliance: An investigation using confirmatory factor analysis in a nested design. Psychoanalysis Quarterly 1995; 63: 636–643.
63. Marmar CR, Horowitz MJ, Weiss DS, Marziali E. The development of the Therapeutic Alliance Rating System. In: Greenberg LS, Pinsof WM, eds. The psychotherapeutic process: A research handbook. New York: Guilford Press; 1986.
64. Kokotovic AM, Tracey TJ. Working alliance in the early phase of counseling. Journal of Counseling Psychology 1990; 37(1): 16–21.
65. Tryon GS, Kane AS. Client involvement, working alliance, and type of therapy termination. Psychotherapy Research 1995; 5(3): 189–198.
66. Gelso CJ, Carter JA. Components of the psychotherapy relationship: Their interaction and unfolding during treatment. Journal of Counseling Psychology 1994; 41(3): 296–306.
67. Bachelor A, Salame R. Participants' perceptions of dimensions of the therapeutic alliance over the course of therapy. Journal of Psychotherapy Practice and Research 2000; 9: 39–53.
68. Krupnick J, Sotsky SM, Simmens A, Moyer J, Elkin I, Watkins J, et al. The role of the alliance in psychotherapy and pharmacotherapy outcome: Findings in the National Institute of Mental Health treatment of depression collaborative research program. Journal of Consulting and Clinical Psychology 1996; 64: 532–539.
69. Kivlighan DM, Shaughnessy P. Patterns of working alliance development: A typology of client's working alliance ratings. Journal of Counseling Psychology 2000; 47(3): 362–371.

70. Tracey TJ, Ray PB. The stages of successful time-limited counseling: An interactional examination. Journal of Counseling Psychology 1984; 31: 13–27.
71. Golden BR, Robbins SB. The working alliance within time-limited therapy. Professional Psychology: Research and Practice 1990; 21(6): 476–481.
72. Horvath AO, Marx RW. The development and decay of the working alliance during time-limited counselling. Canadian Journal of Counselling 1991; 24(4): 240–260.
73. Stiles WB, Glick MJ, Osatuke K, Hardy GE, Shapiro DA, Agnew-Davies R, et al. Patterns of alliance development and the rupture-repair hypothesis: Are productive relationships U-shaped or V-shaped? Journal of Counseling Psychology 2004; 51(1): 81–92.
74. Strauss JL, Hayes AM, Johnson SL, Newman CF, Brown GK, Barber JP, et al. Early alliance, alliance ruptures, and symptom change in a nonrandomized trial of cognitive therapy for avoidant and obsessive–compulsive personality disorders. Journal of Consulting and Clinical Psychology 2006; 74(2): 337–345.
75. Wallner Samstag L, Muran JC, Safran JD. Defining and identifying ruptures in psychotherapy. In: Charman D, ed. Core concepts in brief dynamic therapy: Training for effectiveness. Hillsdale: Lawrence Erlbaum Associates; 2004. p. 187–214.
76. Alexander F, French TM. Psychoanalytic therapy: Principles and application. New York: Ronald Press; 1946.
77. Weiss J, Sampson H, Group. TMZPR. The psychoanalytic process: Theory, clinical observations, and empirical research. New York: Guilford Press; 1986.
78. Safran JD, Muran JC. The resolution of ruptures in the therapeutic alliance. Journal of Consulting and Clinical Psychology 1996; 64(3): 447–458.
79. Safran JD. Breaches in the therapeutic alliance: An area for negotiating authentic relatedness. Psychotherapy: Theory, Research and Practice 1993a; 30: 11–24.
80. Safran JD, Muran JC. Has the concept of the alliance outlived its usefulness. Psychotherapy 2006; 43: 286–291.
81. Jones E. Therapeutic action: A guide to psychoanalytic therapy. Northvale, NJ: Jason Aronson; 2000.
82. Safran JD. The therapeutic alliance rupture as a transtheoretical phenomenon: Definitional and conceptual issues. Journal of Psychotherapy Integration 1993; 3: 33–49.
83. Safran JD, Crocker P, McMain S, Murray P. The therapeutic alliance rupture as a therapy event for empirical investigation. Psychotherapy: Theory, Research and Practice 1990; 27: 154–165.
84. Safran JD. Breaches in the therapeutic alliance: An area for negotiating authentic relatedness. Psychotherapy: Theory, Research and Practice 1993; 30: 11–24.
85. Strupp HH. Success and failure in time-limited psychotherapy. Further evidence (Comparison 4). Archives of General Psychiatry 1980; 37: 947–954.
86. Rennie DL. Clients' deference in psychotherapy. Journal of Counseling Psychology 1994; 41(4): 427–437.
87. Regan AM, Hill CE. Investigation of what clients and counselors do not say in brief therapy. Journal of Counseling Psychology 1992; 39: 168–174.
88. Hill CE, Thompson BJ, Cogar MC, Denman DW. Beneath the surface of long-term therapy: Therapist and client report of their own and each other's covert processes. Journal of Counseling Psychology 1993; 40(3): 278–287.
89. Rhodes R, Hill CE, Thompson B, Elliot R. Client retrospective recall of resolved and unresolved misunderstanding events. Counseling Psychology 1994; 41: 473–483.
90. Hill CE, Nutt-Williams E, Heaton KJ, Thompson BJ, Rhodes RH. Therapist retrospective recall impasses in long-term psychotherapy: A qualitative analysis. Journal of Counseling Psychology 1996; 43(2): 207–217.
91. Castonguay LG, Goldfried MR, Wiser S, Raue PJ, Hayes AM. Predicting the effect of cognitive therapy for depression: A study of unique and common factors. Journal of Counseling and Clinical Psychology 1996; 64(3): 497–504.

92. Piper WE, Azim H, Joyce AS, McCallum M. Transference interpretations, therapeutic alliance, and outcome in short term individual psychotherapy. Archives of General Psychiatry 1991; 48: 946–953.
93. Piper WE, Ogradniczuk JS, Joyce AS, McCallum M, Rosie JS, O'Kelly JG, et al. Prediction of dropping out in time-limited, interpretive individual psychotherapy. Psychotherapy 1999; 36(2): 114–122.
94. Critchfield KL, Henry WP, Castonguay LG, Borcovec TD. Interpersonal process and outcome in variants of cognitive–behavioral psychotherapy. Journal of Clinical Psychology 1999; 63(2): 31–35.
95. Henry WP, Strupp HH. The therapeutic alliance as interpersonal process. In: Greenberg AOHLS, editor. The working alliance: Theory, research and practice. A. O. Horvath & L. S. Greenberg ed. New York: Wiley; 1994. p. 51–84.
96. Strupp HH. The Vanderbuilt Psychotherapy Studies: Synopsis. Journal of Consulting and Clinical Psychology 1993; 61: 431–433.
97. Foreman SA, Marmar CR. Therapist actions that address initially poor therapeutic alliances in psychotherapy. American Journal of Psychiatry 1985; 142: 922–926.
98. Lansford E. Weakenings and repairs of the working alliance in short-term psychotherapy. Professional Psychology: Research and Practice 1986; 17(4): 364–366.
99. Muran JC. A relational approach to understanding change: Multiplicity and contextualism in a psychotherapy research program. Psychotherapy Research 2002; 12(2): 113–138.
100. Rice LN, Greenberg LS. Patterns of change: Intensive analysis of psychotherapy process. New York: Guilford; 1984.
101. Safran JD, Greenberg LS, Rice LN. Integrating psychotherapy research and practice: Modeling the change process. Psychotherapy: Theory, Research and Practice 1988; 25: 1–17.
102. Safran JD, Muran JC, Samstag LW. Resolving therapeutic alliance ruptures: A task analytic investigation. In: Horvath AO, Greenberg LS, eds. The working alliance: Theory, research, and practice. New York: Wiley; 1994. p. 225–255.
103. Muran JC, Safran JD, Samstag LW, Winston A. Evaluating an alliance-focused treatment for personality disorders. Psychotherapy: Theory, Research, Practice, Training 2005; 42(4): 532–545.
104. Samstag LW, Muran JC, Samstag LW, Winston A. Evaluating alliance-focused intervention for potential treatment failures: A feasibility study and descriptive analysis. Psychotherapy: Theory, Research, Practice, Training 2005; 42(4): 512–531.
105. Benjamin J. The bonds of love. New York: Pantheon Books; 1988.
106. Mitchell SA. Relational concepts in psychoanalysis: An integration. Cambridge, MA: Harvard Universities Press; 1988.
107. Winkelman E, Safran JD, Muran JC. The development and validation of the rupture resolution questionnaire (RRQ). New York: Beth Israel Medical Center, NY; 1998.
108. Proskurov B. Psychometric properties of the Rupture Resolution Questionnaire (RRQ). New York: The New School for Social Research; 2006.

# Chapter 10
# Affect-Focused Techniques in Psychodynamic Psychotherapy

Marc J. Diener and Mark J. Hilsenroth

## Introduction

In a review of the research literature contrasting psychodynamic–interpersonal (PI) and cognitive–behavioral (CB) treatment, Blagys and Hilsenroth [1, 2] identified seven techniques/processes that distinguished PI from CB therapies. In particular, PI treatments contained greater frequency of emotion focus and encouraged patients to express their feelings. This affect-focused process garnered the most evidence for distinguishing PI from CB [1, 2], suggesting a heightened attention in psychodynamic treatments to patient emotions. These findings also point to the next research step, namely investigating the utility of this potentially significant psychodynamic process.

The present chapter explores the importance of affect-focused techniques in psychodynamic therapy from a number of perspectives. We begin with a review of relevant theory concerning affect focus in dynamic treatments. Next, we consider empirical research bearing on both the relevance of these techniques in psychodynamic therapy in general and indications for context-specific use of such techniques. Finally, we highlight the clinical implications of these studies by integrating the research findings with clinical examples of therapeutic interventions. We attempt throughout to underscore the applied relevance of the empirical research findings in a coherent and user-friendly manner.

This chapter is based in part on the doctoral dissertation of the first author. Earlier versions of this chapter were presented at the North American Society for Psychotherapy Research, Newport, RI (2003, November) and the Society for Psychotherapy Research, Rome, Italy (2004, June). We thank Dr. Matthew Blagys for his assistance in reviewing the literature for relevant studies. We are grateful to Dr. Jared DeFife for permission to use his Effect Size Calculator computer software.

M.J. Diener
American School of Professional Psychology, Argosy University/Washington DC,
1550 Wilson Blvd., Suite 600, Arlington, VA 22209
e-mail: mdiener@argosy.edu

R.A. Levy, J.S. Ablon (eds.), *Handbook of Evidence-Based Psychodynamic Psychotherapy*,
DOI: 10.1007/978-1-59745-444-5_10, © Humana Press 2009

## Theory

Many theorists have focused their attention on developing a *definition* or *categorization* of affect, and detailing its relationship to other psychological constructs such as cognition, motivation, drives, primary process, or object relations [3–10]. Nevertheless, the treatment implications of these often meta-psychological theories are not always explicitly articulated. As a result, the following brief review concentrates specifically on the history of an *affective treatment focus* in psychodynamic therapy.

In Breuer and Freud's original formulation [11], they posited that verbalization of a traumatic event would lead to a release of affect and thereby free the patient from the bonds of hysteria [12]. The term "abreaction" refers to this specific affective expression *process*, whereas "catharsis "denotes the *outcome* of this process [13, 14]. Breuer and Freud argued that hysterical symptoms develop when an experience produces intense affect that cannot be discharged through the normal means of reflex actions (such as crying, talking about the incident) or gradual decay brought about by the connection of the affect to conscious material [15]. Thus, Freud came to believe that this pent up affect needed to be released verbally by hypnotically suggesting to the patient to remember unconscious material [15].

However, as Freud's theory evolved and he shifted from hypnotic suggestion to psychoanalysis, Freud also replaced the emphasis on the cathartic method with a greater emphasis on patient resistance [12]. Freud essentially made the following two major modifications to the cathartic method: (1) he dropped the requirement of using hypnosis and (2) he reorganized the significance of patient affect in his theory of change. In place of hypnosis, Freud shifts to an emphasis on analysis of patient resistance to free association [12]. And, instead of considering affective release to be the main mechanism of change, Freud considered the development of insight to be primary.

Still, patient affect retains some degree of significance in Freud's later theory, particularly in his discussion of transference. Freud [16] defined transference as the template (or templates) that guides an individual's erotic life. Freud's distinction between the positive and negative transferences or between affectionate and hostile *feelings,* respectively, provides a crucial link between emotions and transference. He further argued that manifestations of the unconscious transferences make the patient's emotional impulses more immediate and manifest, allowing them to be properly interpreted [16].

We should note, however, that in one of his last papers, Freud's [17] description of the therapeutic process seems to once again highlight the importance of affect in a way that makes affective experiencing appear primary (as in his original formulation in [11]):

> ...[T]he work of analysis aims at inducing the patient to give up the repressions (using the word in the widest sense) belonging to his early development and to replace them by reactions of a sort that would correspond to a psychically mature condition. With this

purpose in view he must be brought to recollect certain experiences *and the affective impulses called up by them which he has for the time being forgotten...*. [H]e produces ideas, if he gives himself up to 'free association', in which we can discover allusions to the repressed experiences *and derivatives of the suppressed affective impulses* as well as reactions against them. And, finally, there are hints of repetitions *of the affects belonging to the repressed material* to be found in actions performed by the patient...[T]he relation of transference, which becomes established towards the analyst, is particularly calculated to favor *the return of these emotional connections.* (pp. 257–258; emphases added).[1]

Alexander and French [19] outlined the primacy of a corrective emotional experience, explaining that genetic (i.e., historical) insights are significant only in so far as they facilitate this corrective emotional experience. They highlighted two fundamental aspects of the corrective emotional experience, namely the exposure to previously intolerable emotional situations (corresponding to the "emotional" component of the corrective emotional experience) in a positive, healing relationship (corresponding to the "corrective...experience" component of the corrective emotional experience). These two components, Alexander and French [19] explain, yield two outcomes that are therapeutically significant. First, "the therapist has an opportunity to help the patient both to see intellectually and to *feel* the irrationality of his emotional reactions" [19, p. 67; emphasis in original]. This is important presumably because the patient gains insight and understanding into his/her distorted subjective reaction to the therapist (similar to Freud, but with perhaps stronger emphasis on the significance of the emotional experience). But, Alexander and French [19] underscore the importance of a *second* result of the experience, one that sets their approach apart from Freud's:

At the same time, the analyst's objective, understanding allows the patient to deal differently with his emotional reactions and thus to make a new settlement of the old problem. The old pattern was an attempt at adaptation on the part of the child to parental behavior. When one link (the parental response) in this interpersonal relationship is changed through the medium of the therapist, the patient's reaction becomes pointless. (p. 67)

According to Alexander and French [19], the patient's maladaptive tendencies originally emerged as a way of dealing with dysfunctional parental behavior. When the therapist, therefore, interacts with the patient in a more positive manner, the patient's maladaptive patterns are no longer necessary, and they disappear.

Affective focus in self-psychology centers around the disruption-restoration process. Inevitably, the patient's experience of his/her relationship with the therapist (which previously had positively impacted the patient's sense of self) takes a turn for the worse as a result of failures on the part of the therapist.

---

[1] See Freud's [18] discussion of the evolution of his technique, where he explained that the underlying purpose of the various interventions he proposed was "to fill in gaps in memory...to overcome resistances due to repression" (p. 148).

When the therapist intervenes and offers the patient an explanation of what has happened (including reference to etiological factors) in an empathic manner, a healing process termed "transmuting internalization" will be set into motion. Empathically offering an explanation of the disruption leads the patient to feel emotionally accepted [20].

Wachtel [21] proposed the use of exposure (to warded-off thoughts, wishes, and *feelings*) to help the patient overcome his/her anxiety-based difficulties. He maintained that this is, in fact, the *purpose* of therapy, rather than the more classical analytic understanding of therapy as helping the patient uncover and renounce infantile wishes and feelings. Wachtel [21] explained that interpretations, although useful as well for clarifying meaning and conveying the therapist's understanding of the patient, are the primary vehicles of exposure in psychodynamic psychotherapy. Wachtel [21] added that mere exposure to the feared experience does not suffice to yield change, since a traumatic exposure can simply confirm the patient's fears. Instead, the therapist must pay attention to and facilitate the patient's sense of mastery and experience of safety in order to effect change.

Related to this approach, McCullough [22] suggested that psychopathology is the result of conflicts (or fears) about feelings, or "affect phobia." More specifically, pathology arises when activating, adaptive feelings (or impulses) are obstructed by defenses (maladaptive thoughts, feelings, or behaviors) and anxieties (inhibitory affects such as anxiety, guilt, shame, and pain). Broadly speaking, McCullough's approach to treatment consists of systematic desensitization of the underlying affect phobia. The systematic desensitization can be divided into interventions that (1) facilitate gradual exposure to the adaptive feelings and (2) prevent the usual defensive response of avoiding the conflict. This general outline of systematic desensitization of the affect phobia yields the following three specific treatment objectives: (1) defensive restructuring, (2) affect restructuring, and (3) restructuring images of self and other. In *defense restructuring*, the therapist helps the patient (a) recognize his/her defensive avoidances and then (b) relinquish them. The defense restructuring objective, therefore, comprises the second component of the broader technique of systematic desensitization, namely response prevention. In *affect restructuring*, the therapist works to facilitate (a) emotional experience and (b) emotional expression, both of which gradually expose the patient to the feared emotion (i.e., the exposure component of systematic desensitization). In *restructuring images of self and other*, the therapist attempts to provide these internal images with more positive valences. This is accomplished by exposing the patient to more benign and positive feelings of himself/herself and others while also pointing out the fears/anxieties that work against such feelings [22].

Fosha's [23] Accelerated Experiential–Dynamic Psychotherapy (AEDP) in many ways parallels the general treatment approach offered by McCullough [22]. Fosha's [23] AEDP can be considered an integrative approach to therapy, which maintains a relational, psychodynamic framework while including components of experiential therapy. In broad terms, AEDP's goal is to facilitate "new emotional experiences." This goal is actualized by drawing on what Fosha calls "core affective experiences." These core affective experiences are the crux of the therapeutic process and are made up of a number of components, including emotions, relational experiences, self states, visceral body states, and the transformation process itself. Core affective experiences result from an intermediate step termed "state transformations." State transformation refers to the process of significant, qualitative shift from one psychological state to another (these states consist of everything we would consider psychological, such as arousal, attention, motivation, affect, cognition, and communication). Overall then, AEDP seeks to facilitate state transformation, which in turn leads to core affective experience in an emotionally engaged relationship [23].

Shear and colleagues [24] outline a "dynamically informed," emotion-focused therapy for treating panic disorder. This treatment includes a psychoeducational component, which offers information about panic disorder and the relevance of emotion, as well as an analysis of emotional reactions and their consequences. In this second component, the therapist and the patient identify triggers to panic symptoms and other unexplained emotional reactions, the personal meaning of these triggers in the context of previous (interpersonal) experiences, and strategies that the patient employs to manage the unexplained emotional reaction. The goal of treatment is to decrease symptoms by increasing awareness and adaptive management of negative emotional reactions [24].

## Research on the Utility of Affect-Focused Techniques in Psychodynamic Psychotherapy

Of the various theorists that we have reviewed, the only one who has subjected his/her concepts (regarding an affective treatment focus) to empirical evaluation is McCullough.[2] McCullough and colleagues [26] examined the relationship between an affective focus and outcome in a study of 16 patients with specific Axis II disorders[3] who received 1 of 2 forms of brief psychodynamic therapy, either short-term dynamic psychotherapy (STDP) or brief adaptation-oriented psychotherapy (BAP). Both of these forms of brief dynamic therapy employ techniques derived from Mann, Malan, Sifneos, and Davanloo, although STDP contains a relatively more active and confrontational therapeutic stance. In BAP, therapists identify and explore maladaptive relationship patterns (past, present, and in the patient–therapist relationship), whereas

---

[2] Shear and colleagues [25] present data comparing CBT, emotion-focused psychotherapy, and imipramine for patients with panic disorder; however, only outcome data are reported with no process ratings utilized to examine specific effects of emotion-focused techniques.

[3] The larger sample of 42 patients, from which the current study was drawn, had to meet criteria for compulsive, avoidant, dependent, passive-aggressive, histrionic or mixed personality disorder and could not have an Axis II diagnosis of paranoid, schizoid, schizotypal, narcissistic, or borderline personality disorder.

STDP therapists are more likely to confront patient defenses as they manifest in the therapy and to evoke affective patient responses. Videotape review of sessions was used to ensure adherence to therapy manuals. The authors found that ratings (made by independent judges) of any of three therapist interventions (interpretations of patient–therapist relationship, interpretations of significant other relationships, and clarifications), *which was followed by* patient-affective response, correlated $r = 0.51$, $p = 0.05$, $N=16$ with a composite outcome score (average of residual gain scores across four outcome measures, i.e., the Social Adjustment Scale and three Target complaints) [26]. These results suggest that therapists consider interventions that facilitate patient-affective response. More specifically, therapists may improve their effectiveness by designing their interpretations and/or clarifications in a manner that is likely to result in a patient-affective response. Similarly, Porter (as cited in [27]) found that patients had better outcomes when interpretations were followed by experienced affect in contrast to a defensive response.

The results of McCullough et al. [26] and Porter (as cited in [27]) focus specifically on the therapeutic impact of affective-evoking *interpretations* and/ or *clarifications*. Hill et al. [28], however, studied the potential impact of *various* forms of interventions that were related to patient-affective response. In this study, therapists[4] provided brief psychotherapy (maximum 20 sessions). Clients were five females with problems of self-esteem and relationship issues, three of whom were diagnosed as primarily dysthymic, and one was diagnosed as primarily cyclothymic. Clients reviewed a tape of each session and rated their reactions (up to five) to each therapist speaking turn using the *Client Reactions System* (40 nonmutually exclusive categories, later reduced to 21 relatively independent categories). A proportion was calculated by dividing the total number of reactions for each category by the total number of reactions identified by the client. Pre–post changes were measured by the average change score on eight self-report measures [28].

Results indicated that client ratings of having "a greater awareness or deepening of feelings or could express my emotions better" after therapist interventions were associated ($r = 0.81$, $p > 0.10$, $N = 5$) with greater pre–post changes in outcome, although this correlation was not statistically significant (due to the small sample size) [28]. These findings suggest that a positive relationship with outcome emerges when therapist interventions foster awareness or increased experience of emotions and/or help patients express their emotions better.

Hilsenroth and colleagues [29] used a larger sample than Hill et al. [28], and the analyses yielded statistically significant findings. In this study, 21 patients with Axis I diagnosis of a depressive spectrum disorder (major depressive disorder, depressive disorder not otherwise specified, dysthymic disorder, or

---

[4] Therapists rated themselves as more psychoanalytic ($M = 3.75$, SD = 0.50) than humanistic ($M = 2.75$, SD = 0.96) or behavioral ($M = 1.50$, SD = 0.58) on five-point scales [28].

adjustment disorder with depressed mood) were treated with 1–2 times weekly short-term psychodynamic psychotherapy that was informed (but not pre-scribed) by four treatment manuals [21, 30–32]. Several patients received an Axis II diagnosis or subclinical personality disorder features. Active supervision was provided to the therapists throughout the study and incorporated video-tape review of sessions. Treatment fidelity was ensured by the analysis of ratings on the Comparative Psychotherapy Process Scale (CPPS) [33] completed by two judges coding the subscales independently in random order. Outcome was assessed by reliable change indices of a number of variables, including the depression subscale of the SCL-90-R and the total number of major depressive episode (MDE) symptoms [29].

Hilsenroth et al. [29] found that the CPPS item entitled "Therapist encourages patient to experience and express feelings in the session" was sig-nificantly related to outcome as measured by the reliable change index of MDE depressive symptoms ($R = 0.62$, $R^2 = 0.39$, $p = 0.003$, $N = 21$). In addition, the CPPS item entitled "Therapist addresses the patient's avoidance of important topics and shifts in mood" correlated significantly with the patient-rated reli-able change index of the Symptom Checklist-90-Revised Depression Subscale ($R = 0.51$, $R^2 = 0.26$, $p = 0.02$, $N = 20$) [29]. These findings, taken together with the results of Hill et al. [28], suggest the therapeutic importance of *general* facilitation of patient-affective experience and expression (i.e., not limited to use of interpretations or clarifications that are associated with patient affect). Additionally, results from Hilsenroth et al. [29] suggest that positive therapeutic change is associated with therapist efforts at addressing or attending to fluctua-tions in patient affect, i.e., "avoidance of important topics and shifts in mood" rather than simply ignoring this in-session process. These findings are consis-tent with the results of McCullough et al. [26] who demonstrated a *positive* association between interventions followed by patient *affect* and outcome, and a *negative* association between interventions followed by patient-*defensive* response (i.e., patient attempts to avoid difficult issues) and outcome. In other words, patients did better when therapist interventions lead to patient-affective responding, and patients did less well when therapist interventions lead to patient's trying to avoid difficult issues. Taken together, the results of Hilsen-roth et al. [29] and McCullough et al. [26] point to the utility of both encoura-ging patient emotional experience/expression and attending carefully to patient avoidance of particular feelings/issues.

Jones and colleagues [34] investigated brief, 16-session psychodynamic psy-chotherapy in private practice settings of 30 patients from an archival data set collected by the Mt. Zion Psychotherapy Research Group. Two judges rated randomly presented verbatim transcripts of hours 1, 5, and 14 of the treatments using the Psychotherapy Process Q-Set (PQS). Outcome was assessed in various ways, including an Overall Change Rating (nine-point scale), averaged across ratings made by the patient, therapist, and clinical evaluator [34].

Results indicated a statistically significant relationship between outcome and item "T[herapist] comments on changes in P[atient]'s mood or affect"

$(r = 0.31, p < 0.05, N = 30)$ [34]. This finding parallels the results of Hilsenroth et al. [29] noted above, which indicated that the item "Therapist addresses the patient's avoidance of important topics and shifts in mood" correlated significantly with patient-rated outcome. In addition, this finding is consistent with the results of McCullough et al. [26] described above, which demonstrated a *negative* association between outcome and therapist interventions leading to patient avoidance of difficult feelings/issues. The convergence of findings on this process variable suggests that it may be a particularly robust clinical intervention and highlights the importance of explicitly addressing patient in-session affect and process.

Caspar and colleagues [35] examined three cases (one excellent outcome, one moderate outcome, and one poor outcome) selected from the same Mt. Zion research project archival data set utilized in Jones et al. [34] using the Patient Experiencing Scale (EXP) on 3-min segments of patient speech immediately before and after therapist interpretations. The raters were blind to where the segment occurred in therapy, what interpretation the segment was connected to, and whether it was a pre- or postinterpretation segment. The assignment of outcome status (i.e., excellent, moderate, or poor) was determined by ratings on "standard psychotherapy outcome measures" [35, p. 311], including patient ratings of change and ratings completed by therapists and independent judges [36]. To facilitate comprehension of Caspar et al. [35], we (the authors) calculated the correlation between outcome and mean experiencing ratings. The correlation between outcome and postinterpretation experiencing ratings was $r = 0.87$, $p = 0.33$, $N = 3$ and the correlation between outcome and residual experiencing ratings was $r = 0.98$, $p = 0.12$, $N = 3$. These correlations, although nonsignificant (a result of the small sample size), are consistent with the findings of McCullough et al. [26] and Porter (as cited in [27]), which pointed to the therapeutic utility of interpretations/clarifications, which is followed by increased patient-affective response.

Strupp [37, 38] reported data on two pairs of two patients each (one patient in each pair was considered successful and one was considered unsuccessful) from the Vanderbilt Psychotherapy Project who received time-limited psychoanalytic psychotherapy. Outcome data included scores on the Depression, Psychasthenia, and Social Introversion scales of the MMPI rated by patients at intake and at termination, global change ratings completed by patients, therapists, and clinical judges, and Target Complaint ratings completed by patient, therapist, and clinical judges at intake and termination. Process variables included a number of items from the Vanderbilt Psychotherapy Process Scale (VPPS), which assessed therapist facilitation of patient affect [37, 38]. We (the authors) calculated a correlation between therapist facilitation of patient affect (mean of various items from the VPPS) and outcome (mean of change scores calculated from the raw intake and termination outcome data described above), $r = 0.59$, $p > 0.10$, $N = 4$ (Fisher and Yates; as cited in [39]). These results suggest a positive (although nonsignificant, due to the small sample size), large effect [40] relationship between therapist facilitation of patient affect and improvement over the course of therapy.

Coady [41] studied nine clients from a larger cohort [42] who received time-limited (20 sessions) individual psychodynamic therapy and who were described as "relatively well-functioning psychiatric outpatients" [41, p. 262]. Clients were assigned to either the "Good Outcome" category or the "Poor Outcome" category based on factor change scores on a one-factor solution generated from three outcome measures (Derogatis Symptom Index, Beck's Mood Scale, and Weissman's Social Adjustment Scale) [41, 43]. Categorical process ratings were made of whether the therapist communication focused on client affect, specifically "Therapist references to client feelings as they pertained to any aspect of the client's life or the therapy situation." These process ratings were made blind to the outcome status and were applied to the first 200 verbal behavior units of session three for each client. Results indicated that, although not statistically significant (sample size was small with $N = 9$), therapists of clients with good outcomes had a higher percentage of communication focused on client affect ($M = 17.2$, SD $= 6.7$) compared to therapists of clients with poor outcome ($M = 10.3$, SD $= 13.8$) [41]. These findings suggest that therapists may improve outcomes by assuring that out of the various techniques they employ, at least some of the time (about 17% of their verbal behavior) they discuss patient feelings that occur either in the therapeutic relationship or more generally in the patient's life.

Ablon and colleagues [44] studied 17 participants who met criteria for panic disorder and who received an average of 21 sessions of naturalistic psychotherapy by clinicians who self-identified as psychodynamic. External raters used the *PQS* [45] to describe the 12th session after listening to audiotapes. Results [44] indicated that treatment, in fact, contained greater cognitive–behavioral process than psychodynamic process. Still, psychodynamic and interpersonal process predicted outcome more than cognitive-behavioral process. In addition, the following items correlated with the SCL-90-R, controlling for pretreatment scores: "Therapist emphasizes patient's feelings to deepen them" ($r = 0.70$, $N = 17$), "Therapist draws attention to feelings patient regards unacceptable" ($r = 0.43$, $N = 17$), "Therapist focuses on patient's feelings of guilt" ($r = 0.34$, $N = 17$).

Thus far, we have focused on results that suggest either the *general* utility of facilitating patient affect or the *specific* importance of therapist *interpretations/ clarifications*, which are followed by patient-affective response (compared to patient-defensive response). We have not, however, delineated guidelines for determining which clinical situations are particularly suitable for an affective treatment focus. In this context, the results from a number of other studies are particularly important. Gaston and Ring [46] studied 10 subjects who received brief dynamic therapy as part of a larger controlled outcome study of behavioral, cognitive, and brief dynamic therapy for older individuals (between the ages of 60 and 80) with major depressive disorder [46, 47]. Therapists used the manual developed by Horowitz and colleagues [48]. Outcome measures included the Beck Depression Inventory and the Hamilton Rating Scale for depression, both of which were completed pre- and posttreatment. Scores on these measures were used to dichotomize the participants into a group of improved patients ($n = 5$) and a group of unimproved patients ($n = 5$). Therapist interventions were rated using the Inventory of Therapeutic Strategies (ITS) for sessions 5, 10, and 15. The ITS contains 19 items rated on a five-point Likert-type scale from "no emphasis" to "major emphasis," and the ITS intention category "exploratory" has an "emotions" content subcategory. Clinical judges rated the alliance using the California Psychotherapy Alliance Scale (CALPAS) for sessions 5, 10, and 15 [46].

Results indicated that, contrary to expectations, therapists of unimproved patients emphasized emotions ($M = 1.07$, $SD = .67$) more than did therapists of improved patients ($M = .48$, $SD = .39$). Gaston and Ring [46] report that this difference was statistically significant ($t = -2.94$, $p < 0.005$). However, this is true because although there were 10 patients, they assigned $N = 30$, arguing that there were 30 total observations (three sessions rated for each of 10 patients). If, however, we assign $N = 10$ and use the $M$s and $SD$s to calculate $r$, we find that $r = -.52$,[5] $p > 0.10$ (Fisher and Yates; as cited in [39]). Although nonsignificant, an $r$ of $-0.47$ is a moderate effect size [40] and still warrants attention. Gaston and Ring [46] performed additional analyses,[6] which indicated that therapists utilized the general category of exploratory strategies (which includes the "emotion" subcategory) with improved patients who had stronger alliances ($r = 0.65$, $df = 13$, $p < 0.01$), whereas no significant relationship was found between the use of exploratory strategies and alliance with unimproved patients ($r = -0.30$, $df = 13$, $p > 0.05$) [46].[7] This suggests that therapist exploration of patient affect may indeed be related to improvement, but only in the context of a sound therapeutic alliance.

Additional guidelines for the context-specific use of affect-focused techniques may be derived from Horowitz and colleagues [50]. In this study, 52 patients suffering from stress-response syndromes received 12 sessions of time-limited dynamic psychotherapy. Treatment integrated the principles of Mann, Malan, and Sifneos with contributions from Horowitz's own research group. Outcome was assessed in a number of ways including outcome ratings by patient, therapist, or independent clinician. Therapist action was measured in a number of ways including (a) mean value on the Action Checklist across hours 2, 5, 8, and 11 of pooled ratings of three judges, (b) ratings made by the therapist using the Therapist Action Scale after session 4, and (c) mean value of therapist ratings on the Therapist Action Scale across all 12 sessions. Clinical evaluators rated the patients using the self-concept rating scale, which assesses the coherence and stability of experience of the self and others [50].

---

[5] This calculation was done using software developed by DeFife [49].

[6] Once again, these analyses were performed with the assumption that $n = 15$ for each of the two patient groups (i.e., improved and unimproved) rather than $n = 5$.

[7] The difference between these two correlations was statistically significant, $z = 2.67$, $p < 0.01$ [46].

Results indicated that neither of the following therapist actions was significantly related to adjusted outcome: "Reliving feelings of affect-laden ideas in immediate in-treatment situation encouraged," "Termination reactions and feelings discussed." However, an interaction effect from a hierarchical regression analysis suggested that increased "Reliving feelings of affect-laden ideas in immediate in-treatment situation encouraged" lead to more positive outcomes for patients with higher levels on the self-concept dispositional variable (and less positive outcomes for patients with lower levels on the self-concept dispositional variable; $\Delta R2 = 0.07$, $p > 0.05$; Horowitz, personal communication, October 22, 2003) [50]. These results indicate that for patients who have more coherent and stable experiences of self and others, therapist interventions that facilitate immediate reliving of emotions in sessions may lead to better outcomes. In addition, it also suggests that caution may be indicated in facilitating such emotional experiences with patients who have less coherent and stable experiences of self and others.

Foreman and Marmar [51] evaluated a small subset of six female patients (who had high initial negative contributions to the alliance, determined by independent judges' review of videotapes from hour 2 of treatment) from the original Horowitz et al. [50] publication. One judge rated each therapy using a therapist action list (which included an item measuring emphasis of therapist addressing problematic feelings in the therapist–patient relationship and another item measuring emphasis of therapist addressing problematic feelings in patient–other relationships) for relative presence or absence of each action after reviewing summaries of pre- and posttherapy evaluations, process notes, and videotape segments of 3–6 h of therapy in each case. Patients were designated as having "excellent," "good," or "poor" outcomes based on change scores on measures of symptoms and social functioning rated by patients, therapists, and independent evaluators [51]. We (the authors) calculated a correlation between outcome and the mean of the two affect-focused therapist action items, which yielded $r = 0.89$, $p = 0.02$, $N = 6$. These results suggest that, at least for patients who have high initial negative contributions to the alliance, therapist emphasis on problematic feelings in the therapist–patient relationship and in patient–other relationships is associated with greater improvement.

Anderson and colleagues [52] present data from 30 patients randomly selected from the Vanderbilt II psychotherapy research project [53] who received time-limited dynamic psychotherapy [54]. Transcriptions of the third session for each patient were analyzed and the middle 15 min were split into 25 thought units each with highest and lowest frequency of affective adjectives. These units were then analyzed with a microprocess computer, corrected by two coders, for measures of cognitive and affective speech. Patients were divided into "good" and "poor" outcome categories using a composite measure of four outcome ratings. Results indicated that patients of therapists who used *fewer* cognitive words in *high*-affect segments had better outcomes. These results suggest that therapists need to capitalize on the opportunities afforded by high-affect segments, and that therapists may do well to avoid a cognitive focus during these moments [52].

Two studies [55, 56] present data that highlight the utility of therapist facilitation of *specific* affects or specific *types* of affects. Mintz [55] investigated 18 patients who received brief psychoanalytic psychotherapy originally reported in Malan's [57, 58] books. Outcome variables included global ratings of improvement and ratings of symptomatic improvement. Additionally, for the purpose of several analyses, patients were divided into groups of "no improvement" and "any improvement" by dichotomizing outcome ratings. One of the process variables reported in [55] is interpretation of "negative transference." Malan defines transference as "feelings that are neurotically based" [57, p. 31] and an interpretation as "an intervention in which the therapist suggests or implies an emotional content in the patient over and above what the patient has already stated" [57, p. 236]. The correlation between *continuous* outcome ratings and therapist interpretation of negative transference was significant for three out of seven correlations. When outcome ratings were *dichotomized*, the relationship with therapist interpretation of negative transference was significant in all three point-biserial correlations [55]. These results suggest that patient improvement is associated with therapist interpretation of patients' *negative* feelings directed toward the therapist.

Piper et al. [56] studied 21 patients who received psychoanalytically oriented, short-term psychotherapy as part of a larger comparative outcome study [59]. Outcome variables included an "Overall Usefulness" rating by therapists at the end of treatment. Process variables included ratings averaged across eight sessions of interpretations of patient conflictual anxiety (a component of the Therapist Intervention Rating System or TIRS). Results indicated a statistically significant correlation between interpretations of patient conflictual anxiety (percent out of total interventions) and usefulness ratings of the treatment, $r = 0.59$, $p < 0.01$, $N=21$ [56]. These findings suggest that specific focus by the therapist on patient conflictual anxiety is associated with more useful treatments. This conclusion is consistent with data from Mintz [55], which pointed to the utility of facilitating experience/expression of *negative* affect in general.

A recent meta-analysis [60] examined the relationship between therapist affect focus and patient outcomes in 10 independent samples of short-term dynamic therapy, yielding an overall average weighted effect size of $r = 0.30$, $p < 0.01$, 95% confidence interval $= 0.11$–$0.48$. Moderator analyses indicated that studies utilizing multiple outcome constructs demonstrated a statistically significant relationship between affect focus and outcome, whereas studies with a single or unclear outcome construct did not. In addition, methodological quality of individual studies was not related to the size of the effects, although use of audio/videotape for supervision yielded the largest positive correlation ($r = 0.29$). These findings indicate that across various studies and samples, therapist facilitation of patient-affective experience and expression correlates with patient improvement in psychodynamic psychotherapy, particularly when investigators define outcome in a multidimensional manner. In addition, results point to the utility of close observation of actual techniques using audio/videotape review during supervision sessions.


## Clinical Implications

Overall, results from research on dynamic psychotherapy ([26, 28, 29, 34, 35, 37, 38, 41, 44, 60], Porter as cited in [27]) converge on the utility of facilitating affective experience/expression. This suggests that therapists intervene in ways that (a) increase patients' awareness of their emotions, (b) deepen patients' in-session emotional experience, and (c) help patients express their feelings.

Next, we provide several examples of interventions and therapeutic principles based on the above research findings to facilitate the assimilation of the empirical results into everyday clinical practice. The following interaction provides an example of a therapist intervention that increases the patient's *awareness* of his/her emotions, one of the therapeutic processes found by Ablon et al. [44] and Hill et al. [28] to be positively correlated with outcome:

| | |
|---|---|
| *Therapist* | What's it like for us to talk about this in here? |
| *Patient* | Fine, no problem (loudly). |
| *Therapist* | Well, I noticed that your voice changed when we were talking about it, and I wonder what you are feeling right now? |
| *Patient* | I'm feeling fine, just trying to explain what happened with me and my wife. |
| *Therapist* | Yes, you're making a great effort to help me understand what exactly took place. At the same time, I often find that when someone's voice gets louder like that, then maybe they're describing something that can be uncomfortable. Is that the case for you right now? |

In terms of facilitating patient's emotional *expression* [28, 29], the therapist may respond in one of the following ways to a patient who has been crying:

| | |
|---|---|
| *Therapist 1* | If these tears could speak, what would they say? |
| *Therapist 2* | What are the feelings right now, in your body, that you're crying? |
| *Therapist 3* | Tears can mean different things for different people or even for the same person at different times. What do you think your tears mean now? |

Therapists should remain wary, however, of intervening too quickly when a patient begins crying, so the patient does not interpret this intervention as suggesting discomfort with the patient's sadness. In fact, taking the time to "sit with" the sadness can indicate the therapist's concern and ability to tolerate strong negative affect. In addition, this therapeutic decision can inhibit the temptation to intellectualize the patient's affective experience (as per [52]).

Many of the above examples highlight therapist interventions in response to overt displays of patient emotion (e.g., patient's tears or fluctuation in tone of voice). However, other research we reviewed suggests the importance of a more proactive approach where the therapist intentionally devises interventions such as *interpretations* and *clarifications* in ways that result in patient-affective response ([26, 35], Porter, as cited in [27]). The following therapeutic interchange illustrates the use of such an interpretation:

| | |
|---|---|
| *Patient* | You won't believe what my idiotic boss said to me the other day! I stopped by her office to drop off my completed project and as I handed it to her, she said, "It's about time." I wanted to yell at the top of my lungs at that witch! It was all I could to stop myself from punching her right in the face! |
| *Therapist* | I imagine that your boss's statement may have been particularly hurtful, especially given your history of being criticized by important people in your life. Perhaps some of that anger can also protect you from the disappointment of being criticized time and again by others whom you turn to for support. |

Another example of an interpretation designed to increase patient affect would be the following:

| | |
|---|---|
| *Therapist* | I've noticed that you seem to respond angrily to any perception that others, including myself, might abandon you. It makes me realize how upsetting and maybe frightening this all must be for you. |

Other research reviewed above [26, 29, 34] suggests that therapists explicitly address shifts in patient emotion during session. The following interaction illustrates this type of therapeutic intervention:

| | |
|---|---|
| *Patient* (*in a monotone*) | So I met this guy and we had a great time and we'll probably go out again... |
| *Therapist* | When you first came in here today, you seemed particularly revved upped and excited. But now, as we talk about your date last night, I noticed you've become quiet and you seem pretty distant from what you're discussing. How do you understand that? |

Another example of addressing shifts in patient emotion would be the following:

| | |
|---|---|
| *Therapist* | I realize that discussing your relationships with your family members makes you uncomfortable. At the same time, though, I can't help but notice that you seem calmer now than before. |

Other research [55, 56] highlighted the importance of facilitating experience/ expression of negative affect, particularly negative feelings toward the therapist and/or conflictual anxiety. The following interchange illustrates such an intervention that combines an attention to negative transference and conflictual anxiety:

| | |
|---|---|
| *Patient* | I'm really sorry for being late again. I just got stuck in the worst traffic. In any case, I've had a whopper of a week... |
| *Therapist* | Before we get into the events of your week, I'd like to bring us back a bit to your first comment about being late. As you pointed out, it seems like it's been harder to make it on time over the last few weeks. |
| *Patient* | You're right. I keep trying to get here on time, but I don't seem to be having much luck. |
| *Therapist* | You know sometimes I find that when people are late it's worth looking into because this could be communicating something. Do you think that might be the case here? |
| *Patient* | No, it's not like I'm *angry* with you or anything. In fact, *overall* you have been quite helpful to me. |
| *Therapist* | When you mentioned that I've been helpful to you *overall*, it makes me wonder about when there might be some times that I'm not as helpful. |
| *Patient* | Well, maybe just that you wait for me to bring things up and never start the session yourself. |

The therapist and the patient continue to discuss the patient's frustration in some detail. Afterwards, the therapist remarks:

| | |
|---|---|
| *Therapist* | I really appreciate your sharing some things about our work that irritate you. It's not an easy thing to do. In fact, talking about these feelings might make anyone nervous or uncomfortable, so it is understandable to put the focus on something else instead, like other events going on in your life. |

The question of *when* or *under what circumstances* to utilize affect-focused techniques in order to maximize their effectiveness can be discerned from the results of other studies previously reviewed. Results from Horowitz's research [50] (Horowitz, personal communication, October 22, 2003) suggest that facilitating in-session patient affect can be useful for patients who have more coherent and stable experiences of self and others. In addition, it also suggests that caution may be indicated in facilitating such emotional experiences with patients who have less coherent and stable experiences of self and others. As an example of the former, consider a patient who has the capacity to think of others as having both positive and negative attributes. With such a patient, a therapist might make the following interventions:

Therapist 1        I noticed that you just looked away for a moment and I'm wondering what emotions you're experiencing right now?

Therapist 2        You seem less engaged today than usual. I'm wondering if we're getting close to some feelings that might be intense and even scary, too?

Moreover, consider a patient who demonstrates difficulty in integrating positive and negative attributes of other people, often seeing them as "all good" or "all bad." In a particular session, the therapist looks away for a moment and the patient responds with a significant verbal attack:

Patient            I can't believe you're not paying any attention to me! You're just like everyone else! You just want to take my money and you don't care about the things I'm saying. It makes me furious to think that I trusted you this far and only now I'm getting to really know you!

In this instance, the therapist decides that although he certainly will acknowledge his actions and explore the patient's interpretation of them, it seems that encouragement of increased affective expression would be detrimental, as it will likely derail the patient and increase her disorganization. Instead, he chooses to explore the shift in the patient's experience of the therapeutic relationship (which precipitated the increased negative affect).

Therapist          You're right, I did look away for a second, and it seems like it really bothered you. At the same time, I'm noticing that your impression of me seems to have changed quite dramatically from even a few minutes ago. Does that fit with your experience of what happened?

Patient            Yeah, I just got so angry at you for ignoring me!

Therapist          Yes, you did, and I think we've seen this happen before when your feelings are so strong that you feel entirely negative and it makes it difficult to experience any positive feelings in that relationship.

Results from Gaston and Ring [46] suggest that an additional consideration in deciding whether to use affect-focused techniques is the strength of the therapeutic alliance. In the context of a strong therapeutic alliance, affect-exploratory techniques can be useful in promoting patient improvement. This suggests that therapists pay careful attention to developing the therapeutic alliance, resolve therapeutic ruptures [61], and utilize affect-focused techniques when the therapist feels that the alliance is healthy. Consider the following example from an initial session. The patient has been having some difficulty in pulling together her thoughts into a coherent narrative of the events, leading up to her seeking treatment.

| | |
|---|---|
| *Therapist* | Take your time... I'd really like to get a sense of what brings you here today. You know, it's normal for people to be anxious during a first session. |
| *Patient* | Anxious... I'm not anxious...what makes you think that? Maybe *you're* the one who is anxious? |
| *Therapist* | (Realizing that the therapeutic alliance is currently very weak) Well, you're right. That is part of what I'm feeling. When I meet people for the first time, I usually do feel some nervousness about how things will go and also an interested excitement about getting to know them better and the kind of work we might do together. So, you might have picked up on that. Does that make sense to you? Do you feel some nervous energy in here? |

The therapist and the patient continue to process their interaction and the session subsequently proceeds more smoothly. In the context of perceiving a stronger alliance, the therapist later makes the following remarks in response to the patient's report of a number of tragic losses in her life:

| | |
|---|---|
| *Therapist* | The death of loved ones can often leave us with lots of different feelings to try and make sense of. What was that like for you after all of those losses? |
| *Patient* | Awful...I felt so alone and helpless, looking for someone to turn to but realizing that they were all gone. |

To summarize, we outline a number of emotion-focused techniques with empirical support, including increasing patient awareness of his/her emotions and facilitating patients' emotional experience/expression by paying attention to and discussing specific patient indicators such as crying, changes or shifts in patient mood, and behaviors that suggest patient discontent with the therapist/ therapy (e.g., lateness). Therapists are advised to make specific reference to these patient indicators, reflect to the patient their presumed emotional significance, and discuss the underlying emotions in detail. In addition, therapists are encouraged to frame their interpretations/clarifications in a manner that increases patient affect, which can be done by pointing out unexpressed patient feelings while simultaneously indicating that these feelings are understandable in the context of the patient's life. Therapists should consider the specific relational history of the patient and utilize affect-focused techniques with greater frequency/intensity for patients with more stable experiences of self and others. The therapeutic alliance deserves significant consideration to identify and resolve therapeutic ruptures, paving the way for increased therapeutic use of affect-focused techniques. These interventions are devised to increase the patient's curiosity toward his/her unacknowledged feelings and permit their gradual experience as well as their adaptive expression.

## Conclusion

Theoretical expositions of therapeutic technique and process converge with the results from psychotherapy research, underscoring the importance of an affective focus in dynamic therapy. More specifically, results suggest that therapists increase their patients' emotional awareness, deepen patients' in-session affective experience, and facilitate patient's emotional expression. Research has linked these *general* techniques with outcome improvements, as well as when therapists specifically design their interpretations/clarifications to increase patient affect. Additionally, results suggest that therapists pay particular attention to in-session process and shifts in patient emotion as well as facilitate experience and expression of affect in the "here-and-now" [32, p. 139] of the therapeutic relationship. These affect-focused techniques appear particularly suited for patients with more coherent and stable experiences of self and others and/or in the context of a healthy therapeutic alliance. These findings not only buttress contemporary developments in dynamic therapy but also point to the utility of particular affect-focused techniques in guiding clinical intervention.

## References

1. Blagys, M. D. and Hilsenroth, M. J. (2000) Distinctive features of short-term psychodynamic–interpersonal psychotherapy: A review of the comparative psychotherapy process literature. *Clinical Psychology: Science and Practice* **7**, 167–188.
2. Blagys, M. D. and Hilsenroth, M. J. (2002) Distinctive features of short-term cognitive-behavioral psychotherapy: An empirical review of the comparative psychotherapy process literature. *Clinical Psychology Review* **22**, 671–706.
3. Arlow, J. A. (1990) Emotion, Time, and the Self. In R. Plutchik and H. Kellerman (Eds), *Emotion: Theory, research, and experience: Vol. 5. Emotion, psychopathology, and psychotherapy* (pp. 209–229) New York: Academic Press, Inc.
4. Basch, M. F. (1976) The concept of affect: A re-examination. *Journal of the American Psychoanalytic Association* **24**, 759–777.
5. Kellerman, H. (1990) Emotion and The Organization of Primary Process. In R. Plutchik and H. Kellerman (Eds), *Emotion: Theory, research, and experience: Vol. 5. Emotion, psychopathology, and psychotherapy* (pp. 89–113) New York: Academic Press, Inc.
6. Kernberg, O. F. (1990). New Perspectives in Psychoanalytic Affect Theory. In R. Plutchik and H. Kellerman (Eds), *Emotion: Theory, research, and experience: Vol. 5. Emotion, psychopathology, and psychotherapy* (pp. 115–131) New York: Academic Press, Inc.
7. Plutchik, R. (2000) *Emotions in the practice of psychotherapy: Clinical implications of affect theories* Washington, DC: American Psychological Association.
8. Sandler, J. (1983) On the psychoanalytic theory of affects: A historical and developmental review. *Israel Journal of Psychiatry and Related Sciences* **20**, 81–94.

9. Spezzano, C. (1993) *Affect in psychoanalysis: A clinical synthesis* Hillsdale, NJ: The Analytic Press.
10. Stein, R. (1991) *Psychoanalytic theories of affect* New York: Praeger.
11. Breuer, J., and Freud, S. (n. d.) On the psychical mechanism of hysterical phenomena: Preliminary communication. *Studies on Hysteria*, 3–17. New York: Basic Books. (Original work published 1893).
12. Moore, B. and Fine, B. (Eds) (1990) *Psychoanalytic terms and concepts* New Haven: The American Psychoanalytic Association and Yale University Press.
13. Butler, S. F. and Strupp, H. H. (1991) The Role of Affect in Time-Limited Dynamic Psychotherapy. In J. D. Safran and L. S. Greenberg (Eds), *Emotion, psychotherapy and change* (pp.83–112) New York: The Guilford Press.
14. Strupp, H. H. (1967) *An introduction to Freud and modern psychoanalysis* New York: Barron's Educational Series, Inc.
15. Strachey, J. (1966) Editor's Introduction. In J. Breuer and S. Freud (1893–1895), Studies on hysteria *The standard edition of the complete psychological works of Sigmund Freud* **2**, ix–xxviii. London: Hogarth Press.
16. Freud, S. (1958) The dynamics of transference. In J. Strachey (Ed. and Trans.) *The standard edition of the complete psychological works of Sigmund Freud* **12**, 97–108. London: Hogarth Press (Original work published 1912).
17. Freud, S. (1964) Constructions in analysis. In J. Strachey (Ed. and Trans.) *The standard edition of the complete psychological works of Sigmund Freud* **13**, 257–269 London: Hogarth Press (Original work published 1937).
18. Freud, S. (1958) Remembering, repeating and working through (Further recommendations on the technique of psycho-analysis II). In J. Strachey (Ed. And Trans.) *The standard edition of the complete psychological works of Sigmund Freud* **12**, 145–156. London: Hogarth Press (Original work published 1914).
19. Alexander, F. and French, T. M. (1946) *Psychoanalytic therapy: Principles and applications* New York: The Ronald Press Company.
20. Wolf, E. S. (1988) *Treating the self: Elements of clinical self psychology* New York: The Guilford Press.
21. Wachtel, P. L. (1993) *Therapeutic communication: Knowing what to say when* New York: The Guilford Press.
22. McCullough, L. and Andrews, S. (2001) Assimilative integration: Short-term dynamic psychotherapy for treating affect phobias. *Clinical Psychology: Science and Practice* **8**, 82–97.
23. Fosha, D. (2002) The activation of affective change processes in Accelerated Experiential-Dynamic Psychotherapy (AEDP). In F. W. Kaslow (Editor-In-Chief) and J. J. Magnavita (Vol. Ed.) *Comprehensive handbook of psychotherapy: Vol. 1, Psychodynamic/object relations* (pp. 309–343) New York: John Wiley and Sons, Inc.
24. Shear, M. K., Cloitre, M., and Heckelman, L. (1995) Emotion—focused treatment for panic disorder: A brief, dynamically informed therapy. In J. P. Barber and P. Crits-Christoph (Eds) *Dynamic therapies for psychiatric disorders (Axis I)* (pp. 267–293) New York: Basic Books.
25. Shear, M. K., Houck, P., Greeno, C., and Masters, S. (2001) Emotion—focused psychotherapy for patients with panic disorder. *American Journal of Psychiatry* **158**, 1993–1998. (pp. 101–121) Washington, DC: American Psychological Association Press.
26. McCullough, L., Winston, A., Farber, B. A., Porter, F., Pollack, J., Laikin, M., Vingiano, W., and Trujillo, M. (1991) The relationship of patient–therapist interaction to outcome in brief psychotherapy. *Psychotherapy* **28**, 525–533.
27. McCullough, L. (2000) The cross pollination of research and practice: The honeybee, the unicorn and the search for meaning. In S. Soldz and L. McCullough (Eds), *Reconciling empirical knowledge and clinical experience: The art and science of psychotherapy* (pp. 101–121) Washington DC: American Psychological Association Press.

28. Hill, C. E., Helms, J. E., Spiegel, S. B., and Tichenor, V. (1988) Development of a system for categorizing client reactions to therapist interventions. *Journal of Counseling Psychology* **35**, 27–36.
29. Hilsenroth, M. J., Ackerman, S. J., Blagys, M. D., Baity, M. R., and Mooney, M. A. (2003) Short term psychodynamic psychotherapy for depression: An examination of statistical, clinically –significant, and technique specific change. *Journal of Nervous and Mental Disease* **191**, 349–357.
30. Book, H. E. (1998) *How to practice brief psychodynamic psychotherapy: The core conflictual relationship theme method* Washington, DC: American Psychological Association.
31. Luborsky, L. (1984) *Principles of psychoanalytic psychotherapy: A manual for supportive-expressive treatment* New York: Basic Books.
32. Strupp, H. H. and Binder, J. (1984) *Psychotherapy in a new key; A guide to Time-Limited Dynamic Psychotherapy* New York: Basic Books.
33. Hilsenroth, M. J., Blagys, M. D., Ackerman, S. J., Bonge, D. R., and Blais, M. A. (2005) Measuring psychodynamic–interpersonal and cognitive–behavioral techniques: Development of the Comparative Psychotherapy Process Scale. *Psychotherapy: Theory, Research, Practice, Training* **42**, 340–356.
34. Jones, E. E., Parke, L. A., and Pulos, S. (1992) How therapy is conducted in the private consulting room: A multivariate description of brief psychodynamic treatments. *Psychotherapy Research* **2**, 16–30.
35. Caspar, F., Pessier, J., Stuart, J., Safran, J. D., Samstag, L. W., and Guirguis, M. (2000) One step further in assessing how interpretations influence the process of psychotherapy. *Psychotherapy Research* **10**, 309–320.
36. Silberschatz, G., Fretter, P. B., and Curtis, J. T. (1986) How do interpretations influence the process of psychotherapy? *Journal of Consulting and Clinical Psychology* **54**, 646–652.
37. Strupp, H. H. (1980a) Success and failure in time-limited psychotherapy: A systematic comparison of two cases: Comparison 2 *Archives of General Psychiatry* **37**, 708–716.
38. Strupp, H. H. (1980b) Success and failure in time-limited psychotherapy: Further evidence: Comparison 4 *Archives of General Psychiatry* **37**, 947–954.
39. Gravetter, F. J. and Wallnau, L. B. (2000) *Statistics for the behavioral sciences* Stamford, CT: Wadsworth.
40. Cohen, J. (1988) *Statistical power analysis for the behavioral sciences* (2nd Edn) Hillsdale, NJ: Lawrence Erlbaum Associates.
41. Coady, N. F. (1991) The association between complex types of therapist interventions and outcomes in psychodynamic psychotherapy. *Research on Social Work Practice* **1**, 257–277.
42. Marziali, E. (1984) Three viewpoints on the therapeutic alliance: Similarities, differences, and associations with psychotherapy outcome. *Journal of Nervous and Mental Disease* **172**, 417–423.
43. Coady, N. F. (1991) The association between client and therapist interpersonal processes and outcomes in psychodynamic psychotherapy. *Research on Social Work Practice* **1**, 122–138.
44. Ablon, J. S., Levy, R. A., and Katzenstein, T. (2006) Beyond brand names of psychotherapy: Identifying empirically supported change processes. *Psychotherapy: Theory, Research, Practice, Training* **43**, 216–231.
45. Jones, E. E. (2000) *Therapeutic action: A guide to psychoanalytic therapy* Northvale, NJ: Jason Aronson, Inc.
46. Gaston, L. and Ring, J. M. (1992) Preliminary results on the Inventory of Therapeutic Strategies. *Journal of Psychotherapy Practice and Research* **1**, 135–146.
47. Thompson, L. W., Gallagher, D., and Steinmetz Breckenridge, J. (1987) Comparative effectiveness of psychotherapies for depressed elders. *Journal of Consulting and Clinical Psychology* **55**, 385–390.
48. Horowitz, M. J., Marmar, C., Krupnick, J., Wilner, N., Kaltreider, N., and Wallerstein, R. (1984) *Personality Styles and Brief Psychotherapy* New York: Basic Books.

49. DeFife, J. (2008) Effect Size Calculator [Computer software].
50. Horowitz, M. J., Marmar, C., Weiss, D. S., DeWitt, K. N., and Rosenbaum, R. (1984) Brief psychotherapy of bereavement reactions: The relationship of process to outcome. *Archives of General Psychiatry* **41,** 438–448.
51. Foreman, S. A. and Marmar, C. R. (1985) Therapist actions that address initially poor therapeutic alliances in psychotherapy. *American Journal of Psychiatry* **142,** 922–926.
52. Anderson, T., Bein, E., Pinnell, B., and Strupp, H. H. (1999) Linguistic analysis of affective speech in psychotherapy: A case grammar approach. *Psychotherapy Research* **9,** 88–99.
53. Strupp, H. H. (1993) The Vanderbilt Psychotherapy Studies: Synopsis. *Journal of Consulting and Clinical Psychology* **61,** 431–433.
54. Henry, W. P., Strupp, H. H., Butler, S. F., Schacht, T. E., and Binder, J. L. (1993) Effects of training in time-limited dynamic psychotherapy: Changes in therapist behavior. *Journal of Consulting and Clinical Psychology* **61,** 434–440.
55. Mintz, J. (1981) Measuring outcome in psychodynamic psychotherapy: Psychodynamic vs symptomatic assessment. *Archives of General Psychiatry* **38,** 503–506.
56. Piper, W. E., Debbane, E. G., deCarufel, F. L., et al. (1987) A system for differentiating therapist interpretations from other interventions. *Bulletin of the Menninger Clinic* **51,** 532–550.
57. Malan, D. H. (1975) *A study of brief psychotherapy* New York: Plenum.
58. Malan, D. H. (1976) *Toward the validation of dynamic psychotherapy: A replication* New York: Plenum.
59. Piper, W. E., Debbane, E. G., Bienvenu, J. P., & Garant, J. (1984) A comparative study of four forms of psychotherapy. *Journal of Consulting and Clinical Psychology* **52,** 268–279.
60. Diener, M. J., Hilsenroth, M. J., and Weinberger, J. (2007) Therapist Affect Focus and Patient Outcomes in Psychodynamic Psychotherapy: A Meta-Analysis. *American Journal of Psychiatry* **164,** 936–941.
61. Safran, J. D., and Muran, J. C. (2000) *Negotiating the therapeutic alliance: A relational treatment guide* New York: The Guilford Press.

# Chapter 11
# Affect-Focused Short-Term Dynamic Therapy

## Empirically Supported Strategies for Resolving Affect Phobias

**Leigh McCullough and Molly Magill**

## Introduction

The field of psychotherapy research is in the process of solving a great puzzle. To date, differing therapies have often demonstrated similar effectiveness, and no factors have been identified that consistently capture a large portion of the variance in improvement [1, 2]. Therapeutic alliance accounts for about 22% of the variance in outcomes [2] and patient characteristics at admission an additional 20–25% [1], leaving more than half of the variance somewhat of a mystery.

What factors remain obscured in the complex and mysterious other half of the psychotherapy process? Are there powerful curative factors that have not yet been identified or are some interventions not yet powerful enough? Do we lack the proper methods to accurately capture the mechanisms that promote change or do change mechanisms need to be more context-specific and better tailored to the patient? Finally, are there mysterious, treatment-specific mechanisms that remain to be discovered?

Affect may be one of these mysterious variables. Although considered a contributor to change in many theoretical orientations and a common factor in some research studies, research on affect in psychotherapy has been equivocal. This chapter will describe a quest to explore the power of affect in psychotherapy, to better operationalize this complex and confusing construct, and to report on relevant research that might shed some light on aspects of affect that have not been previously examined.

## The Focus on Affect in Short-Term Dynamic Psychotherapy

Short-term dynamic psychotherapy (STDP) theory hypothesizes that most patients' problems can be traced to conflicts or fears surrounding feelings [3–8]. The central premise is that psychodynamic conflict can be thought of as

L. McCullough
Harvard Medical School, and Modum Bad Research Institute, 3370 Vikersuad, Norway
e-mail: leigh@hms.harvard.edu

R.A. Levy, J.S. Ablon (eds.), *Handbook of Evidence-Based Psychodynamic Psychotherapy*, DOI: 10.1007/978-1-59745-444-5_11, © Humana Press 2009

a fear about feeling, or "Affect Phobia," and fears of feeling (both conscious and unconscious) underlie most, if not all problems that patients present [8]. For example, for the problem of unresolved losses, an underlying affect conflict or "phobia" might be: "If start crying, I'm afraid I'll never stop!" For the problem of victimization or abuse, the underlying affect phobia might be: "I can't possibly feel anger because I'd feel too guilty, afraid, or undeserving." For the problem of isolation or loneliness, an affect phobia could be: "I closed my heart years ago, and I'll never let myself be hurt like that again." And for the problem of low self-esteem the affect phobia often takes the form: "I feel too ashamed to feel self compassion or self worth."

Viewing psychodynamic conflicts as Affect Phobias allows therapists to treat the conflicted feelings described above as any standard phobia would be treated – by exposure and response prevention (e.g., [9]), to be discussed below. Patients are encouraged to gradually experience increasing levels of previously avoided affect (a process of exposure) while reducing anxiety or other inhibitory affects (such as guilt, shame, or pain) to a manageable level (thus preventing the avoidant response). The goal is to help patients face, tolerate and put into perspective the previously unbearable and warded-off affects.

## The Historical Roots of the Concept of "Affect Phobia"

The historical roots of "Affect Phobia" have emerged from the integration of "what works" in psychotherapy, such as gestalt therapy (for deepening the experience of feelings); cognitive therapy (CT) approaches (to restructure maladaptive cognitions), interpersonal interventions (to restructure relationships), and self-psychology (in restructuring the self-image). However, the central roots of Affect Phobia are based in psychodynamic theory, examining *defenses* that protect the self from painful affects through *anxieties* that block feeling and learning theory (for *exposure* to warded off feelings, and *response prevention* of defensive avoidance.) These latter two theoretical contributions will be focused on below.

## Psychodynamic Roots of Affect Phobia

Psychodynamic theory provides:

1. A description of intrapsychic components
2. The etiology of psychopathology
3. A description of how problem behavior originates from the resulting conflict

The strong focus on affect in therapy emerged from movements in the psychoanalytic community that began to emphasize more short-term, affect-focused models of treatment. Originally, Freud [10] hypothesized that neuroses were attempts to avoid unpleasant unconscious experiences, and though not often stated explicitly, much of the "unconscious" material involved exposure to feelings contained in fantasies. Wanting to shorten the increasingly lengthy process of psychoanalysis, writers such as Ferenczi and Rank [62] shifted from therapist passivity to therapist activity, and proposed a number of strategies intended to shorten analysis. Alexander and French [11] extended a number of these short-term techniques, such as imposed time limitations, focus on the patient–therapist relationship, and an unrelenting experiencing of the *focal affective conflict,* to facilitate deeper and lasting change. Working with Michael and Enid Balint, Malan [12, 3] continued the focus on feeling. In Malan's words "the aim of every moment in every session is to put the patient in touch with as much of his true feelings as he can bear" [3, p. 84]. Davanloo [4] was also influential and contributed methods for strong confrontation of defenses to unearth warded-off emotions. Growing research in the mother–infant laboratories has supported the focus on feelings (e.g., [13–15]) and demonstrated that infants are born with a broad repertoire of feelings (e.g., sorrow, joy, interest, fear, disgust) that need guidance, but not restriction. Tomkins' [16, 17] theory of emotion provided the foundation for our affect theory.

Further work on Tomkins theory, as described in Ekman and Davidson [18] offered support for the categorization of feelings that are used in the Affect Phobia model: (1) activating affects such as grief, anger, fear that produce flight, joy (including joy or tenderness toward others), and excitement, and (2) inhibitory affects such as guilt, shame, emotional pain, and the "freezing" form of fear/anxiety.

As a result of these clinical and research contributions, emotions have begun to be considered theoretically central in psychodynamic theory, and no longer viewed as drive derivatives, but as primary motivational forces [19].

Thus, according to an updated version of Freudian conflict theory (initially described by Malan in 1979 and operationally defined by McCullough [6] and McCullough and colleagues [8], psychodynamic conflict results from conflicts surrounding feelings. It is, in essence, the opposing affective components of our motivational system. The *inhibitory* forces of anxiety, shame, guilt, or pain are acquired in early life as a result of subjectively experienced faulty attunement or neglectful or abusive interactions with caretakers, whether intentional or unintentional. *These inhibitory affects* then thwart the use of natural, healthy *activating* feeling responses such as grief, assertion, closeness, or self-esteem. Common examples of these "Affect Phobias" are guilt over anger, embarrassment about crying, pain over closeness, or shame about oneself. When adaptive activating emotional responses are blocked by inhibition, less adaptive and defensive responding will take their place. Thus, when there is guilt over anger, blocking healthy limiting setting, passivity, depression, or anxiety might result. When there is shame over crying, blocking healthy grief, overeating, pathological mourning, irritation, or again, depression can occur. These maladaptive symptoms, though unpleasant are just a few of the myriad and multiply determined ways we avoid the even more unpleasant conflicts about emotions.

## Learning Theory Roots of Affect Phobia

Learning theory provides:

1. Redefinition of "unconscious conflicted feelings" as "phobic stimuli."
2. Mechanism of change – desensitization of the phobic stimuli by exposure and response prevention.

Several integrative theorists have proposed ways that psychodynamic and learning principles can work together. Cautela's [20] theory of covert conditioning was the initial impetus in the development of the Affect Phobia concept [21]. Cautela taught that the principles of reinforcement and extinction could impact on internal or covert behaviors such as thoughts or feelings, just as they do on overt behaviors.

Theorists such as Dollard and Miller [22], Stampfl and Levis [23], and Feather and Rhoads [24] believed that anxiety is aroused by the experience of a specific drive or impulse, and the behavioral technology of desensitization through exposure and prevention of avoidance can be applied to drive-related imagery underlying the avoidance behavior. Dollard and Miller pointed out that Freud [25] had observed that anxiety can be steadily weakened by extinction (p. 241). In 1977, Paul Wachtel published *Psychoanalysis and Behavior Therapy*, in which he began an integration of psychodynamic and learning theories and explored fears of feelings as a form of phobia. Far before research data supported the idea, Wachtel wrote that intellectual insight in the absence of emotional arousal was inevitably "therapeutically fruitless" [26].

All of these theorists agreed that feelings, or the "efforts to gratify wants and needs," could become repressed by anxieties. Each believed that reduction of inappropriate anxiety is central to bringing therapeutic change in problems, and that reduction could be achieved by exposure and response prevention. Each believed that neurotic problems developed from fear learned in childhood, causing problems in later life. The Affect Phobia model thus emerged from two main sources: (1) the intensive affect-focused short-term psychodynamic psychotherapy that sought active interventions to accelerate patient change and (2) the integrative theorists seeking commonalities between psychodynamics and behavior therapy. All of these approaches share a primary change agent: expose and desensitize patients to frightening feelings or "Affect Phobias."

## Research on Affect in Psychotherapy

During the last decade, affective responding in therapy has received mixed reviews from research on its efficacy. Studies on affect can be divided into those focusing on total affective arousal, positive affect, and negative affect. According to Orlinsky et al. [27], studies of total affective arousal in response to therapist interventions showed an association to improvement for half of studies reviewed while half showed no association to outcome, and none showed a relationship to negative outcome. Further, four studies showed a relationship to outcome for patients' experience of positive feelings and 20 of 50 studies of negative affect demonstrated significant findings with either positive or negative associations to outcome. Orlinsky concluded that "experiencing distressing and negative emotions during sessions has strong effects that can be for good or ill depending on how effectively therapists deal with them" [27, p. 345].

A recent meta-analysis paints a somewhat clearer picture with respect to the benefit of eliciting affect in psychotherapy. To overcome some of the ambiguity in previous affect studies, Diener, Hilsenroth and Weinberger [61] selected the most methodologically sound research, and only 10 out of more than 700 studies met criteria for inclusion. Therapist facilitation of affect was significantly associated with outcome, but the effect size was small ($r = 0.30$). As findings suggest, and this chapter will discuss, much of the ambiguity with affect research, may not be due only to methodological issues, but also due to confounds in affect constructs.

As Orlinsky et al.'s [28, 27] review noted, the study of affect has focused on positive and negative modes. Unfortunately, this categorization does not take into consideration the many different functions affect can serve. All affects can function in a positive, relieving, constructive manner, and all affects can be used in a negative and destructive way. The resulting complexity and overlap in functioning maybe be one of the largest factors leading to confounds in research results.

## Activating and Inhibitory Affects

A categorization that offers greater potential for identifying change operations in psychotherapy is the distinction between activating affects and inhibitory affects. Affects may function to *motivate action* (assertion, grief, closeness, confidence) or to *motivate inhibition of action* (shame, anxiety). In addition, affects can be used maladaptively to motivate defensive avoidance (weepiness that is depressive rather than resolving or anger that is aggressive rather than assertive). The depressive or aggressive forms of these feelings are unlikely to correlate with improvement while their adaptive counterparts (grief, assertion) should lead to problem resolution.

The activating and inhibitory categories are supported by a number of researchers and theorists. Gray [29] proposed a theory of two motivational systems, which he called the Behavioral Activation System (BAS) and the Behavioral Inhibition System (BIS). Fowles [30, 31] demonstrated that heart rate reflects activity of the BAS, and electrodermal responses reflect activity of the BIS. Wilhelm and Roth [32] demonstrated that both the BAS and BIS are activated during in vivo exposure to fearful events.

Konorski [33] and Dickinson and Dearing [34], also proposed a bimodal categorization of "aversion and attraction." Lang and his colleagues [35] continued this work by identifying two basic motivational systems that they labeled *appetitive* and *defensive*. These systems were further linked to specific brain regions that support activation and inhibition.

In recent years, there has been a growing literature on the behavioral activation and inhibition systems. Carver and White [63] have developed scales to test these constructs that are well validated. Sutton and Davidson [36] showed that right versus left prefrontal brain activity correlated with the BIS and BAS, respectively. They also demonstrated that prefrontal EEG activity was not significantly correlated with positive affect or negative affect scales. Such research supports the validity of this bimodal motivational system of activation and inhibition.

The Affect Phobia model is based on the premise that psychodynamic conflict results from opposition between *activating and inhibitory affects* that underlie behavioral activation and inhibition. The universal principle of psychodynamic therapy [3] is stated as "defenses and anxieties block the expression of true feeling." In other words, phobias can occur in response to external stimuli, or to internal or interoceptive cues such as affects. Thus, in an affect phobia, anxieties are the *inhibitory feelings* that block the expression of true or *activating feelings*. When these two systems are in conflict, defenses emerge as a "compromise response" (in psychodynamic language) or as a "phobic avoidance response" (in learning theory terms).

The benefit of translating dynamic principles into learning theory principles is that one may draw on abundant behavioral research on behavior change. Principles of exposure and response prevention may be explicitly utilized to resolve these conflicts between activating and inhibitory feelings similar to the processes described in Foa and McNally [37] or Barlow [38]. The fundamental change agents involve (1) exposure to and transforming of the activating affective experience (the bodily experience of anger, grief, compassion, and so on) and (2) response prevention by reducing the amount of associated anxiety, guilt, shame or pain, and related avoidant defenses. Moreover, direct exposure is to the *physiological arousal of an adaptive form of the affect*. Desensitization does not occur in response to exposure to thoughts about feelings, words about feelings, or general fantasies or images about feelings. It is essential that the affect be experienced in the body for desensitization to occur.

## Main Treatment Objectives in the Treatment of Affect Phobias

This affect-focused form of STDP emphasizes four main areas of intervention (see [8] for a more thorough discussion):

- *Gaining Insight* – Restructuring of defenses by identifying patterns of avoidance of unconscious conflicted feelings, how they started in early life, and their present day costs and benefits.

- *Exposure to and Expression of Feeling* – Restructuring activating affects by exposure until inhibition is reduced and affects can be tolerated and expressed to others in a well-modulated and adaptive manner.
- Regulation of Inhibitory Affects – Anxiety, guilt, shame, and emotional pain are brought within normal limits to allow more flexible experience and expression of activating feelings.
- Restructuring the sense of self and others – Maladaptive inner images of self and others are altered by reduction of shame attached to self-image and exposure to positive self-feelings, as well as appropriate feelings toward others.

## Methods and Procedures used to Study Affect Phobias

This specific model of therapy has been submitted to two randomized controlled clinical trials (RCTs). The first RCT was conducted at Beth Israel Medical Center in New York City [39, 40]. Sixty-four patients were randomly assigned to two forms of short-term psychotherapy (STOP: Short Term Dynamic Pschotherapy; high confrontation vs. BAP: Brief Adaptive Psychotherapy; moderate confrontation of defenses) and a waiting list control group ($N = 17$). The second RCT was conducted at the Norwegian University of Science and Technology in Trondheim, Norway. Here, 50 subjects were randomly assigned to this STDP model or to CT (Cognitive Therapy) [41].

In both studies, patients who met criteria for one or more Cluster C personality disorders and Axis I disorders of depression or anxiety were randomized to 40 sessions of therapy. Therapists were experienced, full-time clinicians and supervised by experts in the therapy modality. Outcomes were assessed in terms of symptom distress (SCL-90 [42]), interpersonal problems [43], and, in the Svartbert et al. study, core personality dysfunction (MCMI [44]) administered at admission, midphase, at termination and 1.5- to 2-year follow-up. Both of these clinical trials generated videotapes of therapy sessions that could be studied to identify change processes and two intensive programs of process research followed. Several instruments were developed and psychometrically validated in an attempt to discover the treatment mechanisms that led to improvement.

## *The Psychotherapy Interaction Coding System*

The Psychotherapy Interaction Coding (PIC) System (McCullough, L., 1987, The Psychotherapy Intervention Codes (PIC). Unpublished manuscript available at www.affectphobia.com.) was designed to capture the minute-by-minute interaction of therapist interventions and client responses in psychotherapy sessions. Therapist interventions included questions, information, self-disclosure, clarification, confrontation, directives/advice, support, and interpretation. Patient response modes included defensive, affective, and cognitive responding. The

PIC System was a beginning attempt to assess not only therapist interventions but the impact of therapy on the patient in terms of patient response to specific interventions. Thus the PIC System can be used as both a process and a "micro-outcome measure." The interventions are operationally defined in terms of discrete behaviors to permit comparisons across different forms of therapy.

## *The Achievement of Therapeutic Objectives Scale*

The ATOS Scale furthered the methodology for assessing the impact of therapy on patients, by rating from 0 to 100 the amount of therapy that the patient is "absorbing." In other words, the ATOS scale rates the degree to which the patient has "taken-in" the specific objectives of psychotherapy. For example, how much does a patient (1) gain insight by recognizing maladaptive defensive behaviors; (2) show motivation for change by giving up maladaptive behavior, (3) experience activating and inhibitory affects in the session; and (4) express the feeling in relationships outside of therapy. Thus, the ATOS scale measures the degree of impact of therapy on the patient (ATOS; [8]). [1] ATOS scale ratings are made for each 10-min segment of each session and are correlated with various residual measures of pre–post change at termination and follow-up of treatment. The ATOS scale is psychometrically strong, with five reliability studies [45], and one validity study [46] .

## Outcome Research on STDP

Both clinical trials have shown that STDP is an effective treatment for Axis II, Cluster C personality disorders, and according to guidelines suggested by Cohen [47], the effect sizes are strong.

## *Results of the BIMC RCT*

The results of the Beth Israel Medical Center (BIMC) Study (Table 11.1) demonstrated strong improvement at termination in symptoms and interpersonal functioning for both groups. The effect size on the SCL-90 for the high-confrontation group was 0.96 and the low-confrontation group was 1.11. For

---

[1] A website for more information on the Affect Phobia treatment model can be accessed at www.affectphobia.com. This web-site also includes (1) information about videotaping of psychotherapy, (2) the manual for the ATOS for assessment of psychotherapy process on videotape or transcripts, and 3) Psychotherapy Assessment Checklist (PAC Forms – a patient self-report form) to help determine *Diagnostic and Statistical Manual* (DSM) diagnoses and assess patient pretreatment characteristics as well as therapy outcome.

**Table 11.1** Comparison of effect sizes of change in two clinical trials of affect-focused short-term psychotherapy and a meta-analysis of short-term dynamic therapy (STDP)

| Study type / No. of subjects/$R$ × length / Assessment Periods | Symptoms (SCL-90) | | | Social adjustment (IIP/SAS-R) | | |
|---|---|---|---|---|---|---|
| **BIMC Study** Winston et al. [68, 69] RCT: $N=32 + 32/40$ sessions Controls = 17 | STDP High confrontation | BAP Low confrontation | Control Waiting list control | STDP High confrontation | BAP Low confrontation | Control Waiting list control |
| Pre- to posttreatment | 0.96 | 1.11 | 0.46 | 0.80 | 0.70 | −0.07 |
| Pretreatment to follow-up | 0.65 | 0.63 | 0.25 | 0.97 | 0.97 | 0.36 |
| **Trondheim Study** Svartberg et al. [41] RCT: $N=25 + 25/40$ sessions | STDP | CT | Control | STDP | CT | Control |
| Pre- to posttreatment | 0.65 | 0.73 | – | 0.58 | 0.74 | – |
| Pretreatment to follow-up | 0.87 | 0.95 | – | 1.00 | 1.09 | – |
| **STDP Meta-Analysis** Leichsenring, et al. [48] Meta-analysis, 17 studies | STDP | CT | Control | STDP | CT | Control |
| Pre- to posttreatment | 0.90 | 1.04 | 0.12 | 0.80 | 0.92 | 0.21 |
| Pretreatment to follow-up | 0.95 | 0.97 | – | 1.19 | 1.05 | – |

interpersonal functioning, effect size change on the Inventory of Interpersonal Problems (IIP) was 0.80 for the high-confrontation group and 0.70 for the low-confrontation group. At 1.5-year follow-up, the effect size of symptom gains were maintained (due to the large variance in scores the drop to 0.65 and 0.63, respectively, was not significant and interpersonal functioning was improved [ES (effect size) = 0.97, both groups]. Overall, there were no significant differences in the high- versus low-confrontation group due to large variance in scores. The waiting list control group results were not significantly associated with improvement in outcome.

## Results of the Trondheim RCT

As shown in Table 11.1, both CT and STDP demonstrated strong improvement at termination in symptoms on the SCL-90 (STDP: ES = 0.65; CT: ES = 0.73) and interpersonal functioning on the IIP (STDP: ES = 0.58; CT: ES = 0.74). At 2-year follow-up, these gains were not only maintained, but also slightly improved for symptom change on the SCL-90 (STDP: ES = 0.87; CT: ES = 0.95) as well as for interpersonal functioning (STDP: ES = 1.00; CT: ES = 1.09). Overall, there were no statistically significant differences between STDP and CT on any measure across follow-up.

Based on the results of both studies, STDP has been shown to be an effective treatment for patients with Cluster C personality disorders. The effect sizes in both these clinical trials are strong, but not quite as strong as a meta-analysis of short-term psychotherapy (see Table 11.1) conducted by Leichsenring and others [48]. This may be due to the more the difficult to treat Axis II, Cluster C disorder population included in these two RCTs.

## Process Research on STDP

### BIMC Process Research Results: Confrontation of Defenses

The initial process studies in the 1980 s focused on the efficacy of the "anxiety-provoking" model of STDP. Strong confrontation of defenses was hypothesized to lead to increased affective responding and better outcomes. However, using the PIC System, a series of studies from the BIMC lab demonstrated that *supportive*, *empathic*, and *clarifying* methods generated more affect than did *confrontive* interventions. Salerno and colleagues [49] demonstrated that the higher total frequencies of therapist confrontation of defenses in the patient–therapist relationship did not predict improvement at outcome. A subsequent study [50] examined confrontations sustained over 1–9 minutes, hypothesizing that it was the *continued confrontation* that would "break through" the defenses to underlying feeling. Again, and counter to expectations, continued confrontation did *not* predict improvement, thus adding to the growing aware-ness of the need for a graded and empathic procedure for identifying and giving up maladaptive forms of defenses, as well as becoming more flexible and mature in using our defenses to guide underlying affects.

In exploratory analyses of the coding data, it was noted that confrontations given along with a supportive or empathic statement by the therapist [51] resulted in a greater likelihood of expression of affect. A higher rating of therapist alliance, especially in lower functioning or more resistant patients, resulted in a better probability of improvement at outcome [51]. Patients seemed to be much more able to take in the painful information contained in a therapist's confrontation or interpretation when it was paired with a state-ment, which reflected understanding or care. In hindsight it may seem obvious, but the "conventional wisdom" of short-term psychotherapy at that time strongly encouraged provoking anxiety to achieve a "breakthrough" to feeling (e.g., Davanloo's, *anxiety-provoking* methods).

Next, Joseph [52] compared all therapist interventions (e.g., questions, clar-ifications, confrontations, interpretations, self-disclosure, support) in their rela-tive capacity to elicit defensive versus affective responding. Like Makynen [50] and Salerno and associates [49], Joseph demonstrated that confrontation elicited more defensive behavior than any of the other eight interventions. Furthermore, clarification was the only intervention that significantly elicited affect. Appar-ently, the therapist listening carefully and reflecting back what the patient said prepared the patient to respond in a less defensive and more open and affective manner. Studies such as these, supporting empathy and clarification over con-frontation thus called into question the techniques of early forms of STDP for altering defenses, which often involved a heavy barrage of confrontation. How-ever, the therapist stance remained active, focused, and involved, and thus continued to differ markedly from the more classical psychoanalytic approach.

In the years that followed this research, we learned to use confrontation with a gentler touch. We now think that it was not confrontation per se that was the problem in eliciting affect, but that confrontations in the anxiety-provoking forms of STDP were used too strongly, too often, and too soon. With lower functioning patients, we now precede the confrontation of defenses with build-ing of the self-structure and increasing self-compassion, so that when confron-tations are given, they are not experienced as attacking. Sometimes, we blend confrontations with supportive statements (e.g., "This may have been the best you knew to do at the time [*support*], but do you see how you are always avoiding conflict now? [*conf*]"). Or, in other cases, we might include a recogni-tion of the patients' strengths with the confrontation, to help it be better received (e.g., "On one hand you have achieved a great deal in the professional world [*strength*], but the stories you tell of your personal life suggest that you might be sabotaging opportunities for closeness by demanding perfection from others [*conf*] What do you think?"). Such statements allow us to move as rapidly as possible with the uncovering process, but the supportive components help to protect as well as strengthen the patients' vulnerabilities around their sense of self. Patients often exclaim, "I am so relieved that you help me remember my strong points, when I am having to look at all these stupid things that I have been doing!" At which point the therapist might respond by saying, "Why call it stupid?" "Wasn't it the best you knew to do at the time?"

Thus, we have learned that a "spoonful of sugar" helps the confrontive medicine go down. Our clinical experience has taught us that the uncovering process is not only *not* lengthened in this process, but therapy moves much more smoothly, and gentler confrontations avoid therapy ruptures. Consequently, there is a need for a new thrust of research on these more evolved forms of confrontations. We suspect that the outcome, in eliciting affect, might be improved.

## BIMC Process Research Results: Affect Experiencing

Three studies at BIMC supported the need for sustained experiencing of feeling, while one study did not. Porter [53] demonstrated that the overall frequency of patient feeling did *not* correlate with improvement and the overall frequency of defenses did not predict poorer outcomes. These finding ran counter to theory, intuition, and clinical experience. However, a later study demonstrated that patient affect and defense are only predictive of outcome *when in response to therapist intervention* [54]. This study emphasized the importance of understanding context in relation to patient response. Taurke and colleagues [55] demonstrated that the greater the ratio of overall expressed affect to defense, not only in response to therapist intervention, the greater the improvement at outcome. Patients who improved the most changed from experiencing one episode of expressed affect per every five defensive responses at admission, to one affective response for every two defensive responses at termination. Moreover, the five least improved patients showed no change in the 1/5 affect/defense ratio shown at admission. These studies provided pivotal support for Malan's [3] assertion that lowering defensiveness in relation to affective expression will contribute to improvement in outcome.

Viewed as a whole, the BIMC process studies underscored the need for techniques to elicit affective expression and for overcoming the defensive obstacles to affective expression, but with gentler methods than initially thought. The objectives in the short-term Anxiety-Regulating Treatment of Affect Phobias described in this chapter have thus evolved from empirical evidence.

## The Intensive Process Analysis of the Trondheim Psychotherapy Research Program

Since 2001, the TPRP has been involved in the intensive process analyses of ATOS-coded videotapes from the Svartberg and Stiles RCT. These studies provide the opportunity to evaluate the change processes in STDP, and carry further the research begun at BIMC. Many areas of research are underway that include (1) ATOS variables in relation to outcome, (2) defense mechanisms and outcome, (3) differential responding across diagnostic categories, and (4) the relationship of specific affects to outcome. Process research is labor intensive so it will be many years to collect the necessary data. This chapter reports the preliminary results on three ATOS variables in relation to patient outcome.

The Trondheim program focuses on later sessions to identify factors that occur as a result of a growth process during treatment. Thus, sessions 6 and 36 of a 40-session treatment were rated. ATOS variables were levels of inhibitory feelings, activating feelings, and adaptive sense of self. Data were available from videotapes for 23 of 25 subjects in both CT and STDP. Missing data was due to corrupted videotapes or unrecorded sessions. We hypothesized that activating affect and sense of self would increase over time, while inhibitory affect would decrease over time, and that the mean levels of these variables late in therapy (e.g., at session 36) would be predictive of improvement. An averaged standardized composite outcome score was created and ranked patients according to those who were most to least improved on (1) combination of symptoms, (2) interpersonal relationships, and (3) character pathology (SCL-90 + IIP + MCMI-C/3). A standardized composite admission score was computed in the same manner and used as a covariate. Each ATOS variable was entered into a hierarchical regression with two covariates; a composite outcome premeasure and alliance ratings by the patient at session 4 (Working Alliance Inventory; Horvath and Greenberg [64].

## Trondheim Process Research Results: Activating Affect

As Table 11.2 shows, the average level of activating affect in the STDP group at session 6 was 29.4 (SD = 12.7; range = 8–52). By session 36 the average level of activating affect increased 9.2 points to 38.6 (SD = 16.0; range = 10–70). The cognitive group was quite similar to the STDP group at session six with an average level of activation of feeling at 30.4 (SD = 10.5; range = 15–52). By

**Table 11.2** Mean ATOS levels of activating and inhibitory affect and sense of self at sessions 6 and 36: and relationship to composite outcome score at termination in short-term dynamic therapy (STDP) and cognitive therapy (CT)

| ATOS variables and session number | ATOS levels in STDP | ATOS levels in CT |
|---|---|---|
| Activating affect: session 6 | 29.4 (SD = 12.7) | 30.4 (SD = 10.5) |
| Activating affect: session 36 | 38.6 (SD = 16.0)[*] | 32.5 (SD = 17.1) |
| Inhibitory affect: session 6 | 57.8 (SD = 16.7) | 56.2 (SD = 15.2)[**] |
| Inhibitory affect: session 36 | 46.9 (SD = 17.9) | 44.37 (SD = 15.1)[**] |
| Sense of self: session 6 | 34.7 (SD = 12.9) | 36.4 (SD = 13.3) |
| Sense of self: session 36 | 48.0 (SD = 21.4)[§] | 48.5 (SD = 16.7)[§] |

Relationship to composite outcome score:
[*]$p = 0.03$; [**]$p = 0.000$.
[§]$p = >0.01$, only when both CT and STDP groups were combined. Association with outcome was not significant for each group separately.

session 36, activating affect in the CT group had increased on average only 2.5 points to 32.5 (SD = 17; range = 5–64). In addition, Table 11.2 indicates that level of inhibitory affect at session 6 was significantly associated with outcome in the cognitive group, but not in the STDP group. This finding is in line with other research that shows that CT achieves symptom change quickly because it focuses on symptoms early in treatment. Interpersonal and dynamic models show similar change, but achieve that change later in treatment (e.g., [56]).

Figure 11.1 shows an excerpt of the activating affect scale thus placing these ratings in clinical terms. Both groups at session 6 were at the top edge of the *slight affective arousal* level (i.e., minimal or barely visible signs of feelings). By session 36, the STDP patients averaged an increase to the top of the *low affective arousal* level and nearly to the 41–50 *low-moderate arousal* level. The cognitive group increased only 2.5 points in 30 sessions (indeed their focus was not on this form of feelings) and activating affect in CT no longer was significantly associated to outcome at session 36. The low-moderate level refers to "mild feelings with much holding back." Surprisingly, this relatively low level of activating affect was significantly associated with outcome in the STDP group and captured 8% of the variance in outcome. In this regression, alliance remained the stronger factor with the expected 22% of the variance, and the pretreatment composite received 17%.

## Trondheim Process Research Results: Inhibitory Affects

The average level of inhibitory affect in the STDP group at session 6 was 57.8 (SD = 16.7; range = 28–91) and by session 36 this level had dropped 10.9 points

| 51–60 | Moderate affective arousal. Moderate feeling; moderate duration/moderate holding back, e.g. tearing up, moderate anger, some tender feelings as shown in face/vocal tone/body. Imagery or memories with moderate emotional content. Some relief. |
|---|---|
| 41–50 | Low-moderate affective arousal. Mild feeling with much holding back shown in face, vocal tone or body, e.g. briefly tears up, raises voice a little in anger, or says a few tender words for short duration, speaks openly. Imagery or memories with some emotional content. Mild relief. |
| 31–40 | Low affective arousal. Low, quickly passing experience of feeling shown in face, vocal tone or body; e.g. clenching fist, sighs, grimaces, choking up, slight sadness/anger/care for self but quickly stopped. Imagery or memories with low emotional content but appears very restrained/held back/constricted. A little relief. |
| 21–30 | Slight affective arousal. Minimal or barely visible/audible signs of feeling of short duration shown in face, vocal tone or body. May report slight change in internal bodily state. Imagery/memories have only slightest expression of feeling. Almost no relief. |
| 11–20 | No affective arousal, BUT bland verbal report of feeling. Almost no expression on face. Flat/dull/bland tone of voice, stiff or barely moving body. Patient may sense a change in internal bodily state, but is unsure whether it is a feeling or not. Only bland, unfeeling report of images or memories with emotional content. No relief. |

**Fig. 11.1** Excerpts of levels of activating affect on ATOS

to 46.9 (SD = 17.9; range = 20–89). Again the cognitive group was quite similar to the STDP group at session 6 with an average level of inhibitory affect of 56.2 (SD = 15.2; range 17–84) and by session 36, inhibitory affect had decreased on average 11.9 points to 44.37 (SD = 15; range = 12–68).

The inhibitory affect ratings on the ATOS (Fig. 11.2) show that both CT and STDP patients demonstrated a *moderate* level of inhibitory feelings (i.e., "anxiety, guilt, shame or pain was visibly evident in body language, vocal tone, or verbal report"). Both groups dropped between 11 and 12 points to a *low-moderate* level of inhibition (41–50). However, decrease in inhibitory affect was significantly associated with improvement only in the cognitive group ($p = 0.001$) and not in the STDP group. In CT, inhibitory affect captured 22% of the variance in outcome, and exceeded that of the alliance (17%).

It was unclear why decrease in inhibition was not related to outcome in the STDP group, until we rated a few tapes at session 16 and 26. In the CT group, inhibition appears to drop steadily throughout treatment, but in the STDP group, anxiety rose to high levels in session 16 tapes, in response to confrontation of defenses, and then dropped to and remained at low levels as activating affect emerged. This rise, then fall, in the inhibitory affects may be the reason that inhibitory feeling in STDP did not directly correlate with outcome, but we must await further data collection to confirm preliminary findings.

Nevertheless, the very positive results of the CT reduction in anxiety call into question, once again, the value of the STDP's use of confrontation to provoke anxiety. Further research is needed to see if a similar rapid reduction in anxiety would improve outcomes in STDP. It is interesting to imagine what the effects on outcome would be in *both groups* if levels of anxiety or shame could be reduced to levels even lower than we see in this study. The association with

| 71–80 | **Strong Inhibition**. Strong inhibitory affects. Much shakiness, hesitation, sighing or guardedness in tone of voice or non-verbal behavior. Restrained, withdrawn non-verbal behavioir. Very much discomfort. |
|---|---|
| 61–70 | **Much Inhibition**. Much inhibitory affect. Much shakiness, hesitation, sighing or guardedness in tone of voice. Some restraint or withdrawal in non-verbal behavior. Much discomfort. |
| 51–60 | **Moderate Inhibition**. Moderate inhibitory affects with moderate weakness in vocal tone; bodily movement vs restraint (moderate shakiness/hesitance/sighing, guardedness, slowness). Moderate discomfort. |
| 41–50 | **Low-moderate inhibition**. Some inhibitory thoughts or feelings. More fullness than shakiness/hesitation/sighing or guardedness in vocal tone or behavior. Less than moderate discomfort. |
| 31–40 | **Low inhibition**. Low inhibition. Only slight shakiness/hesitance/sighing/guardedness in voice or restraint in bodily movement. Low discomfort. |
| 21–30 | **Little inhibition.** Minimal or fleeting inhibition. Tone of voice or non-verbal behavior suggests a little discomfort . |

**Fig. 11.2** Excerpts s of levels of inhibitory affect on the ATOS

outcome in the cognitive group is already very strong. How much of the variance in outcome would be demonstrated if inhibition could be reduced to the low (31–40) or minimal (21–30) level in both groups?

## Trondheim Process Research Results: Sense of Self

The average level of positive sense of self at session 6 in the STDP group was *low-moderate* or 34.7 (SD = 12.9; range = 29–40). By session 36 the average level of sense of self had increased 13.2 points to 48.0 (SD = 21.4; range = 38–58). The CT group at session 6 had a *low-moderate* level of sense of self of 36.4 (SD = 13.3; range = 30–42). By session 36, sense of self had increased 12.1 points to 48.5 (SD = 16.7; range = 42–55).

Patients in both groups were rated on the ATOS (Fig. 11.3) as having a "somewhat maladaptive sense of self." Thirty sessions later, both groups had improved to a level of "mixed maladaptive and adaptive view of self." By the end of treatment, patients, on average, were approaching the next level indicating a "slightly more adaptive than maladaptive sense of self." This is an important accomplishment in a relatively short time. Some of the most exciting work in brief therapy is the active, focused work directly on feelings about the self. At session 6, the level of sense of self was not related to outcome. By session 36, the level of sense of self in both CT and STDP approached significance in relationship to outcome (STDP, $p = 0.065$, CT, $p = 0.085$). When the two

---

\61–70  **Somewhat adaptive sense of self:** Some pride in own strengths, and some affirming of own wants and needs. Some ability to acknowledge and accept limitations. Some compassion and self acceptance, but moderate self-blame or shame present.

51–60  **Mixed adaptive/maladaptive view of self:** Slightly more adaptive than maladaptive view of self. Slightly more pride than shame in self. Compassion & self-acceptance slightly greater than devaluation or grandiosity. Only moderately affirming of own wants and needs. Only a little more compassion and self-acceptance than self-blame or shame.

41–50  **Mixed maladaptive/adaptive view of self:** Slightly more maladaptive than adaptive view of self. Slightly more shame than pride in self. Devaluation or grandiosity is slightly stronger than self-compassion or acceptance of limitations. Only moderately affirming of own wants and needs. Slightly more self-blame and shame than compassion for self.

31–40  **Somewhat maladaptive sense of self:** Some shame in self. Minimal pride in own strengths. Somewhat affirming of own wants and needs in relation to others. Somewhat able to acknowledge and accept limitations. Some compassion and self-acceptance of self regarding limitations, but more self-blame or shame.

21–30  **Very maladaptive sense of self:** Much shame in self. Little pride/some grandiosity. Almost no affirming of wants and needs. Minimal ability to acknowledge and accept limitations and minimal ability to control impulses. Minimal compassion and self acceptance of self regarding limitations. Much self-blame or shame.

---

**Fig. 11.3** Excerpts of levels of image of the self on ATOS

groups were combined, the level of sense of self was associated with the composite outcome ($p = 0.009$) and captured 8% of the variance. In this regression analysis, alliance accounted for 16% and the pretreatment composite outcome measure (explained on p. 261) accounted for for 29.5% of the variance in outcome. Although it is commonly believed that the self-image does not change quickly, this data shows that within 30 sessions the sense of self improved on average, from being more maladaptive to close to being more adaptive, and that it significantly contributed to outcome.

As with the two affect variables, it is interesting to speculate what percent of the variance would be captured by change in sense of self if the average level of patients' self-image could be brought up just one level on the ATOS (61–70) "somewhat adaptive sense of self," that includes "some pride in oneself, some affirming of one's needs, some compassion or self-acceptance").

In summary, the preliminary ATOS data tell us that, first, a low-moderate ATOS level of activating feelings is associated with improvement in the STDP group. This finding is in line with STDP theory – exposure to feeling leads to resolution of the conflicted affect. Second, a low-moderate level of inhibitory feelings (e.g., anxiety, guilt, shame, pain) is very strongly associated with improvement at outcome in the CT group. Again, these results are in line with what is observed clinically as CT focuses more on reduction of anxiety or shame. Also, a lowered ATOS level of inhibitory feeling in session 36 captured more of the variance (27%) than alliance (17%). Finally, a near to moderate ATOS level on sense of self in both groups combined is significantly associated with improvement. It is well known that therapies of different names may rely on the same underlying mechanisms of change [35, 57–60]. Yet, the effects of activating and inhibiting affects show quite different and theoretically consistent pathways that ultimately arrived at the same level of outcome in CT and STDP groups.

It is important to remember that this data is based on two sessions out of a total of 40 and that these are preliminary analyses on specific treatment groups. We do not yet know if one session is representative of the beginning or end of treatment, or if a larger percentage of sessions are required to accurately capture what is taking place. In the coming years we will continue rating several thousand sessions on a number of different instruments with the objective of more clearly identifying the main ingredients of psychotherapy. However, these finding are consistent with STDP theory and lend support that we are moving in the right direction.

## Future Directions for Practice and Research

These preliminary process findings may offer guidance for training of therapists. In the 31–40 range of low-moderate affective responding, there remains much unprocessed grief, and much untapped anger or compassion for self. What if patients could be exposed to slightly higher levels of feeling? What if therapist skill could improve so that their capacity to elicit patients' conflicted feelings increases? These are the challenges we face as psychotherapists. Instruments such as the ATOS give feedback on patient growth and change, and may thus be of help in developing greater mastery of therapeutic skills.

Future research will explore what levels of affect experiencing and self-restructuring are optimal for change. At this point, we hypothesize that a high moderate level (ATOS rating of 61–70) would be optimal exposure (full feeling but not so high to be disorienting or overwhelming) and if attained, might capture a large and significant proportion of the variance in outcome. Additional work is underway to rate the initial evaluation session as well as sessions 16 and 26 so that we will be able to analyze changes across time. Many other process studies are planned and others are underway in the Trondheim program as well.

## Case Illustration of Objectives and Intervention in Resolving Affect Phobias

### *The Melancholic Grandmother*

The following is an illustration of how Affect Phobia objectives and interventions have been used in the treatment of a 69-year-old married woman who reported "lifelong depression," "misery" since early childhood and "countless" unsuccessful therapies over many decades. In clinical practice, the vast majority of Affect Phobias concern a few basic feeling categories (e.g., grief, anger/assertion, closeness, and positive feelings toward the self).

In the first 10 sessions in this treatment, dramatic change resulted from the exposure to feelings she had never felt in her 40 years of previous therapy. The therapist focused on compassion for herself, and grief over losses in her life. She was initially quite resistant and skeptical, but the therapist persisted, and by session 5, she no longer felt that she was a "bad seed." She began to see that her perfectionist and critical parents had crippled her spirit early in her life. She reported crying in therapy for 40 years, but this was likely a helpless, hopeless, weepiness, and not a resolving grief process. In the early treatment sessions, the therapist focused on exposure to self-compassion as well as identifying her self-attacking defenses.

## Objective: Gain Insight into Maladaptive Patterns (Identify Defenses)

Gaining insight refers to helping the patient become aware of unconscious defensive reactions as soon as they happen, and exploring their underlying feelings, origins in the past, and maintenance in current relationships

## Interventions

- A compassionate and collaborative therapist stance
- Regulating anxieties and shame associated with growing insight of defenses
- Validating defensive patterns as natural and once needed

*The therapist works with defenses beginning with a discussion on what it would be like to grieve in the session:*

| | |
|---|---|
| *Patient* | I am careful about my public personae. I am very aware of what other people might be thinking of me. |
| *Therapist* | Let's try to look at that. We need to make you comfortable with all kinds of feelings. What might I be thinking of you if you came here and just cried your eyes out? *(The therapist uses the real relationship to help the patient face and bear her shame over expressing sadness.)* |
| *Patient* | I don't know. |
| *Therapist* | Can we sit with it for just a moment and see *(holding the patient on blocks to grief).* |
| *Patient* | [tearful] I think it is because I have cried so much and it does not get me anywhere. |
| *Therapist* | Yes, that would be frightening wouldn't it? *(compassionate and validating stance)* |
| *Patient* | And [pause] I'll never stop, maybe *(anxiety about the grief).* |
| *Therapist* | That fear is so common *(anxiety regulation – the therapist calms the patient's anxiety by normalizing the experience).* The problem is that people stick their toe in the pool of grief, get scared, and pull out *(validating defense).* They don't know to go through it and come out the other side. That is what I am here to help guide you through *(anxiety regulation – psycho education about the treatment process).* |
| *Patient* | But I have been doing this for years [laughs]. |
| *Therapist* | And this is what keeps you in a chronic low-grade depression; it must be worked through *(identifying the costs of the defenses).* |

## Objective: Relinquish Maladaptive Patterns (Response Prevention)

Identifying the costs of defenses will build motivation for their relinquishing.

## Interventions

- An active therapist stance
- Noting the costs of defenses
- Regulating anxieties associated with giving up

*The therapist begins to look more closely at the origins of defensive patterns, while gently challenging self-attacking belief systems and guiding the patient toward motivation for change:*

| | |
|---|---|
| Patient | I think … I was born with a kink loose somewhere. |
| Therapist | There are clear things that I'm hearing with your feelings of perfectionism, and "never good enough" and so forth … |
| Patient | Yes. "Something's wrong with me" [sighs]. |
| Therapist | Rather than "What was wrong with the situation under which you learned these habits?"(*anxiety regulation – challenging the self-attacking, shameful beliefs*) |
| Patient | I guess I am rather moralistic. [pause] But other people have gone through greater odds and come out fine. |
| Therapist | … Can you see how there's no compassion for yourself? (*continually identifying self-attacking defense*) No work will be done unless this [self attack] gets out of the way. On one hand you say, "There is something wrong with me," or "I was born with a kink loose," but you describe yourself as an intelligent and feisty child – who had parents holding you back. And that is just a tragic thing. (*The therapist attempts to elicit grief and self-compassion in the patient for her plight.*) |
| Patient | they told me "The best was none too good." |
| Therapist | Their moralistic and perfectionistic standards were laid on you, and can you see how you are holding on to them, tight! (*Confronting the defenses and identifying developmental origins*). We need to help you to treat yourself like you treat your grandchildren. What would you say to them if they make a mistake? (*Self-restructuring – changing perspectives to begin to improve her sense of self.*) |
| Patient | I would be so gentle with them…but [pausing and covering face] …I am not worth it. |
| Therapist | You are not worth it? Let's stay with that [pause]. What brings that pain right there? (*actively focusing on exposure to grief*) |

| | |
|---|---|
| *Patient* | [Sobs with her face covered by her hands]. I don't know why I am not worth it. I really do believe that deep down there is something horrible in me. (*From the repeated therapist challenges, she begins to realize the destructiveness of her self-attack.*) |
| *Therapist* | The issue that hovers around your life is this enormous lack of compassion for self that you have carried for all these years. (*Gently pointing out self attacking defenses.*) |

*Although the patient moves closer to experiencing the grief associated with the costs of defenses, her self-attacking beliefs remain. Next, self-restructuring works to bring the patient closer to motivational stages, that is, readiness to begin facing core affect phobias.*

### *Objective*: Restructure the Sense of Self (Build Strength for Affect Exposure)

Through graduated exposure to positive feelings toward the self and adaptive feelings toward others, patients become increasingly able to bear conflicted affects.

### Interventions:

- A compassionate therapist stance
- Identifying self attacking thoughts, feelings and behaviors
- Exposing patients to positive, compassionate feelings toward the self and from others, including he therapist.

*Continued ...*

| | |
|---|---|
| *Patient* | I just can't imagine ever feeling good about myself. |
| *Therapist* | If you had another woman sitting here, telling the story of her life and that she carried, for 65 years, that she was not a good person, what would you say to her? From your heart, what would you say? (*changing perspectives and exposure to compassionate self-feelings*). |
| *Patient* | [sigh] I would tell her "be yourself, your real self," and I would probably cry. |
| *Therapist* | Tell me why you would cry for her (*focus on exposure to feeling of compassion*). |
| *Patient* | Because it is such a waste of life, think of all the waste [gazing off, silence]. |

| | |
|---|---|
| *Therapist* | What is going on for you now? What do you think I feel, seeing you, hearing this story today? (*exposure to the positive feelings of the therapist – Socratic questioning*). |
| *Patient* | [looks away – *shame*] It feels very juvenile. |
| *Therapist* | Very juvenile? How do you mean? (*focusing on continued self-attack*) |
| *Patient* | My thought is, "Oh hell, grow up!" |
| *Therapist* | You can see it intellectually and know you want to stop, but emotionally it's hard (*a validating, compassionate stance*). Your emotions are conditioned patterns, like cigarettes or drinking, and needing reworking. (*The therapist then decides to change the patient's perspective by using her own feelings.*) What do you sense that I am I feeling when I am hearing this story? (*actively focusing on exposure to therapist compassion – Socratic questioning*). |
| *Patient* | Well, I hope you have a plan [laughs]. (*Response is intellectual rather than emotional.*) |
| *Therapist* | Yes, that is in my mind. But, what is in my heart? (*Focusing on the feeling.*) |
| *Patient* | I don't know [looks down]. (*Defensive avoidance.*) |
| *Therapist* | Can you let yourself go there for a moment? (*Holding focus on therapist compassion.*) |
| *Patient* | My instinct is to say "what a wimp" [laughs nervously– *and attacks self-critically*]. |
| *Therapist* | You do not criticize this (*imaginary*) other woman, but instead, you turn the attack on yourself (*identifying self-attack*). And I will catch that every time. But, I just had a strong reaction toward you, and I want you to try to pick it up. What is in me? (*actively staying with exposure to therapist compassion – Socratic questioning. The therapist will not acknowledge her feelings, until the patient has searched within herself to sense the therapist's response*). |
| *Patient* | [timidly] I hope sympathy? |
| *Therapist* | You bet there is sympathy! (*Once offered, it is strongly supported.*) But not only that...I had this aching feeling thinking about it, and it is heartache (*shared affect*). The word...heartache came up. A little bit of tears, a real sad feeling in my body (*modeling identification of feelings*). Yet I am not living what you are going through. It is a real tragedy how you have suffered all your life, and there is that grief in you somewhere about these losses. I am going to shine a spotlight on it, and you can too, until you can't bear to hurt yourself any longer. How does that sound? |
| *Patient* | [with a slight raising of the eyes] ....Hopeful. |

*The process of restructuring defenses and feelings toward the self often takes time and repetition depending on the intensity of the presenting conflicts, the rigidity of the patient's defenses, and the degree of the patients strengths. In this case, the work of actively and consistently desensitizing her phobias to grief and self-compassion began within the first five treatment sessions. The carefully considered use of therapist feelings has been a powerful tool to impact on sense of self. We learn who we are from others responses to us.*

## Objective: Exposure to activating affect with graduated intensity (Exposure)

The therapist draws from Gestalt and experiential strategies as well as from a variety of cognitive, behavioral, and psycho-educational interventions employed in step-wise desensitization in doses that the patient can bear.

## Interventions

- Active therapist stance
- Graduated exposure to feared affect in imagery, memory or fantasy
- Focus on emotional experiencing in bodily arousal
- Preventing defensive avoidance ("Stay with the feeling in your body")
- Modulate anxieties ("What's the hardest part of feeling the grief?")

*Session 10: Here, the therapist guides the patient in grieving the losses of childhood – the loss of nurturance and parental compassion.*

| | |
|---|---|
| *Patient* | I am sad. So damn it, I want to work this out, get over it. (*She has become highly motivated.*) |
| *Therapist* | Just stay with that (*encouraging exposure to feeling*). |
| *Patient* | [struggling] I can't [pause]. I really can't…[trailing off] |
| *Therapist* | Just try to stay with your body (*preventing defensive avoidance and connecting emotional and bodily arousal*). What hurts the most? (*anxiety regulation*). |
| *Patient* | My body [points to her heart]. |
| *Therapist* | Your heart hurts most? So let's help you sit with the grieving. (*Giving support*) |
| *Patient* | I don't want to stay with the grieving. (*A phobic response to the feeling*) |
| *Therapist* | What is hardest about it? (*Anxiety regulation is used to help her stay with the feeling by exploring her fears about the feeling.*) |

| | |
|---|---|
| *Patient* | It is just such a familiar path. And it comes again, and again, and again [tears up]. |
| *Therapist* | Yes, well let's go with it for a little bit (*response prevention – holding patient on the grief*). Your eyes water and there is so much pain in you right now. [softly] Will you let me look at it with you? |
| *Patient* | [sighs] I don't know what to do with it. |
| *Therapist* | Let's put some words on it for a moment. What are you feeling that could speak for that hurt heart? (*helping patient to label the experience*). |
| *Patient* | It feels like I want my mama; that is what it feels like. |
| *Therapist* | Yes, right. |
| *Patient* | It is so sad [tears up]. |
| *Therapist* | Let yourself float back, way back then (*exposure to grief through imagery*). What ever comes, what memories come? "I want my mama." It is such a deep part of all of us. What did you long for most from her? (*continues imagery of longing for her mother*). |
| *Patient* | [tearful] Hugs [And she begins to cry]. |

*The process is best characterized by graduated steps, the Grandmother's "toe is dipped in the waters of grief." Affect work is often characterized by brief moments of affect followed by defense restructuring and anxiety regulation. Later, the patient experiences a much fuller and deeper grieving process as described below. Successful resolution of affect phobias typically involves much repletion of the same affect-laden images.*

| | |
|---|---|
| *Therapist* | Let's imagine that she could love you (affect exposure – *imagining the action tendency*). Let's create an ideal mother. |
| *Patient* | She would just hold me. |
| *Therapist* | And how would she hold you? (*affect exposure – provide rich detail to images*). |
| *Patient* | Just hug me, I guess [looks down]. |
| *Therapist* | Are you kind of detached from this part? (*pointing out defensive resistance*). |
| *Patient* | Yes, I can't possibly imagine that happening in real life. |
| *Therapist* | But right now see if you can imagine an ideal mother (*affect exposure – holding patient on focus of receiving care for self*). |
| *Patient* | [sighs] So a real mother would have put her arms around me and told me that it was going to be all right? |
| *Therapist* | And she would have rubbed you a little bit and held you tight? And how would that make you feel to have somebody there saying that? |

| | |
|---|---|
| *Patient* | [with a sad voice] That would feel so good. |
| *Therapist* | Yes, how does it feel in your body if you really let yourself go deep into that (*connecting image to bodily experience*)? She is holding you; she might be resting her head on your head. Stroking your hair. Where do you feel it in your body? |
| *Patient* | [starts to cry deeply] |
| *Therapist* | Just stay with that. [silence, patient crying] |
| *Patient* | It makes my heart ache [covers eyes and sobs]. I have never felt so alone. [sobs deeply] …I think I am still grieving the loss of a mother I never had. |

*This session was rated on the ATOS, Her level of experiencing of grief was in the high 70's, ebbing and flowing for over 40 min. Her level of inhibitory feeling was in the 70–80 range (her great pain over the profound neglect in childhood, and her shame about herself.) She continued the grief process until the shame and pain were reduced and she felt a more compassionate, and accepting stance toward herself. The adaptive grief she was exposed to resulted in a lifting of her depression, discontinuance of her antidepressant medication, and as best described in the following examples, a new way of experiencing herself and the world.*

| | |
|---|---|
| *Patient* | My daughter came to visit and she said, "Mom! You're better!" "You're really better!" |
| *Therapist* | So what do you think is the shift? |
| *Patient* | The depression lifting. |
| *Therapist* | What do you think made the depression lift? What aspect of what we did? |
| *Patient* | I got deeper into what was reality, instead of telling the same old story of complaining and feeling sorry for myself. You did not let me get away with that [laughs]. |
| *Therapist* | What was the same old story? |
| *Patient* | You know, that I was constantly criticized and never fully praised. (*This patient spent 30 + years in therapy telling the "same old story!" She knew what was wrong; the intellectual stories were told, but she had never focused so intently on the associated feelings.*) |
| *Therapist* | What did we do different here? |
| *Patient* | We went deeper. You did not let me off the hook. |

*Finally, here in a discussion of her day*

| | |
|---|---|
| *Patient* | I was early, so I drove a different route. While driving, I thought how beautiful everything looks. The houses are wonderful, the sun is wonderful, spring is coming and [pause]. It is different; I really am different! |

*At one and a half year follow-up she was able to maintain these gains and stay off antidepressant medication. She then had many crises in the coming years, including her husband's increasing illness, and a tragic death of an adult child, but she coped better than expected, and throughout the difficulties, never again felt herself to be a "bad seed."*

## Conclusion

It has been said repeatedly that research does not influence clinical practice. However, this treatment model has been developed and repeatedly revised, always closely guided by research findings. Research has been the architect as well as the demolition squad of the affect phobia treatment model. The data has often challenged us in unexpected ways but remembering that "the data is our friend" has guided us well and led to a more nuanced understanding of underlying processes.

Twenty-five years of process research has pointed us to affect as the primary change agent in short-term psychotherapy; possibly stronger than insight or motivation for treatment, and now, some forms of affect restructuring may be, in some instances, a stronger factor than the therapeutic alliance. If we improve our therapeutic skills, the affect variables may capture more variance and may challenge the alliance factor even further. These results suggest that the interventions taught in this chapter can be said to be evidence-based, and may lend support to specific factors at work in short-term psychotherapy.

Finally, emerging therapists or seasoned clinicians can feel more confident that the empirical evidence is pointing to feeling as a prime focus in for resolution of patient symptoms, interpersonal problems, and character pathology. So:

*Don't forget to follow the affect!*

## References

1. Wampold, B. (2001). *The great psychotherapy debate*. New Jersey: Lawrence Erlbaum.
2. Lambert, M.J. & Ogles, B.M. (2004) Chapter 5. The efficacy and effectiveness of psychotherapy. In M. Lambert (Ed.), *Bergin and Garfield's handbook of psychotherapy and behavior change* (5th edition), New York: John Wiley & Sons, Inc., 139–193.
3. Malan, D.M. (1979). *Individual psychotherapy and the science of psychodynamics*. London: Heineman-Butterworth Press.
4. Davanloo, H. (Ed.) (1980). *Short-term dynamic psychotherapy*. New York: Jason Aronson.
5. Davanloo, H. (1988). The technique of unlocking of the unconscious: Part I. *International Journal of Short-Term Psychotherapy, 3*(2), 99–121.
6. McCullough, L. (1991). Davanloo's short-term dynamic psychotherapy: A cross-theoretical analysis of change mechanisms. In R. Curtis & G. Stricker (Eds.), *How people change: Inside and outside of psychotherapy*. New York: Plenum Press, 59–79.
7. McCullough, L. (1999). Short-term psychodynamic therapy as a form of desensitization: Treating affect phobias. *In Session: Psychotherapy in Practice 4*(4), 35–53.

8. McCullough, L., Kuhn, N., Andrews, S., Kaplan, A, Wolf, J. & Hurley, C.L. (2003). *Treating affect phobia: A manual for short-term dynamic psychotherapy.* New York: Guilford Press.

9. Foa, E. and Kozak, M.J. (1986). Emotional processing of fear: Exposure to corrective information. *Psychological Bulletin 99*(1), 20–35.

10. Freud, S. (1956). Turnings in the ways of psychoanalytic therapy. In E. Jones (Ed.), *Collected Papers,* Vol. 2, London: Hogarth Press, 392–402.

11. Alexander, F. & French, T.M. (1946). *Psychoanalytic therapy: Principles and applications.* New York: Ronald Press.

12. Malan, D.M. (1963). *A study of brief psychotherapy.* New York: Plenum.

13. Stern, D.N. (1995). *The motherhood constellation.* New York: Basic Books.

14. Stern, D.N. (1985). *The interpersonal world of the infant: A view from psychoanalysis and developmental psychology.* New York: Basic Books.

15. Stern, D.N. (1977). *The first relationship: mother and infant.* Cambridge, Mass.: Harvard University Press.

16. Tomkins, S.S. (1962). *Affect, imagery, and consciousness: Vol. I. Positive affects.* New York: Springer.

17. Tomkins, S.S. (1963). *Affect, imagery, and consciousness: Vol. II. Negative affects.* New York: Springer.

18. Ekman, P. & Davidson, R. (1994). *The nature of emotion.* New York: Oxford University Press.

19. Eagle, M. (1984). *Recent developments in psychoanalysis. A critical analysis.* New York: McGraw Hill.

20. Cautela, J.R. (1977). Covert conditioning: Assumptions and procedures. *Journal of Mental Imagery, 3, 53–64.*

21. Cautela, J.R & McCullough L. (1977). Covert conditioning: A learning theory perspective on imagery. In J.L. Singer & K.S. Pope (Eds.) *The power of the human imagination.* New York: Plenum Press, 227–254.

22. Dollard, J. & Miller, N.E. (1950). *Personality and psychotherapy: An analysis in terms of learning, thinking, and culture.* New York: McGraw-Hill.

23. Stampfl, T.G. & Levis, D.J. (1967). Essentials of implosive therapy: A learning-theory based psychodynamic behavioral therapy. *Journal of Abnormal Psychology, 72,* 496–503.

24. Feather, B.W. & Rhoads, J.M. (1972). Psychodynamic behavior therapy: II: Clinical aspects. *Archives of General Psychiatry,* 26, 503–511.

25. Freud, S. (1923). The Ego and the Id. *Standard Edition,* 19, 2–66.

26. Wachtel, P.L. (1977). *Psychoanalysis and behavior therapy: Toward an integration.* New York: Basic Books.

27. Orlinsky, D.E., Ronnestad, M.H. and Willutzki, U. (2004). Fifty Years of Psychotherapy Process-Outcome Research: Continuity and Change. In Michael Lambert (Editor) *Bergin and Garfield's handbook of psychotherapy and behavior change:* (5th Edition), New York: John Wiley & Sons, 307–390.

28. Orlinsky, D., Grawe, K. & Parks, B.K. (1994). Process and outcome in psychotherapy – noch einmal. In S.L. Garfield & A.E. Bergin (Eds.), *Handbook of psychotherapy and behavior change* (4th edition), New York: John Wiley & Sons.

29. Gray, J.A: (1975). *Elements of a two-process theory of learning.* New York: Academic Press.

30. Fowles, D.C., (1980). The three arousal model. Implications of Gray's two-factor learning theory for heart rate, electrodermal activity, and psychopathy. *Psychophysiology, 17*(2), 87–104.

31. Fowles, D.C. (1988). Psychophysiology and psychopathology. A motivational approach. *Psychophysiology, 25*(4), 373–391.

32. Wilhelm, F.H. & Roth, W.T. (1998). Taking the laboratory to the skies: Ambulatory assessment of self-report, autonomic, and respiratory responses in flying phobia. *Psychophysiology, 35*(5), 596–606.
33. Konorski, J., (1967). *Integrative activity of the brain: An interdisciplinary approach.* Chicago: University of Chicago Press.
34. Dickinson, A. & Dearing, M.F. (1979). Appetitive-aversive interactions and inhibitory processes. In: A. Dickinson & Boakes, R.A. (Eds.) *Mechanisms of learning and motivation.* Hillsdale, NJ: Erlbaum, 203–231.
35. Lang, P., P.J., Bradley, M.M. & Cuthbert, B.N: (1998). Emotion, motivation, and anxiety: Brain mechanisms and psychophysiology. *Biological Psychiatry, 44:* 1248–1263.
36. Sutton, S.K. & Davidson, R. (1997). Prefrontal Brain Asymmetry: A biological substrated of the behavioral approach and inhibition systems.*Psychological Science, 8,* 204.
37. Foa, E. & McNally, R.J. (1996). Mechanisms of change in exposure therapy. In R. M. Rapee (Ed.), *Current controversies in the anxiety disorders.* New York: The Guilford Press, 229–343.
38. Barlow, D.H. (Ed.) (2002). *Anxiety and its disorders: The nature and treatment of anxiety and panic.* New York: The Guilford Press.
39. Winston A, McCullough L, Trujillo M, Pollack J, Laikin M, Flegenheimer W & Kestenbaum, R. (1991) Brief psychotherapy of personality disorders. *Journal of Nervous and Mental Disease, 179*(4), 188–193.
40. Winston, A., Laikin, M., Pollack, J., Samstag, L.W., McCullough, L. & Muran, J.C. (1994). Short-term psychotherapy of personality disorders. *American Journal of Psychiatry, 151*(2), 190–194.
41. Svartberg M., Stiles, T. & Seltzer, M. (2004). A randomized controlled trial of the effectiveness of short term dynamic psychotherapy and cognitive therapy for cluster C personality disorders. *Journal of Consulting and Clinical Psychology, 161,* 810–817.
42. Derogatis, L.R. (1983). *SCL-90-R: Administration, scoring & procedures manual-II for the revised version and other instruments of the psychopathology rating scale series* (2nd edition). Towson, MD: Clinic Psychometric Research.
43. Horowitz, L.M., Rosenberg, S.E., Baer, B.A., Ureno, G. & Villasenor, V.S. (1988). Inventory of interpersonal problems: psychometric properties and clinical applications. *Journal of Clinical and Consulting Psychology, 56,* 885–892.
44. Millon, T. (1984). Millon clinical multiaxial inventory (3rd edition). Minneapolis, MN: National Computer Services.
45. McCullough, L., Larsen, A.E., Schanche, E., Andrews, S., Kuhn, N., Hurley, C.L., et al. (2004). *Achievement of therapeutic objectives scale.* Short-Term Psychotherapy Research Program at Harvard Medical School. Can be downloaded from www.affectphobia.com.
46. Carley, M. (2006). The validity of the achievement of therapeutic objectives scale. Dissertation. Fielding Institute. Boston, MA, 2006.
47. Cohen, J. (1988). *Statistical power analysis for the behavioral sciences.* Hillsdale, NJ: Lawrence Erlbaum.
48. Leichsenring, F., Rabung, S. & Leibing, E. (2004). The Efficacy of Short-term pspsychodynamic psychotherpay in specific psychiatric disorders: A meta-analysis. *Archives of General Psychiatry, 61,* 1208–1216.
49. Salerno, M., Farber, B., McCullough, L., Winston, A. & Trujillo, M. (1992). The effects of confrontation and clarification on patient affective and defensive responding. *Psychotherapy Research, 2*(3), 181–192.
50. Makynen A. (1992). The effects of continued confrontation on patient affective and defensive response. Columbia University Teachers' College, May, 1992. *Dissertation Abstracts International, 54-01B.*
51. Foote, J. (1989). Interpersonal context and patient change episodes. New York University, May, 1989. *Dissertation Abstracts International, 51-12B.*

52. Joseph, C. (1988). Antecedents to transference interpretation in short-term psychody-namic psychotherapy (doctoral dissertation, Rutgers University). *Dissertation Abstracts International, May 1988 50-04B.*
53. Porter, F. (1988). The immediate effects of interpretation on patient in-session response in brief dynamic psychotherapy. Columbia University Teachers College, May, 1987. *Dissertation Abstracts International, 48,* 87-24076.
54. McCullough L., Winston A., Farber B., Porter F., Pollack J., Laikin M., Vingiano W. & Trujillo, M. (1991). The relationship of patient-therapist interaction to outcome in brief psychotherapy.*Psychotherapy, 28*(4), 525–533.
55. Taurke, E., McCullough, L., Winston, A., Pollack, J. & Flegenheimer, W. (1990). Change in affect-defense ratio from early to late sessions in relation to outcome.*Journal of Clinical Psychology, 46*(5), 657–668.
56. Coombs, M.M, Coleman, D. & Jones, E.E. (2002). Working with feelings: The impor-tance of emotion in both cognitive-behavioral and interpersonal therapy in the NIMH Treatment of Depression Collaborative Research program. P*sychotherapy: Theory/ Research/Practice /Training, 39*(3), 233–244.
57. Goldfried M.R., Raue P.J. & Castonguay, L.G. (1998). The therapeutic focus in significant sessions of master therapists: A comparison of cognitive behavioral and psychodynamic–interpersonal interventions. *Journal of Consulting and Clinical Psychology, 66,* 803–810.
58. Ablon, J.S. & Jones, E.E. (1998). How expert clinicians' prototypes of an ideal treatment correlate with outcome in psychodynamic and cognitive behavioral therapy. *Psychotherapy Research, 8,* 71–83.
59. Ablon, J.S. & Jones, E.E. (1999). Psychotherapy process in the National Institute of Mental Health Treatment of Depression Collaborative Research Program. *Journal of Consulting and Clinical Psychology, 67,* 64–75.
60. Ablon, J.S. & Jones, E.E. (2002). Validity of Controlled Trials of Psychotherapy: Findings from the NIMH Treatment of Depression Collaborative Research Program. *American Journal Psychiatry, 159,* 775–783.
61. Diener, M.J., Hilsenroth, M.J. & Weinberger, J. (2007). Therapist affect focus and patient outcomes in psychodynamic psychotherapy: A meta-analysis. *American Journal of Psychiatry, 164,* p 936–941.
62. Ferenczi, S. and Rank, O. (1925). *The Development of Psychoanalysis.* New York: Nervous and Mental Disease Publishing Company.
63. Carver, C.S. and White; T.L. (1994). Behavioral inhibition, Behavioral Activation, and Affective Responses to Impending Reward and Punishment: The BIS/BAS Sacles. *Journal of Personality and Social Psychology, (1994). 67,* 319–333, content.apa.org.
64. Horvath, A.O. and Greenberg, L.S. (1989). Development and validation of the Working Alliance Inventory. *Journal of Counseling Psychology, 36,* 223–233.

# Chapter 12
# Factors Contributing to Sustained Therapeutic Gain in Outpatient Treatments of Depression

**Sidney J. Blatt, David C. Zuroff, and Lance Hawley**

It is vital for the mental health disciplines, in this era of public and scientific demands to identify empirically supported treatments (ESTs), to differentiate themselves from other types of health-care providers, to define more precisely the uniqueness of the disorders with which we work, and to identify the central features of the treatments we provide and the dimensions that contribute to constructive and sustained therapeutic change. The disease model, dominant in medical practice and in much of psychiatry, has, at best, limited applicability in the mental health disciplines. Increasingly, questions are raised about the disease model and its focus on manifest behavioral symptoms, inherent in the diagnostic nosological structure of the *Diagnostic and Statistical Manual of Mental Disorders* (DSM-IV), for understanding clinical disturbances in mental health, particularly its failure to recognize subclinical expressions of clinical phenomena [1]. Furthermore, recent research has raised questions about symptom reduction as the primary goal in the treatment of psychological disorders [2]. In addition, though aspects of the doctor–patient relationship play an important role in many medical treatments, recent evidence unequivocally demonstrates the critical role that the therapeutic relationship has in the treatment process of psychological disturbances and psychiatric disorders (e.g., [2–6]).

DSM-IV of the American Psychiatric Association [7] presents a seemingly endless list of separate diseases or disorders and specifies arbitrary threshold values (not established through empirical investigation) for identifying an array of symptoms that define each of these disorders. Because DSM-IV is essentially a-etiological, various pathways are possible for the development of the symptoms associated with each disorder (equifinalilty) and similar etiological factors can contribute to the symptoms associated with different disorders (multifinality). Similar symptomatic patterns may emerge from different etiological pathways and similar etiological factors, depending on a variety of factors and circumstances, which may be expressed in different disorders [8]. As a consequence of this loose (fuzzy)

S.J. Blatt
Department of Psychiatry and Psychology, Yale University, 300 George Street, Suite 901, New Haven, CT 06511, USA
e-mail: Sidney.blatt@yale.edu

R.A. Levy, J.S. Ablon (eds.), *Handbook of Evidence-Based Psychodynamic Psychotherapy*, DOI: 10.1007/978-1-59745-444-5_12, © Humana Press 2009

categorical system, considerable overlap occurs among the symptomatic criteria defining various disorders, contributing to the vexing problem of "comorbidity" in clinical practice and research in which patients often meet criteria for a number of different disorders. This diagnostic confusion makes it difficult to discover etiological factors that contribute to the onset of psychological difficulties or to define precisely which treatments are appropriate for which disorders. These diagnostic problems are particularly apparent in the area of depression, in which difficulties are encountered in establishing meaningful diagnostic distinctions, other than degree of severity, and in understanding the etiological factors that contribute to the onset of depression and in identifying ESTs.

Research findings indicate relatively little success in treating depression [9] either with psychotherapy, medication, or with a combination of these two treatment modalities because of the relatively high relapse rate [10, 11]. Only approximately 20% of the patients in the National Institute of Mental Health (NIMH) sponsored landmark investigation, the Treatment of Depression Collaborative Research Program (TDCRP), for example, were rated as fully recovered – as having a reduction in symptoms at termination without substantial relapse in the 18 months following the termination of treatment [10]. These findings suggest that a broad approach is needed to understand depression, an approach that goes beyond diagnostic classifications based on manifest symptoms, an approach that begins to consider factors that contribute to the onset of depression and attempts to identify, assess, and treat vulnerability factors as well as the symptoms of depression. After an era of predominant focus on diagnoses based on manifest behavioral symptoms and on treatments directed toward reducing these symptoms, investigators are beginning to focus on issues of vulnerability. Ingram and Price [12, p. ix], for example, note that "there is little doubt that the future of clinical research and treatment lies in the study of vulnerability processes." It has become increasingly apparent that it is essential to understand the vulnerabilities that contribute to the onset of depression as well as the factors that contribute to effective treatment that reduces these vulnerabilities and results in long-term, sustained, clinical improvement. The predominant contemporary preoccupation with symptom reduction must be supplemented by concerns about the reduction of vulnerabilities in the treatment process if we are to develop treatments that prevent relapse after the termination of treatment [13].

The extensive relapse rate following the brief treatment of depression with psychotherapy, medication, or a combination of psychotherapy and medication, has led to the realization of the ineffectiveness of brief treatment for depression and the need to either extend the length of treatment or to develop follow-up maintenance programs to reduce relapse rates [14]. Another approach has been to develop alternative treatments that address particularly maladaptive cognitive-affective interpersonal schemas or personality dimensions (e.g., [15–25]) that have been identified as vulnerability factors in depression. Extensive research (see summaries in [19, 26]) clearly indicate that preoccupation with interpersonal relatedness, especially feelings of dependency, as well as intense concerns about self-worth, especially self-critical perfectionism, are important sources of vulnerability to depression. Extensive research demonstrates that these personality factors of dependency/sociotropy and self-critical perfectionism/ autonomy [15, 17, 27, 28] play important roles in the etiology, clinical course, and treatment of depression. These distorted cognitive-affective interpersonal or relational schemas of self and others contribute to the establishment of depressogenic environments (e.g., [19, 30, 31]). Brief treatments of depression, focused primarily on symptom reduction, may temporarily deactivate these maladaptive cognitive-affective interpersonal schemas, but these vulnerabilities are often reactivated by stressful life experiences that occur after the termination of treatment. Thus, systematic research must be devoted to identifying treatments that result in changes in these maladaptive interpersonal schemas and other personality factors that create vulnerabilities to depression [32, 33].

Evidence also increasingly indicates the central role of the therapist and the quality of the therapeutic relationship in the treatment process [6, 34, 35]. The quality of the therapist and the therapeutic relationship has always been central in psychodynamic treatments (e.g., transference and countertransference and the contemporary emphasis on intersubjectivity) and more recently, cognitive-behavioral approaches have begun to consider the role of therapist competence [36] and the therapeutic relationship as important aspects of therapeutic interventions (e.g., [23, 37]). Schema-focused cognitive therapy [25], for example, which shares conceptual similarity with the emphasis on internalization in psychodynamic treatments (e.g., [38–42]), stresses the need to go beyond surface level cognitions and symptoms to explore factors that contribute to change in the relatively stable cognitive-affective interpersonal schemas and personality dimensions in the treatment process in an effort to identify treatments that result in sustained therapeutic change [19, 43–45].

The goal of this paper is to address these issues in the treatment of depression: (1) the relative role of changes in symptoms and vulnerability factors (i.e., cognitive-affective interpersonal schemas and personality features in the treatment process), (2) the relative effectiveness of different types of treatment [i.e., medication and two forms of psychotherapy [cognitive-behavioral therapy (CBT) and interpersonal therapy (IPT)] in the reduction of symptoms and vulnerability factors, and (3) the role of the therapist and the therapeutic relationship in the treatment process. Thus, in this paper we study treatment outcome at termination and at an extended follow-up and compare the contributions of types of treatment, patient factors [19, 46], therapist variables (e.g., [47]) and aspects of the treatment process (i.e., therapeutic alliance) [48, 49] to treatment outcome. We address these issues through summarizing, extending and integrating various analyses that we and our colleagues have conducted on data gathered as part of the remarkably comprehensive data set established by the NIMH-sponsored TDCRP. Though our approach to these issues is through consideration of further analyses of data gathered in a comprehensive study of brief, manual-directed treatments for depression, we believe that these findings have important implications for psychodynamic treatment and we address these implications toward the close of this paper.

# Method

## Treatment of depression in the NIMH-sponsored Treatment of Depression Collaborative Research Program

An extensive and diverse data set on the brief outpatient treatment of serious depression was established by the TDCRP, probably the most extensive and comprehensive randomized clinical trial for the treatment of depression even conducted in psychotherapy research. The empirical data from this research program became available to the scientific community in 1994, after the TDCRP investigators concluded their primary explorations of this remarkable data set.

The TDCRP was a well-designed, carefully conducted, randomized, multi-site, clinical trial comparing 16 weeks of two forms of brief outpatient manual-directed psychotherapy for depression (CBT and IPT) with antidepressant medication (imipramine, the antidepressant of choice at the time of the investigation) with clinical management, and a double-blind placebo, also with clinical management.[1] The TDCRP data set contains extensive and diverse evaluations of patients before, during, and subsequent to treatment. These extensive clinical evaluations were conducted by a PhD-level clinical evaluator (CE) prior to treatment, every 4 weeks during the treatment process, and again at 6, 12, and 18 months following the termination of treatment. Additionally, evaluations and reports were obtained periodically from the therapists and the patients. Extensive periodic evaluations were also conducted on aspects of the therapeutic process:

1. A measure of the patients' experience of the quality of the therapeutic alliance using the Barrett-Lennard Relationship Inventory (B-L RI, 1985) obtained early in the treatment process (after the second treatment session). The B-L RI, based on Rogers' [50–52] assumptions about the necessary and sufficient conditions for treatment, has four scales (Empathic Understanding, Level of Regard, Unconditionality of Regard, and Congruence) that assess the extent to which patients experienced the therapist as empathic and understanding.
2. Systematic ratings of the contributions that patient and therapist make to the therapeutic alliance in the 3rd, 9th, and 15th treatment sessions by Krupnick and colleagues [48] based on videotape recordings of the treatment sessions using a modified version of the Vanderbilt Therapeutic Alliance Scale (VTAS) [53]. Krupnick et al. [48] found that treatment outcome in the

---

[1] The clinical management (CM) component was designed to manage the medications and to "provide a generally supportive atmosphere and to enable the psychiatrist to assess the patient's status." "The manual and training ... include guidelines for providing support and encouragement to the patient and giving direct advice when necessary. This CM component thus approximates a 'minimal supportive therapy' condition" [88].

TDCRP was significantly related to the degree to which the patient was rated as being engaged in the treatment process (e.g., open and honest with the therapist, agreeing with the therapist about tasks, goals, and responsibilities; and actively engaged in the therapeutic task). The therapist contributions factor, however, was not significantly related to therapeutic outcome [48].

Therapeutic progress was evaluated every 4 weeks during treatment, and at three follow-up assessments at 6-month intervals following the termination of treatment by a clinical interview and a self-report measure of depression [the Hamilton Rating Scale for Depression (HRS-D) and the Beck Depression Inventory (BDI), respectively], interview and self-report measures of general clinical functioning [the Global Assessment Scale (GAS) from DSM-IV and the Hopkins Symptom Checklist (SCL-90), respectively], and an interview measure of social adjustment [Social Adjustment Scale] [54]. Though the TDCRP investigators (e.g., Elkin, Parloff, Shea, and Docherty) and their colleagues used the HRS-D as their primary outcome measure (e.g., [55]), Blatt et al. [56] found that the residualized gain scores of these five outcome measures (HRS-D, BDI, GAS, SCL-90, and the SAS) at termination were highly intercorrelated, each loading substantially (>0.70) on a common factor. Blatt et al. [56] converted these five measures to standard scores to construct a composite measure of therapeutic gain that reflected the overall level of clinical functioning, with a particular emphasis on depressive symptoms. In addition, the TDCRP investigators included the Dysfunctional Attitudes Scale (DAS) [57] in their assessment evaluations at baseline and throughout treatment and follow-up. Research (e.g., [58]) indicates that the DAS assesses the two dimensions of vulnerability discussed above (dependency and self-critical perfectionism).

This extensive data set of evaluations of therapeutic outcome and aspects of the therapeutic process enabled us to address fundamental questions about the relative contributions of medication and the two forms of psychotherapy (CBT and IPT) and aspects of the therapeutic alliance to changes in symptoms and in vulnerability to depression. It also enabled us to examine the longitudinal relationship between changes in symptoms and vulnerability factors during treatment process and in the 18-month follow-up period.

In the primary analyses of their data, the TDCRP investigators found "no evidence of greater effectiveness of one of the psychotherapies as compared with the other and no evidence that either of the psychotherapies was significantly less effective than … imipramine plus clinical management" [9, p. 971]. Comparison of the effects of 16 weeks of treatment indicated that though medication (imipramine) resulted in more rapid reduction in symptoms [59]; no significant differences were found in symptom reduction among the three active treatment conditions at termination (e.g., [9]) and at the follow-up assessment conducted 18 months after the termination of treatment [18, 82]. In addition, the TDCRP investigators [10] reported follow-up data that indicated substantial relapse over an 18-month period subsequent to the termination of treatment, especially in the medication conditions.

**Phenomenological Subtypes of Depression**

Dissatisfaction with symptom-based classifications of depression had led several clinical investigators (i.e., [15, 17–19, 27, 28, 60–64]) to differentiate types of depression on the basis of the fundamental concerns that lead individuals to become depressed [65]. These formulations derive from diverse theoretical perspectives (i.e., attachment theory, CBT, psychoanalytic object relations theory). Clinical investigators from both psychodynamic (e.g., [17, 27, 28, 60, 61, 63, 64, 66]) and cognitive-behavioral [15] perspectives identified two major types of experiences that result in depression: (1) disruptions of gratifying interpersonal relationships (e.g., loss of a significant figure) and (2) disruptions of an effective and essentially positive sense of self (e.g., feelings of failure, guilt, and worthlessness). These two types of depressive experiences, anaclitic (dependent or sociotropic) and introjective (self-critical or autonomous) depression, have been studied in a broad range of studies using several well-established scales: the Depressive Experiences Questionnaire (DEQ) [27] (Blatt, S. J., D'Afflitti, J., & Quinlan, D. M. (1979). Depressive Experiences Questionnaire (DEQ). Unpublished research manual, Yale University.) and similar scales such as the Sociotropy-Autonomy Scale [15], the Personal Styles Inventory (PSI) [67], and the DAS [57]. Research results demonstrate important differences between anaclitic and introjective patients in the clinical expression of depression as well as in the early and current life experiences that create these vulnerabilities to depression (see summaries of this research [18, 19, 26, 65, 68, 69]) and in their response to the treatment process [2].

Because prior findings (e.g., [70–73]) demonstrated the value of introducing these patient factors into the study of long-term intensive treatment of both inpatients and outpatients, we explored the role of these patient factors in the brief treatments for depression evaluated in the TDCRP data set. These explorations yielded considerable understanding about the complex interactions among aspects of the treatment, the patients, and the therapeutic process on therapeutic outcome in the brief treatment of depression. The introduction of the anaclitic–introjective distinction into the analyses of the TDCRP data set not only facilitated more effective evaluation of the differential effects of the various forms of treatment (medication and the two forms of brief, manual-directed psychotherapy) on therapeutic outcome as measured by reductions in symptoms and vulnerability factors at termination and follow-up, it also resulted in fuller understanding of the processes of therapeutic change and some of the mechanisms of therapeutic action in the brief outpatient treatment of depression.

## *Anaclitic and Introjective Vulnerabilities in the TDCRP*

In an effort to introduce the anaclitic–introjective distinction into analyses of the data from the TDCRP, we reviewed the initial clinical intake evaluations of patients in the TDCRP. These case reports, however, focused primarily on neurovegative symptoms of depression and lacked substantial descriptions of experiential aspects of the patients' lives. Fortunately, however, patients in the TDCRP had been administered the DAS [57] at intake, throughout treatment, and at follow-up. The DAS [57] is a 40-item questionnaire assessing attitudes presumed to predispose an individual to depression. Factor analysis of the DAS obtained at pretreatment in the TDCRP [74], consistent with prior findings (e.g., [58, 75–77]), identified two major factors in the DAS: (1) need for approval (NFA) and (2) perfectionism (PFT). The first factor taps patient's NFA by others and corresponds to the anaclitic, dependent, or sociotropic form of depression; the second factor, which assesses patients' tendency to set extremely high and unrealistic self-standards and to adopt punitive and critical attitudes toward the self, corresponds to the introjective, self-critical, or autonomous form of depression (e.g., [78–80]; Powers, T. A., Zuroff, D. C., & Topciu, R. (2002), covert and overt expressions of self-criticism and perfectionism and their relation to depression. Unpublished manuscript). Thus, pretreatment DAS scores were used to introduce the anaclitic–introjective personality vulnerability dimensions into further analyses of the TDCRP data set.

# Results

## *Therapeutic Outcome*

Though no significant differences were found among the three active treatments in the TDCRP at termination and follow-up, highly significant relationships were found between pretreatment level of self-critical perfectionism, as measured by the PFT factor of the DAS, and treatment outcome across all four treatment conditions [81]. Introjective qualities, as assessed by the DAS self-critical PFT factor, significantly ($p$'s $= 0.031$–$0.001$) predicted less positive outcome at termination as assessed by the residualized gain scores of all five primary measures of clinical change in the TDCRP across all four treatment groups [81]. Pretreatment PFT also predicted the composite residualized gain score [56] at termination ($r = 0.29$, $p < 0.001$). In contrast, NFA, a measure of anaclitic personality qualities, had a consistent marginally positive relationship to treatment outcome on by all five outcome measures, as well as to the combination of all five residualized gain scores ($p = -0.11$). Thus, while anaclitic interpersonal concerns, as assessed by DAS NFA, tended to facilitate therapeutic gain, pretreatment preoccupation with introjective self-critical perfectionistic issues of self-definition and self-worth, as measured by DAS PFT, significantly impeded response to short-term treatment for depression, whether the treatment was pharmacotherapy (IMI-CM), psychotherapy (CBT and IPT), or placebo (PLA-CM) [81]. Pretreatment PFT also had consistent and significant negative relationships with ratings made by the therapists, by independent CEs, and with ratings by patients at termination of their satisfaction with treatment and with ratings by CEs of their assessments of the patients' clinical condition and need for further treatment at termination and follow-up [82]. Thus, the disruptive effects of pretreatment PFT on treatment outcome were apparent in assessments from multiple perspectives (reports by patients, therapists, and evaluations by independent CEs) at termination, and these disruptive effects persisted even at a follow-up evaluation conducted 18 months after the termination of treatment.

## *Therapeutic Process*

Therapeutic progress in the TDCRP had been assessed every 4 weeks during the 16-week treatment process, and thus it was possible to evaluate when and how PFT disrupted therapeutic progress. Patients at three levels of perfectionism were compared on the composite residualized measure of therapeutic gain at each of the five evaluation points in the treatment process. Repeated measures analysis of variance (ANOVA) of the composite measure (the combination of all five outcome measures) of therapeutic gain indicated a significant perfectionism-by-time interaction, in which the negative effect of pretreatment PFT on therapeutic outcome emerged primarily during the second half of treatment. Only one-third of the sample, those patients with low pretreatment self-critical perfectionism scores, continued to improve in the latter half of treatment. Two-thirds of the patients, those with moderate and high levels of self-critical perfectionism, made no further progress in the last half of the treatment process, beginning between the 9th and 12th treatment session, independent of the type of treatment they had received [83]. These findings suggest that self-critical perfectionist (introjective) patients may be negatively affected by the anticipation of an arbitrary, externally imposed termination. As perfectionistic introjective patients begin to confront the end of treatment, they may experience a sense of personal failure, dissatisfaction, and disillusionment with themselves and the treatment process [83]. Also, because perfectionist (introjective) individuals often need to maintain control and preserve their sense of autonomy [17, 19, 26, 84, 85], they may react negatively to a unilateral, externally imposed, termination date [83]. These issues appear to disrupt the therapeutic progress of a substantial segment (approximately two-thirds) of the patients in the TDCRP in the latter half of the treatment process in all four treatment conditions.

Additional analyses indicated that impact of pretreatment level of perfectionism on therapeutic outcome was mediated primarily by disruptions in the patients' interpersonal relationships both within the treatment process as well as in their social relationships outside of treatment. Zuroff and colleagues [86], using Krupnick et al.'s [48] ratings of the therapeutic alliance, found that the participation of more perfectionistic patients in the therapeutic alliance significantly declined in the latter half of the treatment process (beginning at the 9th session) and that this decline significantly mediated the effect of pretreatment perfectionism on treatment outcome at termination. Shahar et al. [87], furthermore, found that pretreatment perfectionism also led to significant decline in social support outside of treatment that also significantly mediated the relationship of perfectionism to treatment outcome. Using ratings by CEs on the Social Network Form [88] to assess patients' social network, Shahar and colleagues [87] found that patients with high levels of pretreatment self-critical perfectionism reported less satisfying social relationships over the course of treatment and that this disruption in social relationships in turn predicted poorer therapeutic outcome at termination. Thus, perfectionist (introjective) patients appear to experience greater interpersonal difficulty both within and outside the treatment process; they establish a less effective therapeutic alliance [86] and have a more limited social network [87] in the latter half of the treatment process. Consistent with psychoanalytic concepts of transference, these results indicate that disengagement from the therapeutic relationship is paralleled by a similar disengagement of patients from interpersonal relationships in their social network. This disengagement from interpersonal relationships both in the treatment process and more generally, leaves patients vulnerable to stressful life events. Thus, patients with higher pretreatment levels of perfectionism were also more vulnerable to stressful life events during the follow-up period, and this vulnerability led to increased depression [89].

In summary, the distinction between anaclitic and introjective dimensions facilitated the identification of a large segment of the depressed patients in the TDCRP (about two-thirds of the sample) who failed to make progress in the second half of the treatment process and who continued to remain vulnerable in the follow-up period. Thus, the effects of brief treatment for depression were significantly determined by patient dimensions – by pretreatment level of self-critical perfectionism independent of the type of treatment provided. This negative effect of PFT in brief treatment, including medication, stands in contrast with the findings that self-critical perfectionistic introjective outpatients did relatively well in long-term, intensive, psychodynamically oriented outpatient treatment [70, 73], and in psychnamically oriented extended inpatient treatment of seriously disturbed, treatment resistant patients [72] and in a 9-months inpatient treatment program for personality disordered patients [90].

Introjective patients, who emphasize separation, autonomy, control, and independence and concerns about self-worth, did relatively poorly in brief treatment in the TDCRP but had substantial constructive therapeutic response in intensive, exploratory, psychodynamic treatment in both inpatient and outpatient settings. These findings are consistent with findings of Fonagy et al. [91] and the conclusions of Gabbard et al. [92] about the constructive response of introjective patients to long-term psychodynamic treatment. In contrast, dependent, interpersonally oriented anaclitic patients were more constructively responsive to the supportive dimensions of the treatment process and to a therapeutic context in which there is more direct interpersonal interaction

[70, 73]. These findings are consistent with the conclusions of Vermote [90] that personality disordered anaclitic patients were responsive primarily to the supportive aspects of the treatment provided in extended (9 months) inpatient treatment while personality disordered introjective patients were more responsive to the explorations and interpretations of the treatment process.

Future investigations are needed to replicate and extend the findings of the role of anaclitic–introjective distinction in both long-term intensive and brief treatment. Future research should prospectively include the anaclitic–introjective distinction in the research design and evaluate the differential response of these two types of patients to different types of therapeutic intervention.

## Mechanisms of Therapeutic Action

The extensive data gathered as part of the NIMH TDCRP also provided an opportunity to evaluate circumstances within the treatment process that mitigated the negative effects of pretreatment self-critical perfectionism on treatment outcome in the brief treatment of depression. The B-L RI had been administered as part of the TDCRP research protocol to assess the quality of the therapeutic relationship early in treatment (after 2 sessions) and at termination. The B-L RI is based on the views of Rogers [50–52] that the therapist's empathic understanding, unconditional positive regard, and congruence are the "necessary and sufficient conditions" for therapeutic change. Using these formulations, Barrett-Lennard [93] developed four scales (Empathic understanding, Level of regard, Unconditionality of regard, and Congruence) to assess the patient's perception of the therapeutic relationship. Several reviews of research [94–96] indicate acceptable levels of reliability and validity for the B-L RI scales. Prior research, for example, indicated that these scales predict therapeutic change and are related significantly to independent estimates of the therapist's competence [93].

The degree to which patients in the TDCRP perceived their therapists at the end of the second treatment hour as empathic, caring, open, and sincere, as assessed by the B-L RI, had a significant ($p. < 0.05$) positive relationship to therapeutic outcome, as assessed by residualized gain scores of four of the five outcome measures (BDI, SCL-90, GAS, and SAS), as well as by the composite residualized outcome variable [56]. The perceived level of the therapeutic relationship at the end of the second treatment hour, as measured by the B-L RI, was independent of the patients' pretreatment level of DAS perfectionism ($r = -0.09$). Though highly self-critical perfectionist patients appear capable of perceiving their therapists positively, they are relatively less able to benefit from treatment. Surprisingly, the interaction of DAS PFT and B-L RI did not add significantly to the prediction of therapeutic outcome. Exploratory analyses indicated, however, a significant curvilinear (quadratic) component to the interaction between DAS PFT and the BL-RI in predicting therapeutic outcome at termination. The level of B-L RI at the end of the second hour had marginally significant effects on therapeutic outcome at low and high levels of self-critical perfectionism ($p$'s < 0.10 and 0.15, respectively), but the level of the BL-RI significantly ($p < 0.001$) reduced the negative effects of perfectionism on treatment outcome at the midlevel of perfectionism [56].

The TDCRP design also allowed for a comparison of the characteristics of more and less effective therapists. Blatt and colleagues [47], using the composite outcome measure that integrated the five primary outcome variables employed in the TDCRP, aggregated the outcome scores at termination of all the patients seen by each of the 28 therapists who had participated in the TDCRP (10 each providing IPT and pharmacotherapy and eight providing CBT). These 18 MD psychiatrists and the 10 PhD-level clinical psychologists had, on average, more than 11 years of clinical experience. All the therapists received training in the treatment they provided in the TDCRP, and only therapists who met competency criteria participated in the study. Tapes of sessions were reviewed periodically to assure adherence to treatment protocols, and therapists received consultation throughout the study [9].

To explore the contributions of the therapists to treatment outcome, Blatt and colleagues [47] identified three groups of therapists – more, moderately, and less effective therapists – defined by the average therapeutic gain achieved by the patients that each therapist had seen in active treatment in the TDCRP (their residualized composite therapeutic gain score). These therapists had completed a questionnaire assessing aspects of their clinical experiences and their attitudes toward the treatment of depression. Significant differences were found among the groups of therapists, independent of the type of treatment they provided. Differences in therapeutic efficacy were associated with a basic psychotherapeutic orientation about the treatment process. More effective therapists had a more psychological than biological orientation and reported that in their general clinical practice they predominantly used psychotherapy with depressed patients and rarely used biological interventions [i.e., medication and electroconvulsive therapy (ECT)].

The therapists in the TDCRP had been asked to describe their general clinical practice in terms of the percentage of time they usually devoted to psychotherapy alone, to medication alone, and to a combination of psychotherapy and medication. Less effective therapists, somewhat like the more effective therapists, reported that they tended to use psychotherapy alone in their clinical practice (42.1% of the time). More effective therapists responded that they primarily used psychotherapy alone (73.8% of the time) and only occasionally (19.6%) combine their psychotherapy with medication. Moderately effective therapists use primarily medication, either alone (14.4% of the time) or in combination with psychotherapy (56.1%), and relatively rarely use psychotherapy alone (29.4%) in their clinical practice. Thus, the moderately effective therapists appear to be more biologically oriented. Less effective therapists, like the more effective therapists, were primarily interested in psychotherapy, but they more often combined their psychotherapy with the use of medication than did the more effective therapists. Additionally, more effective therapists, compared with moderately and less effective therapists, expected therapy with depressed patients to require more treatment sessions before patients begin to manifest therapeutic change. Also, more effective therapists had significantly ($p < 0.023$) less variability (smaller standard deviation) in therapeutic outcome among the patients they treated and a significantly lower dropout rate than did moderately and less effective therapists. The greater variability in therapeutic outcome among the patients of less effective therapists suggests that the less effective therapists were able to work effectively with only a limited number of patients whereas more effective therapists were able to work effectively with almost all the patients that had been randomly assigned to them for treatment. It is important to stress that these differences among these three levels of effective therapists are particularly impressive because they occurred in a relatively homogeneous group of highly trained and experienced therapists who participated in three well-specified, manual-directed treatment conditions in three independent research sites. Relatively few significant differences were found, however, among the three groups of therapists on their attitudes about the etiology of depression or about the techniques they considered essential for the treatment of depression.

The overall results in the comparison of the more, moderately, and less effective therapists in the TDCRP as well as the impact of the patients' perceived quality of the therapeutic relationship at the end of the second treatment session indicate that qualities of the therapist are important dimensions that influence therapeutic outcome. The results from these analyses of data from the TDCRP are consistent with prior findings [5, 32–35, 48, 97, 98] that therapeutic outcome is significantly influenced by the interpersonal dimensions of the treatment process – by personal qualities of patients and therapists and their ability to establish an effective therapeutic relationship – rather than by the techniques and tactics described in treatment manuals.[2] These findings, consistent with recent extensive literature reviews (e.g., [5, 11, 99–101]), indicate that primary among the factors that contribute to therapeutic gain in

---

[2] Several studies of brief cognitive and pharmacological treatment of depression provide further support for the influence of the patients' personality styles on therapeutic outcome. Peselow, Robins, Sanfilipo, Block, and Fieve [107], investigating the response to pharmacotherapy among 217 depressed outpatients, found that patients with high autonomous–low sociotropic profile on the SAS (introjective patients) responded better to antidepressants than patients who had a high sociotropic–low autonomous profile (anaclitic patients). According to Peselow and colleagues (1992), these findings support Beck's [15] contention that the autonomous form of depression includes endogenomorphic characteristics. Rector, Bagby, Segal, Joffe, and Levitt [108], investigating depressed outpatients treated with either cognitive therapy ($N = 51$) or pharmacotherapy ($N = 58$), found that DEQ self-criticism did not influence the response to medication but did predict poorer response to cognitive therapy. Zettle and colleagues [109, 110] compared the responses of sociotropic and autonomous (anaclitic and introjective) depressed outpatients to individual and group cognitive therapy for depression and found that sociotropic patients had greater therapeutic response in group therapy, while autonomous patients had greater therapeutic response to individual therapy.

the brief outpatient treatment of serious depression is the quality of the therapeutic relationship that the patient and therapist established very early in the treatment process. These findings indicate the importance of the therapeutic relationship and its interaction with patients' pretreatment personality characteristics, especially level of pretreatment self-critical perfectionism, in facilitating some of the processes involved in therapeutic change.

Soffer and Shahar [102] recently entered these various aspects of the treatment process in the TDCRP into a regression analysis and found that these factors accounted for 22% of the variance of therapeutic outcome at termination. Statistically significant predictors of treatment outcome at termination (the residualized composite outcome score) were the level of pretreatment symptoms ($B = 0.20$, $p < 0.05$, accounting for 4% of the total variance), pretreatment self-critical perfectionism ($B = 0.30$, $p < 0.001$, accounting for 9% of total variance), the patient's contribution to the therapeutic alliance in the third treatment session ($B = -0.20$, $p < 0.01$; accounting for 4% of the total variance), and the patient's pretreatment social network ($B = -0.20$, $p < 0.01$; accounting for 4% of the variance). The contribution of the treatments, contrasting the three active treatments with the placebo condition, accounted for only 1% of the total variance and was not a statistically significant predictor of treatment outcome at termination ($B = -0.12$, $p = 0.11$). These findings clearly indicate, at least in the TDCRP, that treatment outcome was significantly influenced by patients' pretreatment personality characteristics, the quality of the therapeutic alliance, and the pretreatment quality of their interpersonal relationships and not by the type of treatment the patients received.


## Sustained Therapeutic Change

The consistently significant negative impact of patients' pretreatment levels of self-critical perfectionism on treatment outcome in the brief treatment for depression in the TDCRP are consistent with an extensive and wide-ranging literature that demonstrates the destructive effects of introjective personality characteristics (e.g., [19, 86, 103]). These findings raise the important question about the relationship between therapeutic change in these personality factors of vulnerability (i.e., self-critical perfectionism) as compared to changes in the symptoms of depression and their differential role in the treatment process. It is important to assess the efficacy of brief treatments for depression in reducing the vulnerability to depressive experiences and the impact of this reduction in vulnerability on symptom relief in the treatment of depression. Hawley et al. [104] addressed these questions in the TDCRP data set by using recently developed advanced statistical procedures (Latent Difference Score Analysis, LDS) for the analysis of longitudinal data. LDS is a structural equation modeling technique for evaluating temporal effects in longitudinal data that combines features of latent growth curve and cross lagged regression models.

Hawley et al. found a significant unidirectional longitudinal relationship between vulnerability in personality organization, as measured by self-critical perfectionism on the DAS, and rate of change in symptoms of depression in the brief outpatient treatment of depression in the TDCRP. Their findings revealed that symptoms of depression diminish rapidly early in therapy, followed by a gradual slowing of therapeutic progress. In contrast, the vulnerability dimension of self-critical perfectionism, gradually diminished throughout treatment and, most importantly, significantly predicted change in symptoms of depression. Their findings indicate that brief treatment in the TDCRP was most effective if it had an impact on the introjective personality factor of self-critical perfectionism, which in turn had an impact on depressive symptoms. These findings suggest that the high degree of relapse in symptom reduction following brief treatment for depression (e.g., [10]) may be the consequence of the primary focus on symptom reduction in these treatments and the failure to address the issue of vulnerability.

Hawley and colleagues [104] also found that the quality of the therapeutic alliance significantly predicted longitudinal change in self-critical perfectionism that, in turn, predicted change in symptoms of depression (see also [13]).[3] Hawley and colleagues concluded that the relationship between vulnerability (self-critical perfectionism) and depression suggests that focus of treatment needs to extend beyond symptom reduction to include the reduction of personality factors that contribute to vulnerability, and that the quality of the therapeutic alliance plays a significant role in the reduction of this vulnerability. The quality of the therapeutic alliance had only an indirect effect on symptom reduction, but the quality of the therapeutic alliance significantly predicted the reduction in personality vulnerability that in turn significantly predicted symptom reduction.

In subsequent LDS analysis, Hawley et al. [105] explored factors that contribute to vulnerability to relapse following the brief treatment of depression in the TDCRP. They found that the report of stressful life events in follow-up assessments, conducted 6, 12, and 18 months after termination, was significantly associated with increased symptoms of depression. However, this only held for those patients receiving medication. This stress reactivity in the follow-up period did not occur in patients who had received psychotherapy (either CBT or IPT). Psychotherapy, as compared to pharmacotherapy, appears to provide patients with enduring adaptive capacities [106] and revisions of maladaptive representations or cognitive-affective schemas of self and of significant others (e.g., [44]) that enable them to cope with the occurrence of stressful life events following the termination of treatment. While medication may lead to more rapid reduction of symptoms [59], it is also associated with greater relapse

---

[3] Similarily, Cox, Walker, Enns, and Karpinski [111] found that changes in level of self-critical perfectionism/autonomy were significantly related to outcome in brief group CBT of patients with generalized social phobia. The extent of change of self-critical perfectionism predicted therapeutic outcome.

[10], possibly because it does not address maladaptive schemas and the diatheses for depression, like self-critical perfectionism, that are sources of vulnerability to subsequent experiences of depression.

These further analyses of data from the TDCRP indicate that in the evaluation of therapeutic gain it is essential to include, in addition to symptom reduction, assessments of change in vulnerability and the development of resilience as expressed in increased adaptive capacities in the ability to manage stressful life events [2, 6, 106] and revisions of maladaptive representations or schemas both at termination of treatment and in extended follow-up assessments. These findings also question the validity of current efforts to identify ESTs by comparing different types of treatment in their relative efficacy and effectiveness in reducing symptoms [2]. Efforts to identify ESTs require a much more complex view of the treatment process, one that needs to adopt a multidimensional longitudinal approach to evaluating the treatment process. An approach is needed that includes other dimensions of the treatment process, especially the quality of the therapeutic relationship and patients' pretreatment characteristics, as well as the impact of these factors on the therapeutic process across a range of outcome measures beyond symptom reduction at termination and later [2]. These findings also have important implications for clinical practice and suggest that treatments need to focus on issues broader than symptom reduction, especially dealing with the personality issues that create vulnerability to dysphoric experiences. These findings also offer some understanding of the limitations of an exclusive reliance on medication in the treatment of depression and the advantages of a psychotherapeutic approach, particularly an approach that appreciates the importance of the therapeutic alliance in the treatment process.

## Implications for Psychodynamic Treatment

It is noteworthy that many of the findings in the further analyses of data that we and our colleagues have conducted on the brief manual-directed treatments for depression evaluated in the NIMH TDCRP yielded results that are very consistent with psychodynamic views about the treatment process. These findings indicate the limitations of symptom reduction as a criterion of therapeutic gain and suggest that the reduction of personality characteristics that create vulnerabilities to stressful life events, such as experiences of rejection and failure, are of equal importance in assessing therapeutic gain. In psychodynamic terms, these aspects of personality structure or personality organization, especially feelings of self-criticism and failure, must be addressed in treatment because they have a critical role in relapse following the termination of treatment. Even further, as the findings of Hawley et al. [104] indicate, symptom reduction during treatment is significantly mediated by a reduction in these personality characteristics of vulnerability. Effective therapy involves primarily a reduction in these vulnerability factors that in turn contributes to symptom reduction during treatment and to a reduction of relapse subsequent to the termination of treatment. This reduction in self-critical perfectionism as a major vulnerability factor appears to be a function of changes in the structural organization and thematic content of patients' cognitive-affective schemas or mental representations of self and of significant others and of their actual or potential interactions [44]. Though medication results in more rapid reduction in symptoms, psychotherapy is much more effective than medication in reducing vulnerability because it facilitates the development of enhanced adaptive capacities and revisions of distorted or impaired cognitive-affective schemas of self and of others.

The therapeutic relationship and qualities of the therapist as well as his or her ability to establish a therapeutic relationship early in the treatment process, more than the brand name of the psychotherapy treatment provided, are essential aspects of the mutative factors that determine therapeutic outcome at termination and at follow-up. Therapeutic outcome is determined by the patient's experience, early in the treatment process, of the therapist as available and understanding which facilitates the patient's constructive participation in the therapeutic alliance throughout the treatment process. The fact that the therapeutic relationship prospectively predicts therapeutic outcome suggests that the therapeutic relationship is a causal factor in the treatment process, (see summaries of this research [18, 19, 26, 65, 68, 69]).

Psychodynamic formulations (e.g., [44, 40]), suggest that internalization may be one of the mechanisms through which the therapeutic alliance contributes to a reduction in the vulnerability factor of perfectionism and to sustained therapeutic progress. The finding that the patient's engagement in the therapeutic relationship mirrors important aspects of the patient's engagement in his or her general social network is noteworthy. The patient's disengagement from the therapeutic relationship and from his or her social network had a significant negative impact on treatment outcome. This parallel process between aspects of the therapeutic relationship and broader social relationships is consistent with psychodynamic concepts of transference. And this disengagement from interpersonal relationships both within and external to the treatment process occurs primarily in highly self-critical perfectionistic (introjective) patients. Thus, patients' pretreatment personality characteristics have a powerful effect on therapeutic outcome – highly self-critical perfectionistic (introjective) patients do relatively poorly in brief treatment in contrast to their responsiveness to long-term, intensive psychodynamically oriented psychotherapy [70, 73, 91, 92]. Conversely, the ability to establish an effective therapeutic alliance is associated with more constructive interpersonal relationships in the patient's social network and both of these constructive interpersonal processes contribute to sustained therapeutic change.

It is noteworthy that these findings from analyses of data from the investigation of brief manual-directed treatments are consistent with psychodynamic formulations about the treatment process. Though future studies need to address interactions among aspects of the patient, therapist, and the treatment process and their impact on multiple aspects of therapeutic outcome (symptoms, vulnerabilities, and adaptive capacities) in different kinds of treatments with patients with other types of difficulties other than depression, these findings on the treatment process in brief manual directed treatment of depression are impressive in their congruence with psychodynamic views of the treatment process. This congruence indicates that psychodynamic principles of treatment are applicable not only in long-term, intensive treatment, but are relevant even in brief manual-directed treatments as well.

# References

1. Luyten, P., & Blatt, S. J. (2007). Looking back towards the future: Is it a time to change the DSM approach to psychiatric disorders? *Psychiatry: Interpersonal and Biological Processes, 70*, 85–99.
2. Blatt, S. J., & Zuroff, D. C. (2005). Empirical evaluation of the assumptions in identifying evidence based treatments in mental health. *Clinical Psychology Review, 25*, 459–486.
3. Barber, J. P., Connolly, M. B., Crits-Christoph, P., Gladis, L., & Sigueland, L. (2000). Alliance predicts patients' outcome beyond in-treatment change in symptoms. *Journal of Consulting and Clinical Psychology, 68*, 1027–1032.
4. Klein, D. N., Schwartz, J. E., Santiago, N. J. Vivan, D., Vocisano, C., & Catonguay, L. G. (2003) Therapeutic alliance in depression treatment: Controlling for prior change and patient characterisitics. *Journal of Consulting and Clinical Psychology, 71*, 997–1006.
5. Wampold, B. E. (2001). *The great psychotherapy debate: Models, methods, and findings.* Mahwah, NJ: Erlbaum.
6. Zuroff, D. C., & Blatt, S. J. (2006). The therapeutic relationship in the brief treatment of depression: Contributions to clinical improvement and enhanced adaptive capacities. *Journal of Consulting and Clinical Psychology, 47*, 130–140.
7. American Psychiatric Association Commission on Psychotherapies (1982). *Psychotherapy research: Methodological and efficacy issues.* Washington, DC: American Psychiatric Association.
8. Luyten, P., Blatt, S. J., van Houdenhove, B., & Corveleyn, J. (2006). Depression research and treatment: Are we skating to where the puck is going to be? *Clinical Psychology Review, 26*, 985–999.
9. Elkin, I. (1994). The NIMH Treatment of Depression Collaborative Research Program: Where we began and where we are now. In A. E. Bergin & S. L. Garfield (Eds.), *Handbook of psychotherapy and behavior change*(4th edition, pp. 114–135). New York: Wiley.
10. Shea, M. T., Elkin, I., Imber, S. D., Sotsky, S. M., Watkins, J. T., Collins, J. F., Pilkonis, P. A., Beckham, E., Glass, D. R., Dolan, R. T., & Parloff, M. B. (1992). Course of depressive symptoms over follow-up: Findings from the National Institute of Mental Health treatment of depression collaborative research program. *Archives of General Psychiatry, 49*, 782–787.
11. Westen, D., Novotny, C. M., Thompson-Brenner, H. (2004). The empirical status of empirically supported psychotherapies: Assumptions, findings, and reporting in controlled clinical trials. *Psychological Bulletin, 130*, 631–663.
12. Ingram, R. E., & Price, J. M. (Eds.) (2002) *Vulnerablity to psychopathology:Risk across the lifespan.* New York: Lippincott, Williams & Wilkins.

13. Luyten, P., Corveleyn, J., & Blatt, S. J. (2005). The convergence among psychodynamic and cognitive-behavioral theories of depression: A critical review of empirical research. In J. Corveleyn, P. Luyten, & S. J. Blatt (Eds.), *The theory and treatment of depression: Towards a dynamic interactionism model* (pp. 95–136). Leuven: University of Leuven Press.

14. Luyten, P., Blatt, S. J., & Corveleyn, J. (2005) Introduction. In Corveleyn, J., Luyten, P., & Blatt, S. J. (Eds.), *The theory and treatment of depression: Towards a dynamic interactionism model* (pp. 5–15). Leuven: University of Leuven Press.

15. Beck, A. T. (1983). Cognitive therapy of depression: New perspectives. In P. J. Clayton, & J. E. Barrett (Eds.), *Treatment of depression: Old controversies and new approaches* (pp. 265–290). New York: Raven.

16. Beck, A. T. (1999). Cognitive aspects of personality disorders and their relation to syndromal disorders: A psychoevolutionary approach. In C. R. Cloninger (Ed.), *Personality and psychopathology* (pp. 411–429). Washington, DC: American Psychiatric Press.

17. Blatt, S. J. (1974). Levels of object representation in anaclitic and introjective depression. *Psychoanalytic Study of the Child, 29*, 107–157.

18. Blatt, S. J. (1998). Contributions of psychoanalysis to the understanding and treatment of depression. *Journal of the American Psychoanalytic Association, 46*, 723–752.

19. Blatt, S. J. (2004). *Experiences of depression: Theoretical, clinical and research perspectives.* Washington, DC: American Psychological Association.

20. Blatt, S. J., & Auerbach, J. S. (2001). Mental representation, severe psychopathology and the therapeutic process. *Journal of the American Psychoanalytic Association, 49*, 113–159.

21. Blatt, S. J, Auerbach, J. S., & Levy, K. N. (1997). Mental representation in personality development, psychopathology and the therapeutic process. *Review of General Psychology, 1*, 351–374.

22. McCullough, J. P. (2003). *Treatment for chronic depression: Cognitive Behavioral Analysis System of Psychotherapy (CBASP).* London: Guilford Press.

23. Linehan, M. M. (1993). *Cognitive-behavior treatment of borderline personality disorder.* New York: Guilford Press.

24. Segal, Z. V. Williams. M. G., & Teasdale, J. D. (2002). *Mindfulness-based cognitive therapy for depression: A new approach to prevention relapse.* New York: Guilford Press.

25. Young, J. E. (1999). *Cognitive therapy for personality disorders: A schema focused approach* (3rd edition). Sarasota, FL: Professional Resource Exchange.

26. Blatt, S. J., & Zuroff, D. C. (1992). Interpersonal relatedness and self-definition: Two prototypes for depression. *Clinical Psychology Review, 12*, 527–562.

27. Blatt, S. J., D'Afflitti, J. P., & Quinlan, D. M. (1976). Experiences of depression in normal young adults. *Journal of Abnormal Psychology, 85*, 383–389.

28. Blatt, S. J., Quinlan, D. M., Chevron, E. S., McDonald, C., & Zuroff, D. (1982). Dependency and self-criticism: Psychological dimensions of depression. *Journal of Consulting and Clinical Psychology, 50*, 113–124.

29. Zuroff, D. C., & Fitzpatrick, D. (1995). Depressive personality styles: Implications for adult attachment. *Personality and Individual Differences, 18*, 253–265.

30. Zuroff, D. C., Mongrain, M., & Santor, D. A. (2004). Conceptualizing and measuring personality vulnerability to depression: Revisiting issues raised by Coyne and Whiffen (1995). *Psychological Bulletin, 130*, 489–511.

31. Hammen, C., Marks, T., Mayol, A., & deMayo, R. (1985). Depressive self-schemas, life stress, and vulnerability to depression. *Journal of Abnormal Psychology, 94*, 308–319.

32. Blatt, S. J., Shahar, G., & Zuroff, D. C. (2002). Anaclitic (sociotropic) and introjective (autonomous) dimensions. In J. C. Norcross (Ed.), *Psychotherapy relationships that work: Therapist contributions and responsiveness to patients* (pp. 306–324). New York: Oxford University Press.

33. Widiger, T. A., & Anderson, K .G. (2003). Personality and depression in women. *Journal of Affect Disorder, 74*, 59–66.

34. Ablon, J. S., & Jones, E. E. (1999). Psychotherapy process in the National Institute of Mental Health Treatment of Depression Collaborative Research Program. *Journal of Consulting and Clinical Psychology, 67*, 64–75.

35. Ablon, J. S., & Jones, E. E. (2002). Validity of controlled clinical trials of psychotherapy: Findings from the NIMH Treatment of Depression Collaborative Research Program. *American Journal of Psychiatry, 159*, 775–783.

36. Shaw , B. F., Elkin, I., Yamaguchi, J., Olmsted, M., Vallis, T. M., Dobseon, K. S., Lowery, A., Sotsky, S. M., Watkins, J. T, & Imber, S. D. (1999). Therapist competence ratings in relation to clinical outcome in cognitive therapy for depression. *Journal of Consulting and Clinical Psychology, 67*, 837–846.

37. Waddington, L. (2002). The therapy relationship in cognitive therapy: A review. *Behavioural and Cognitive Psychotherapy, 30*, 179–191.

38. Blatt, S. J., Auerbach, J. S., & Behrends, R. (in press). Changes in the representation of self and significant others in the treatment process: Links among representation, internalization, and mentalization. In A. Slade and E. Jurist (Eds.), *Representation and mentalization in the treatment process.* New York: Other Press.

39. Behrends, R. S., & Blatt, S. J. (1985). Internalization and psychological development throughout the life cycle. *Psychoanalytic Study of the Child, 40*, 11–39. Translated and reprinted in Arbeitshefte Kinderanalyse.

40. Blatt, S. J., & Behrends, R. S. (1987). Internalization, separation-individuation, and the nature of therapeutic action. *International Journal of Psychoanalysis, 68*, 279–297.

41. Loewald, H. W. (1962). Internalization, separation, mourning, and the superego. *Psychoanalytic Quarterly, 31*, 483–504.

42. Schafer, R. (1967). *Projective testing and psychoanalysis.* New York: International Universities Press.

43. Blatt, S. J. (1995a). Representational structures in psychopathology. In D. Cicchetti, & S. Toth (Eds.), *Rochester symposium on developmental psychopathology: Vol. 6. Emotion, cognition, and representation* (pp. 1–33). Rochester, NY: University of Rochester Press.

44. Blatt, S. J., Stayner, D., Auerbach, J., & Behrends, R. S. (1996). Change in object and self representations in long-term, intensive, inpatient treatment of seriously disturbed adolescents and young adults. *Psychiatry: Interpersonal and Biological Processes, 59*, 82–107.

45. Luyten, P., Blatt, S. J., & Corveleyn, J. (2005). The convergence among psychodynamic and cognitive-behavioral theories of depression: Theoretical overview. In J. Corveleyn, P. Luyten, & S. J. Blatt (Eds.), *The theory and treatment of depression: Towards a dynamic interactionism model* (pp. 67–94). Leuven: University of Leuven Press.

46. Clarkin, J. F., Levy, K. N., Lenzenweger, M. F., & Kernberg, O. F. (2004). The Personality Disorders Institute/Borderline Personality Disorder Research Foundation randomized control trial for borderline personality disorder: Rationale, methods, and patient characteristics. *Journal of Personality Disorders 18*, 52–72.

47. Blatt, S. J., Sanislow, C. A., Zuroff, D. C., & Pilkonis, P. A. (1996). Characteristics of effective therapists: Further analyses of data from the NIMH TDCRP. *Journal of Consulting and Clinical Psychology, 64*, 1276–1284.

48. Krupnick, J. L., Sotsky, S. M., Simmens, S., Moyer, J., Elkin, I., Watkins, J., & Pilkonis, P. A. (1996). The role of the therapeutic alliance in psychotherapy and pharmacotherapy outcome: Findings in the NIMH Treatment of Depression Collaborative Research Program. *Journal of Consulting and Clinical Psychology, 64*, 532–539.

49. Zuroff, D. C., & Blatt, S. J. (2006). The therapeutic relationship in the brief treatment of depression: Contributions to clinical improvement and enhanced adaptive capabilities. *Journal of Consulting and Clinical Psychology, 74*, 130–140.

50. Rogers, C. R. (1951). Client-centered therapy. Boston: Houghton Mifflin.

51. Rogers, C. R. (1957). The necessary and sufficient conditions of therapeutic personality change. *Journal of Consulting Psychology, 21*, 95–103.

52. Rogers, C. R. (1959). A theory of therapy, personality, and interpersonal relationships as developed in the client-centered framework in psychology: A study of science. In S. Koch (Ed.), *Formulations of the person and the social context* (pp. 184–256). New York: McGraw-Hill.
53. Hartley, D. E., & Strupp, H. H. (1983). The therapeutic alliance: Its relationship to outcome in brief psychotherapy. In J. Masling (Ed.), *Empirical studies of psychoanalytic theories*(Vol. 1, pp. 1–27). Hillsdale, NJ: Analytic Press.
54. Paykel, E. S., Weissman, M. M., & Prusoff, B. A. (1978). Social maladjustment and severity of depression. *Comprehensive Psychiatry, 19*, 121–128.
55. Watkins, J. T., Leber, W. R., Imber, S. D., Collins, J. R., Elkin, I., Pilkonis, P. A., Sotsky, S. M., Shea, M. T., & Glass, D. R. (1993). NIMH Treatment of Depression Collaborative Research Program: Temporal course of change of depression. *Journal of Consulting and Clinical Psychology, 61*, 858–864.
56. Blatt, S. J., Zuroff, D. C., Quinlan, D. M., & Pilkonis, P. A. (1996). Interpersonal factors in brief treatment of depression: Further analyses of the National Institute of Mental Health Treatment of Depression Collaborative Research Program.*Journal of Consulting and Clinical Psychology, 64*, 162–171.
57. Weissman, A. N., & Beck, A. T. (1978, August–September). Development and validation of the Dysfunctional Attitudes Scale: A preliminary investigation. Paper presented at the 86th Annual Convention of the American Psychological Association, Toronto.
58. Segal, Z. V., Shaw, B. F., & Vella, D. D. (1987, August). Life stress and depression: A test of the congruence hypothesis for life event content and depressive subtypes. Paper presented at the Annual Convention of the American Psychological Association, Toronto, Canada.
59. Elkin, I., Gibbons, R. D., Shea, M. T., Sotsky, S. M., Watkins, J. T., Pilkonis, P. A., & Hedeker, D. (1995). Initial severity and differential treatment outcome in the National Institute of Mental Health Treatment of Depression Collaborative Research Program. *Journal of Consulting and Clinical Psychology, 63*, 841–847.
60. Arieti, S., & Bemporad, J. R. (1978). *Severe and mild depression: The therapeutic approach.* New York: Basic Books.
61. Arieti, S., & Bemporad, J. R. (1980).The psychological organization of depression. *American Journal of Psychiatry, 137*, 1360–1365.
62. Blatt, S. J., Quinlan, D. M., & Chevron, E. (1990). Empirical investigations of a psychoanalytic theory of depression. In J. Masling (Ed.), *Empirical studies of psychoanalytic theories*, (Vol. 3, pp. 89–147). Hillsdale, NJ: Analytic Press.
63. Bowlby, J. (1988). Developmental psychology comes of age. *American Journal of Psychiatry, 145*, 1–10.
64. Bowlby, J. (1988). *A secure base: Clinical applications of attachment theory.* London: Routledge & Kegan Paul.
65. Blatt, S. J., & Maroudas, C. (1992). Convergence of psychoanalytic and cognitive behavioral theories of depression, *Psychoanalytic Psychology 9*, 157–190.
66. Bowlby, J. (1980). *Attachment and loss: Vol. 3: Loss, sadness and depression.* New York: Basic Books.
67. Robins, C. J., & Luten, A. G. (1991). Sociotropy and autonomy: Differential patterns of clinical presentation in unipolar depression. *Journal of Abnormal Psychology, 100*, 74–77.
68. Blatt, S. J., Quinlan, D. M., Chevron, E. S. McDonald, C., & Zuroff, D. (1982). Dependency and self-criticism: Psychological dimensions of depression. *Journal of Consulting and Clinical Psychology, 50*, 113–124.
69. Blatt, S. J., & Homann, E. (1992). Parent–child interaction in the etiology of dependent and self-critical depression. *Clinical Psychology Review, 12,* 47–91.
70. Blatt, S. J. (1992). The differential effect of psychotherapy and psychoanalysis on anaclitic and introjective patients: The Menninger Psychotherapy Research Project revisited. *Journal of the American Psychoanalytic Association, 40*, 691–724.
71. Blatt, S. J., & Felsen, I. (1993). "Different kinds of folks may need different kinds of strokes": The effect of patients' characteristics on therapeutic process and outcome. *Psychotherapy Research, 3*, 245–259.

72. Blatt, S. J., & Ford, R. (1994). *Therapeutic change: An object relations perspective.* New York: Plenum.
73. Blatt, S. J., & Shahar, G. (2004). Psychoanalysis: For what, with whom, and how: A comparison with psychotherapy. *Journal of the American Psychoanalytic Association, 52,* 393–447.
74. Imber, S. D., Pilkonis, P. A., Sotsky, S. M., Elkin, I., Watkins, J. T., Collins, J. F., Shea, M. T., Leber, W. R., & Glass, D. R. (1990). Mode-specific effects among three treatments for depression. *Journal of Consulting and Clinical Psychology, 58,* 352–359.
75. Cane, D. B., Olinger, L. J., Gotlib, I. H., & Kuiper, N. A. (1986). Factor structure of the Dysfunctional Attitude Scale in a student population. *Journal of Clinical Psychology, 42,* 307–309.
76. Oliver, J. M., & Baumgart, B. P. (1985). The Dysfunctional Attitude Scale: Psychometric properties in an unselected adult population. *Cognitive Theory and Research, 9,* 161–169.
77. Rude, S. S., & Burnham, B. L. (1995). Connectedness and neediness: Factors of the DEQ and SAS dependency scales. *Cognitive Therapy and Research, 19,* 323–340.
78. Blaney, P. H., & Kutcher, G. S. (1991). Measures of depressive dimensions: Are they interchangeable? *Journal of Personality Assessment, 56,* 502–512.
79. Dunkley, D. M., & Blankstein, K. R. (2000). Self-critical perfectionism, coping, hassles, and current distress: A structural equation modeling approach. *Cognitive Therapy and Research, 24,* 713–730.
80. Enns, M. W., & Cox, B. J. (1999). Perfectionism and depressive symptom severity in major depressive disorder. *Behavioral Research and Therapy, 37,* 783–794.
81. Blatt, S. J., Quinlan, D. M., Pilkonis, P. A., & Shea, T. (1995). Impact of perfectionism and need for approval on the brief treatment of depression: The National Institute of Mental Health Treatment of Depression Collaborative Research Program revisited. *Journal of Consulting and Clinical Psychology, 63,* 125–132.
82. Blatt, S. J. (1999). Personality factors in the brief treatment of depression: Further Analyses of the NIMH Sponsored Treatment for Depression Collaborative Research Program. In D. S. Janowsky (Ed.), *Psychotherapy indications and outcomes* (pp. 23–45). Washington, DC: American Psychiatric Press.
83. Blatt, S. J., Zuroff, D. C., Bondi, C. M., Sanislow, C., & Pilkonis, P. A. (1998). When and how perfectionism impedes the brief treatment of depression: Further analyses of the NIMH TDCRP. *Journal of Consulting and Clinical Psychology, 66,* 423–428.
84. Blatt, S. J. (1995). The destructiveness of perfectionism: Implications for the treatment of depression. *American Psychologist, 50,* 1003–1020.
85. Blatt, S. J. (2006). A fundamental polarity in psychoanalysis: Implications for personality development, psychopathology, and the therapeutic process. *Psychoanalytic Inquiry, 26,* 492–518.
86. Zuroff, D. C., Blatt, S. J., Sotsky, S. M., Krupnick, J. L., Martin, D. J., Sanislow, C. A., & Simmens, S. (2000). Relation of therapeutic alliance and perfectionism to outcome in brief outpatient treatment of depression. *Journal of Consulting and Clinical Psychology, 68,* 114–124.
87. Shahar, G., Blatt, S. J., Zuroff, D. C., Krupnick, J., & Sotsky, S. M. (2004). Perfectionism impedes social relations and response to brief treatment of depression. *Journal of Social and Clinical Psychology, 23,* 140–154.
88. Elkin, I., Parloff, M. B., Hadley, S. W., & Autry, J. H. (1985). NIMH treatment of Depression Collaborative Research Program: Background and research plan. *Archives of General Psychiatry, 42,* 305–316.
89. Zuroff, D. C., & Blatt, S. J. (2002) Vicissitudes of life after the short-term treatment of depression: Role of stress, social support, and personality. *Journal of Social and Clinical Psychology, 21,* 473–496.
90. Vermote, R. (2005). Touching inner change. Psychoanalytically informed hospitalization-based treatment of personality disorders. A process-outcome study. Dissertation.

91. Fonagy, P., Leigh, T., Steele, M., Steele, H., Kennedy, R., Mattoon, G., Target, M., & Gerber, A. (1996). The relation of attachment status, psychiatric classification, and response to psychotherapy. *Journal of Consulting and Clinical Psychology*, *64*, 22–31.
92. Gabbard, G. O., Horowitz, L., Allen, J. G., Frieswyk, S., Newson, G., Colson, D. B., & Coyne, L. (1994). Transference interpretation in the psychotherapy of borderline patients: A high-risk, high-gain phenomenon. *Harvard Review of Psychiatry*, *2*, 59–69.
93. Barrett-Lennard, G. T. (1962). Dimensions of therapist responses as causal factors in therapeutic change. *Psychological Monographs*, *76*, (43, Whole No. 562).
94. Barrett-Lennard, G. T. (1985). The Relationship Inventory now: Issues and advances in theory, method, and use. In L. S. Greenberg and W. M. Pinsof (Eds.), *The psychoanalytic process: A research handbook* (pp. 439–476). New York: Guilford Press.
95. Gurman, A. S. (1977). The patient's perception of the therapeutic relationship. In A. S. Gurman & A. M. Razin (Eds.), *Psychotherapy: A handbook of research* (pp. 503–543). New York: Pergamon.
96. Gurman, A. S. (1977). Therapist and patient factors influencing the patient's perception of facilitative therapeutic conditions. *Psychiatry*, *40*, 218–231.
97. Burns, D. D., & Nolen-Hoeksema, S. (1992). Therapeutic empathy and recovery from depression in cognitive-behavioral therapy: A structural equation model. *Journal of Consulting and Clinical Psychology*, *60*, 441–449.
98. Horvath, A. O., & Symonds, B. D. (1991). Relation between working alliance and outcome in psychology: A meta-analysis. *Journal of Couselling*, *24*, 240–260.
99. Lambert, M. J., & Barley, D. E. (2002). Research Summary on the Therapeutic Relationship and Psychotherapy Outcome. In J. D. Norcross (Ed.), *Psychotherapy relationship that work: Therapist contributions and responsiveness to patients* (pp. 17–32). London: Oxford University Press.
100. Luyten, P., Blatt, S. J., van Houdenhove, B., & Corveleyn, J. (2006). Depression research and treatment: Are we skating to where the puck is going to be? *Clinical Psychology Review*, *26*, 985–999.
101. Norcross, J. (2002). *Psychotherapy relationships that work: Therapist contributions andresponsiveness to patients*. New York: Oxford University Press.
102. Soffer, N. and Shahar, G. (in press). Evidence-based psychiatric practice? Long-live the (Individual) difference. *Israel Journal of Psychiatry*, *44*, 301–308.
103. Dunkley, D. M., Zuroff, D. C., & Blankstein, K. R. (2005). Specific perfectionism components versus self-criticism in predicting maladjustment. *Personality and Individual Differences*, *40*, 665–676.
104. Hawley, L. L., Moon-Ho, R. H., Zuroff, D. C., & Blatt, S. J. (2006). The relationship of perfectionism, depression, and therapeutic alliance during treatment for depression: Latent difference score analysis. *Journal of Consulting and Clinical Psychology*, *74*, 930–942.
105. Hawley, L. L., Moon-Ho, R. H., Zuroff, D. C., & Blatt, S. J. (2007). Stress reactivity following brief treatment for depression: Differential effects of psychotherapy and medication. *Journal of Consulting and Clinical Psychology*, *75*, 244–256.
106. Zuroff, D. C., Blatt, S. J., Krupnick, J. L., & Sotsky, S. M. (2003). Enhanced adaptive capacities after brief treatmeant for depression. *Psychotherapy Research*, *13*, 99–115.
107. Peselow, E. D., Robins, C. J., Sanfilipo, M. P., Block, P., & Fieve, R. R. (1992). Sociotropy and autonomy relationship to antidepressants drug treatment response and endogenous-onendogenous dichotomy. *Journal of Abnormal Psychology*, *101*, 479–486.
108. Rector, N. A., Bagby, R. M., Segal, Z. V., Joffe, R. T., & Levitt, A. (2000). Self-criticism and dependency in depressed patients treated with cognitive therapy or pharmacotherapy. *Cognitive Therapy and Research*, *24*, 571–584.
109. Zettle, R. D., Haflich, J. L., & Reynolds, R. (1992). Responsivity to cognitive therapy as a function of treatment format and client personality dimensions. *Journal of Clinical Psychology*, *48*, 787–797.

110. Zettle, D. D., & Herring, E. L. (1995). Treatment utility of the sociotropy-autonomy distinction: Implications for cognitive therapy. *Journal of Clinical Psychology*, *51*, 280–289.
111. Cox, B. J., Walker, J. R., Enns, M. W., & Karpinski, D. C. (2002). Self-criticism in generalized social phobia and reponse to cognitive-behavioral treatment. *Behavior Therapy*, *33*, 479–491.

# Part IV
# The Neurobiology of Psychodynamic
# Theory and Psychotherapy

# Chapter 13
# Neural Models of Psychodynamic Concepts and Treatments: Implications for Psychodynamic Psychotherapy

Joshua L. Roffman and Andrew J. Gerber

## Introduction

Psychotherapy and neuroscience have arrived at an historic crossroad. Since the inception of analytic thinking in the late nineteenth century, its proponents have struggled with the question of how psychotherapy influences brain function – and whether this relationship is relevant to the work or effectiveness of therapy. Despite decades of parallel progress in psychodynamic and neuroscientific research, until recently there was little meaningful interaction between these fields of study. Rather, fierce ideologic and methodologic divisions persisted between investigators of "mind-based" and "brain-based" thinking.

   In the last 10 years, though, a remarkable synergy between these fields has begun to emerge, with powerful (and overwhelmingly positive) implications for the future of psychotherapy. In this chapter, we describe how this transformation has taken place, focusing on the critical role of new technology in understanding brain function. We demonstrate how principles central to dynamic therapy have informed the design, implementation, and analysis of brain imaging experiments, and, conversely, the potential of brain imaging data to further refine and improve the process of psychotherapy. In summarizing the current literature on how psychotherapy affects brain function, we identify the strengths and weaknesses of this scientific undertaking, and discuss ways in which it may ultimately reshape clinical practice.

## *Psychodynamic Therapy and the Brain: A Brief History*

Curiosity about the interface of psychodynamics and brain function stretches as far back as psychoanalysis itself. In 1895 Sigmund Freud embarked upon

J.L. Roffman
Psychiatric Neuroscience Program, MGH-East, Bldg 149, 13th Street, 2nd Floor, Charlestown, MA 02129, USA
e-mail: jroffman@partners.org

R.A. Levy, J.S. Ablon (eds.), *Handbook of Evidence-Based Psychodynamic Psychotherapy*,       305
DOI: 10.1007/978-1-59745-444-5_13, © Humana Press 2009

his Project for a Scientific Psychology (or, as literally translated, "The Psychology for Neurologists"), an attempt to define the unconscious in neurological terms [1]. As mentioned in an April 26, 1895 letter to his friend and confidante Wilhelm Fleiss:

> Scientifically, I am in a bad way; namely, caught up in "The Psychology for Neurologists," which regularly consumes me totally until, actually overworked, I must break off. I have never before experienced such a high degree of preoccupation. And will anything come of it? I hope so, but it is difficult and slow going. [2]

Indeed, having reached the limits of neurologic investigation for his time, Freud abandoned the project in 1896, only to embark on a new ("royal") route to the unconscious through dream analysis. The Project notes were sent privately to Fleiss, and remained unpublished until well after Freud's death. Within the Project, though, Freud developed a prescient, theoretical framework for how neural activity underlies both normal processes (including memory, attention, and judgment) and abnormal ones (hysteria, repression, and displacement).

For the better part of a century, scientific inquiry into the mechanisms of psychotherapy was limited to observational work, often reflecting individual interactions between patients and therapists. This work evolved into a complex and (mostly) internally valid system of psychoanalytic theory and process; however, it failed to integrate with other developments in medical science, and remained entirely distant from the study of neural function [3]. (Of note, there was hardly a complete isolation of psychology and medicine – in fact, efforts in the 1940 s led psychiatrists to consider psychosomatic contributions to many common medical illnesses) [4, 5].

Although a general rapprochement between psychiatry and medicine followed the introduction of psychotropic medications in the 1950s and 1960s [6], the theory and practice of psychoanalysis remained largely isolated. In the years that followed, novel neuroscientific methods shed new light on brain development, memory, psychopathology, and other elements with a close relationship to psychodynamic principles, while at the same time cognitive psychologists developed scientifically rigorous ways to understand these same phenomena. However, it was not until the 1990 s – the "Decade of the Brain" – that brain and psychotherapy investigators truly began to find common ground through scientific collaboration.

In particular, one novel method to understand activity within the living brain – functional neuroimaging – has played a pivotal role in this renewed relationship. For the first time, functional imaging has provided the opportunity to correlate directly cognitive and emotional processes with brain activity profiles, both in healthy individuals and those with psychiatric disorders. As a result, we are newly able to face the challenges that Freud envisioned a century ago, as recalled in a landmark paper by neuroscientist and Nobel laureate Eric Kandel: "Where, if it exists at all, is the unconscious? What are its neurobiological properties? How do unconscious strivings become transformed to enter awareness as a result of analytic therapy?" [5].

## A Lingering Disparity

The availability of new tools to understand brain function, though, has been slower to influence psychotherapy research than it has for cognitive psychology, neuropsychiatry, and psychopharmacology. This is despite the long-held consensus that talk therapies provide substantial relief for many individuals with psychiatric illness, often with similar efficacy and cost when compared to other interventions [7–9]. The extent to which psychotherapy has fallen behind psychopharmacology in this regard is dramatically evident in Fig. 13.1, which summarizes neuroimaging studies of these treatment modalities since 1990 [10].

There are a number of reasons – technical, scientific, historic, even political – why this might be the case. As described throughout this book, psychotherapy research has always been, is now, and will remain a uniquely challenging enterprise. The study of psychodynamic therapy, in particular, does not always lend itself well to the research methods that are commonplace in medicine, and often in other areas of psychiatry [12]. Neuroimaging research provides no exception to this rule. For example: at present, most functional imaging technologies cannot be used to detect meaningful brain activity patterns in individual subjects, who must be grouped together to acquire results that are statistically valid [13]. Yet psychodynamic therapy is a highly individualized

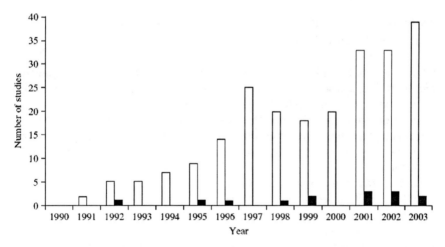

**Fig. 13.1** Imaging/medication (□) and imaging/psychotherapy (■) studies by year. Method: an Ovid MEDLINE search was completed using key words related to neuroimaging (e.g., Pet, fMRI, SPECT) and medication (e.g., psychotropic) to find studies including both neuroimaging and medication between the years 1966 and 2003. Based on the abstracts generated from this search, we selected studies based on four criteria: included studies were published in English between 1990 and 2003, used human subjects, and investigated psychiatric (e.g., depression) rather than neurological (Parkinson's disease) disorders. A similar search was conducted using key words related to neuroimaging and psychotherapy (e.g., psychotherapy, intrapersonal therapy, cognitive-behavioral therapy, and psychodynamic therapy). Figure taken from Roffman et al. [11] © Cambridge University Press, used with permission

treatment that can last months or years; it would therefore be difficult to develop standardized treatment protocols for subjects within a study cohort. However, even for the study of time-limited, manualized psychotherapies, there remain significant obstacles to neuroimaging investigations. Imaging studies are relatively expensive, and with limited support from federal funding sources, cost can be a prohibitive factor. There may also be a bias toward studying the neural mechanisms of medications since they are thought of as a "biological" or "medical" intervention, while some consider psychosocial interventions relatively "soft" [10].

In spite of these complications, the use of neuroimaging has now gained substantial momentum in psychotherapy research, and this investigative approach is now extending into medical, neuroscientific, and sociocultural awareness. It is also becoming clear that these studies have important clinical implications. Understanding how psychotherapy modifies brain function could powerfully influence its perception among new patients who may be weighing it as a treatment option. Furthermore, it is not too audacious to imagine that functional imaging studies, perhaps in concert with other biological markers, could one day be used to guide treatment for individual patients. This would place psychotherapy squarely within the emerging field of individualized medicine, which many consider to be the next revolution in patient care [14].

## Functional Imaging Methods and their Application in Psychotherapy Research

Of course, these kinds of advances will be predicated on neuroimaging studies with rigorous scientific methods and robust findings. Some initial studies of neuroimaging and psychotherapy, discussed later in this chapter, illustrate some of the challenges intrinsic to this kind of research. In this section, we will introduce some basic concepts that are critical to understanding functional neuroimaging, its potential for use in psychotherapy research, and its limitations therein.

Unlike traditional brain images that produce a static picture of brain structure, functional neuroimaging provides a measure of brain activity. The most commonly used functional imaging techniques are positron emission tomography (PET), single photon emission computed tomography (SPECT), and functional magnetic resonance imaging (fMRI) [13]. Both PET and SPECT rely on radioactive tracers that are injected into the bloodstream just prior to imaging. These tracers enter the cerebral blood supply and emit a signal, detectable with a camera placed near the patient's head. As activity increases or decreases in brain regions, blood flow to these regions rises or falls accordingly; the radiotracer signal thus also varies, and for this reason it is considered to be a proxy for the level of neural activity. In other words, PET and SPECT provide a reliable but still indirect measure of neuronal firing [15]. These techniques can be used to measure either resting (baseline) activity, or changes in activity related to a task (which can range from simple finger tapping to complex cognitive or emotional paradigms). PET is more expensive than SPECT but also provides much better spatial resolution. Although the amount of radiation exposure is not considered harmful, it does limit the frequency with which PET and SPECT scans can occur. For example, medical centers generally permit individuals to undergo at most two PET scans per year.

In contrast, fMRI scans do not use ionizing radiation, but rather strong magnetic fields to measure brain activity. In fact, fMRI studies are conducted using the same MRI machines that are used in clinical practice, but with different programming. Like PET and SPECT, the fMRI signal also estimates cerebral blood flow, which shows regional fluctuation based on which parts of the brain are active at a given time. In this case, the signal is generated by measuring relative concentrations of deoxygenated versus oxygenated blood. Exposure to the magnet is safe, except for individuals who have pacemakers or metallic implants in their bodies, who cannot be scanned. The fMRI environment is more restrictive than PET or SPECT, as it involves lying supine and very still within a long tubular structure. However, it is more versatile due to its better temporal resolution, which permits repeated measurements of brain activity every few seconds.

It is important to recognize that brain activity, as measured by these techniques, can reflect several overlapping neural processes related to the subject's current condition. These processes must be carefully identified, and disambiguated to the greatest possible extent when conducting functional imaging analysis. The first such consideration is the general state of the subject: is she disease-free, diagnosed with an illness but currently symptom-free, or actively symptomatic? As we are learning, baseline brain activity profiles can differ substantially based on the presence or absence of psychiatric illness. Second, if a patient is being scanned, when is the scan occurring relative to a treatment intervention? For example, most psychotherapy studies thus far conducted have imaged patients twice: once just before, and once just after completion of the treatment course. By comparing these scans, one can observe a measure of treatment effects; however, in light of the first consideration, it can be difficult to differentiate changes in brain activity that are related to the treatment itself versus those related to the (improved, hopefully) state of the patient's illness. Finally, one must consider what the subject is doing in the scanner – is he resting quietly or engaged in a task? Often, activity in brain regions is compared between these two conditions to give a measure of task-related "activation." Other designs are meant to induce symptoms while the subject is being scanned, so that they may be more readily correlated with brain activity profiles.

## Other Ways to Measure Therapy-Related Changes in Physiology

While functional neuroimaging can provide detailed measures of brain function, imaging techniques can also be costly and logistically difficult to arrange.

Imaging analysis requires the use of complex (and often time-consuming) statistics to convert raw signals into interpretable data. Alternatively, measures of peripheral physiology can provide useful indicators of neural activity, albeit further downstream from brain activation. Psychophysiology techniques can sensitively measure moment-to-moment fluctuations in skin conductance, heart rate, and blood pressure, and do so relatively inexpensively and noninvasively. The great advantage of these techniques, though, is that they can be deployed repeatedly over the course of a treatment, and even *during* treatment sessions. Some investigators have compared psychophysiology measures obtained simultaneously from the patient and therapist as an objective measure of their interaction; for example, Marci and colleagues reported a significant relationship between patient ratings of the therapist's perceived empathy and the concordance of skin conductance between the two during therapy sessions [16].

Even with the availability of these technologies, it is still important for scientific and philosophical reasons to ask the question of why *should* psychotherapy – and psychodynamic psychotherapy in particular – change brain function? One "bottom-up" approach to this question is to examine neural correlates of the building blocks upon which psychotherapy is based. Therefore, before considering the net effect of psychotherapy on the brain function, we will first review evidence that psychoanalytic constructs are themselves associated with meaningful changes in brain activity.

## Experimental Methods and Evidence for Psychoanalytic Constructs

It is widely stated and accepted by friends and foes of psychoanalysis alike that psychoanalytic constructs lack the empirical evidence, in terms of behavior and neurobiology, that is enjoyed by cognitive psychology. This is taken by some as evidence for the intrinsic "untestability" of psychoanalytic hypotheses, often ascribed to the unconscious, subjective, and interpersonal nature of the phenomena central to psychoanalytic theorizing and treatment [17–19]. Others argue that the lack of evidence demonstrates the falsehood of psychoanalytic ideas, or at least, their irrelevance to an empirically based science of the brain and mind [20]. In fact, the story is more complicated than is typically represented by either side in the discussion. Research has been accumulating, with particular growth in the past decade, which supports and elaborates several basic psychodynamic hypotheses related to processes, representations, and relationships [21, 22]. These studies currently focus on phenomena in normal subjects under experimental conditions, as opposed to their action in the therapeutic setting. However, links to therapeutic action are gradually becoming more plausible and it is likely that research will continue to bridge the gap between experimental work and psychoanalytic practice in the coming years.

Neural research on psychodynamic phenomena can broadly be divided into four domains, with significant overlap: (1) memory and learning, (2) affect,

(3) social cognition and relatedness, and (4) processes such as free association and defense mechanisms that reflect the interface between consciousness and unconsciousness. As experimental methodologies have improved, each of these domains has received increasing attention by cognitive neuroscientists, yielding evidence that much important mental functioning goes on outside of awareness. Thus research that did not start out as explicitly "psychodynamic" has pointed back toward an unconscious, representational, and relational mind, and thus toward a recognizably psychodynamic view of mental functioning. Meanwhile, a number of psychodynamic writers have suggested ways in which the accumulating data can be used to inform thinking about psychotherapy [21–26].

## Memory and Learning

Scientists, philosophers, and writers have long appreciated that much of what we know and remember is not in conscious awareness, or even accessible to awareness, at a given moment. Given our reliance on subjective reports of knowledge and memory, it has been difficult to study these phenomena systematically. Freud, based on previous scholarship and his own clinical observations, asserted that a significant portion of possible thoughts are actively excluded from awareness [27]. Due to the objectionable nature of their content, these thoughts are forced to reside in the "dynamic unconscious." However, they continue to exert a significant influence on behavior and conscious processes, including those most relevant to psychotherapy and psychoanalysis. The concept of the dynamic unconscious is often confused, both in and out of the psychodynamic literature, with the "descriptive unconscious," a more inclusive category that includes not only the dynamic unconscious, but also the preconscious (that which is easily accessible by consciousness if one were to focus attention on this) and the nonconscious (that which is inaccessible to consciousness because it has never been symbolized, e.g., procedural knowledge such as how to ride a bicycle) [28].

Over the past several decades, cognitive neuroscientists have developed methods for demonstrating and measuring various systems for memory and learning that have complicated relationships to consciousness (Fig. 13.2) [30–32] (see Fig. 13.1). Particularly relevant to psychodynamic therapy, long-term memory researchers have described an implicit (also called "nondeclarative") memory system, which is not readily accessible to consciousness. The existence of implicit memories was seen by exposing subjects to stimuli so brief that they were not consciously perceived (i.e., subliminal) but yet affected their performance on later tasks. This memory is often described as "associative," though the relationship to the semantic properties that partially define declarative memories is unclear [33–36]. Investigators also found that subjects could be "primed" by consciously perceived information such that later, even when they did not specifically recall the information that they were previously taught, their answers to questions were influenced by having been exposed [37].

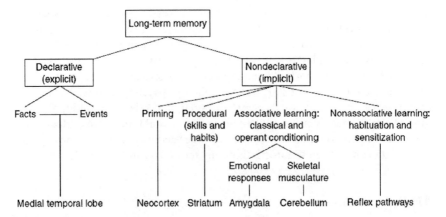

**Fig. 13.2** Forms of long-term memory and associated brain regions. Figure taken from Kandel et al. [29] © McGraw-Hill, used with permission

Other experimental tasks were developed to demonstrate the existence of an implicit procedural memory system in which subjects learned motor or behavioral tasks without developing language to describe what they had learned, and sometimes without even being aware that they had learned something. For example, in the widely used Weather Task, subjects are shown one or more of a set of four symbols and asked, with no prior information, to use them to guess whether it will rain or shine [38, 39]. After responding, they are told whether they are right or wrong and the task is repeated for many trials. Subjects report the subjective experience of guessing at every answer and not learning anything during the course of the task. In fact, unbeknownst to the subject, the correct answer to each trial is calculated based on combinations of fixed probabilities assigned to each symbol. Though subjects feel that they are guessing, their performance improves steadily during the course of the task, demonstrating that they are learning outside of awareness.

Recent functional imaging experiments have demonstrated that the brain regions subserving encoding (i.e., formation) and retrieval of explicit and implicit memory do not fully overlap. Working memory appears to rely heavily on activity in the frontal lobes, primarily in the dorsolateral prefrontal cortex. The formation of long-term declarative memories relies on structures in the medial temporal lobe, most prominently the hippocampus, with involvement from the amygdala and limbic system when significant affects are involved. Formation of implicit memories in priming appears to rely heavily on the frontal lobes, while formation of implicit associative memory may involve the limbic or motor systems, depending on the nature of the memory. Procedural memories formation, such as in the Weather Task, involves components of the basal ganglia, the caudate, and the putamen, if the task is predominantly cognitive, and the cerebellum and brain stem, if the task is motor. Some investigators have suggested that memories related to one's personal history, referred to as "autobiographical memory," may also use a somewhat distinct system, though the evidence remains unclear [40].

The nature of these multiple memory systems has important implications for psychodynamic theory and practice. First, there is substantial evidence that much of learning and memory does take place outside of awareness, raising the possibility for its importance in psychopathology and mental life. Given their functional and anatomical differences, it is therefore important to which memory system a particular learned thought or behavior belongs. For example, a person's expectation of certain responses from a caregiver or significant other (a frequent emphasis in dynamic psychotherapy) may be encoded as an explicit memory, an implicit associative or priming memory, or a procedural memory. Several recent theorists have proposed that the procedural memory explanation is most likely [24], though the more interesting finding might be that all three systems are involved to varying degrees. As each memory system has distinct modes of functioning, properties, and constraints (including capacity and method for change), identification of the role of differing memory systems in psychodynamic work is crucial. For example, it seems likely that patterns of interpersonal relatedness and emotion regulation learned in the first few years of life are encoded in a more procedural (i.e., nonsymbolized) fashion, and therefore are slower to change and less amenable to verbal interpretations (perhaps akin to what is described by some psychodynamic theorists as "pre-oedipal" content). Meanwhile, symptoms based in neurotic conflict that develops later in life may be represented symbolically, despite being unconscious. Such symptoms may be easier to change with accurate and timely pschodynamic interpretations (akin to the so-called Oedipal material).

## Affect

Though psychodynamic thinkers have long emphasized the importance of affect, cognitive neuroscientists initially neglected this area, largely due to the difficulty of measuring or even defining what an affect is (e.g., psychiatrists to this day debate over the definitions of mood and affect, and the extent to which either one can be defined subjectively or by external signs.) Here we will use affect in the broad sense as synonymous with emotion, that is, a mental state with physiologic and psychological components. In recent years, however, affect has become a major topic of research in relation to both psychopathology and normal functioning [41]. The study of fear has been made possible by observing its behavioral correlates in animals. This work led to the identification of the limbic system, particularly the amygdala, anterior cingulate, orbitofrontal, and medial prefrontal cortex, as important in affective processing [42]. Though the study and localization of other affects has been more challenging, there is growing evidence that, at least in humans, affective processing

**Fig. 13.3** The affective circumplex model shows how different affective states may be represented by placement on two continuous and unrelated scales: activation versus deactivation (*y*-axis) and unpleasant–pleasant (*x*-axis). Figure taken from Peterson [22] © Elsevier 2005, used with permission

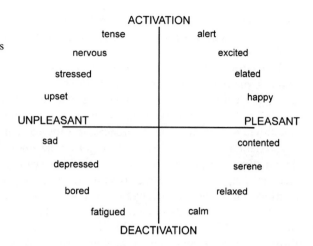

is governed by continuous properties of all affects, rather than relying on a distinct system for each feeling state.

The circumplex model of affect [43, 44] posits that each affect is represented in the brain according to two independent properties: valence (the extent to which the affect is positive or negative) and arousal (the extent to which the affect is seen as stimulating or arousing, Fig. 13.3). Brain systems involved in reward mechanisms, such as dopaminergic areas of the brain stem, are believed to play a role in encoding and processing valence, while systems governing attention and arousal, such as the reticular formation, thalamus, and dorsolateral prefrontal cortex, govern arousal [45]. Since both properties may be salient to the individual, they are processed in common structures such as the amygdala and anterior cingulate, though with increased spatial resolution in our imaging techniques we may learn about subdivisions of these regions relevant to different affective stimuli [46].

Psychodynamic models are concerned with how affects are generated, regulated, and expressed. Thus, neuroimaging findings suggest potential ways to measure affects that are in and out of awareness. Ochsner and colleagues have shown that particular brain regions are involved when subjects consciously manipulate their own affect by reappraising a visual image in a way contrary to an initial impression [47]. Lane argues that engagement of these affect regulation processes, by bringing thoughts and their associated affects into conscious awareness, forms a basic psychotherapeutic mechanism of action. He draws parallels between the hierarchical organization of psychological aspects of emotional experience and their neural substrates, suggesting that engagement of higher level systems leads to better psychological health [25] (Fig. 13.4). Etkin and colleagues further parceled conscious and unconscious awareness of affect by studying activation in the basolateral amygdala in response to fearful faces [48]. They found that when the stimuli are presented subliminally, activity in the basolateral amygdala is related to a subject's baseline trait level of anxiety,

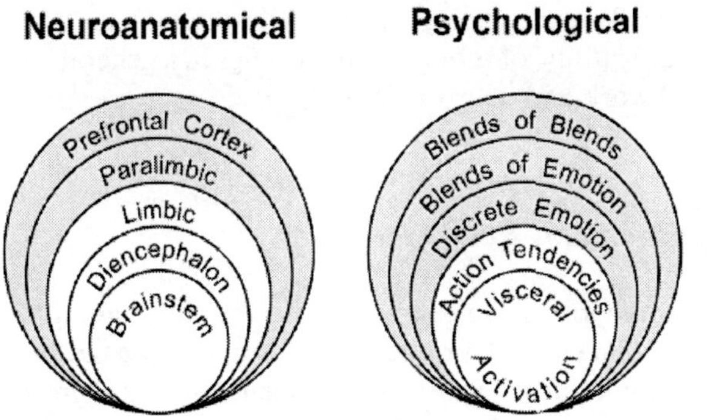

**Neuroanatomical**        **Psychological**

**Fig. 13.4** Lane and Garfield depict hierarchical organization of emotional experience and its neural substrates. Higher levels (larger circles) illustrate mechanisms that add to and modulate lower levels, but do not replace them. A white background for lower level processes indicates an implicit process, whereas a gray background for a higher level process indicates an explicit process. Figure taken from Lane and Garfield [25] © Karnac, London, UK, used with permission

but when stimuli are presented with the subject's conscious awareness, activity in this region is not related to anxiety. This pattern suggests that to understand the conscious representations of affect, we must evaluate not only automatic responses, but also the compensatory responses which depend on the extent to which affect is conscious or unconscious. For example, when using imaging to distinguish between healthy controls and patients with a psychatric diagnosis, one must always keep in mind that observed differences are just as likely to reflect the *compensation* in the individuals with the disorder as they are a core pathological feature of the disorder. Clinicians are familiar with this concept, such as when they note an unusual degree of psychological mindedness in a patient who needed to cope with life difficulties, in comparison with a less psychologically minded healthy individual who was exposed to less stress and thus never needed to develop this capacity.

Lane's typology of affect (see Fig. 13.4) is useful in appreciating the range of affective phenomena that are potentially important in psychopathology and treatment. He cites behavioral and neurobiological evidence for four overlapping categories of affective processes: (1) background feeling, (2) implicit affect, (3) focal attention, and (4) reflective awareness [25]. Background feeling does not require consciousness, but is available on demand. Implicit affect is unconscious. Focal attention is a conscious spotlight on affect, related to reappraisal, as studied by Ochsner. Reflective awareness consists of an appreciation for affect in relation to self and other representations and is perhaps most central to psychodynamic theories. All are likely relevant to psychopathology and mechanisms of change. Across most psychotherapeutic modalities, it is believed that specific attention to problematic thoughts and maladaptive negative feelings helps individuals gain better control over and ameliorate the effects of these mental contents. Lane's typology is an early attempt to frame this kind of "cognitive modification" of thoughts and feelings in a general language relevant to both clinical work and neurobiology.


## Social Cognition and Relatedness

Psychodynamic theorists have long argued for the important role of intrapsychic representations of relationships and interpersonal processes in the basic functioning of the mind. Early cognitive neuroscience and experimental approaches neglected social processes due to the complexity and measurement difficulties inherent to this perspective. However, along with the increasing attention on nonconscious processes and affect, cognitive scientists have also become more interested in the social brain, even coining a new subfield labeled "social cognitive neuroscience." This has been driven by success with animal models, such as Insel's work comparing monogamous and polygamous rodents [49, 50], as well as by functional neuroimaging, with its ability to study complex in vivo processes and associated cognition [51].

Many if not all aspects of the growing social cognitive neuroscience literature are relevant to psychoanalytic theory and treatment. At the most basic level, such research has led to nonanalytic conceptualization and measurement of the neural basis of self versus other representations. Some evidence suggests that person (in psychoanalytic terms, object) representations are processed in distinct regions of the brain (medial prefrontal cortex) [52]. There is even evidence for the possibility of dissociating brain regions involved in processing of self versus other representations [53, 54]. An alternative view is for a neuroanatomical division between processing of data about internal states (typically in the medial part of the frontal lobes) versus external behaviors and properties (typically in the lateral part of the frontal lobes) [55]. Though the exact location of these processes may have little impact on the theories and work of psychoanalytic treatments, such work may shed light on the contrasts between self and object processing and provide tools for studying these crucial systems in association with psychopathology and treatment.

Transference is a relational process hypothesized to be at the core of many clinical phenomena, and even the primary mechanism of change, in psychodynamic treatments [56]. Though there has been research into the effect of transference interpretations on treatment alliance and outcome [57, 58], it was thought to be difficult, if not impossible, to study the neural mechanism of the transference process (as opposed to other known cognitive phenomena).

However, in the early 1990s Susan Andersen developed a behavioral method which she used to demonstrate and probe certain aspects of transference in a population of healthy college students. In her paradigm, subjects participate in two sessions, which they are led to believe are unrelated to one another. In the first session, the subject is asked to provide an equal number of positive and negative short descriptive sentences about one or more (depending on the version of the experiment) significant people (called significant others or "SOs") in their lives. Subjects also select a set of "irrelevant" (i.e., neither descriptive nor counterdescriptive) adjectives in relation to each SO and provide descriptors about a series of famous people. In the second session (carried out at least a month later, so as to prevent the subject from making any connection between the two) the subject is told that he will meet a stranger and is asked, in advance, to memorize a description of that stranger. The stranger (or in some experiments, multiple strangers) described are, in fact, fictitious and their descriptions are constructed in one of three ways: (1) they are created from a semi-random assortment of one of the subject's own SO descriptions (padded with irrelevant descriptors), (2) they are created from a semirandom assortment of a *different* subject's SO description (padded with irrelevants), or (3) they are created from a semirandom assortment of the subject's famous person descriptors.

Andersen demonstrated that though subjects never made the conscious connection between the strangers and their own SOs, their memory for these descriptions, affective response (in and out of awareness), and attributions to the stranger were all significantly influenced by whether the stranger resembled their own significant other or not [59–63]. Work is currently underway by Gerber and Peterson, in collaboration with Andersen, to investigate the neural basis of transference using a modified version of the paradigm suitable for the fMRI environment.

Another perspective on transference is to view it as one example of an individual having to use ambiguous stimuli to make predictions about the future [64, 65]. An incomplete set of information about a person may engage an automatic system that chooses the most likely object representation (usually outside of awareness) and fills in the missing data. Peterson and colleagues have studied the neural basis for viewing bistable percepts such as the Necker cube (where one can see one vertex of a three-dimensional cube either pointing out from the page or pointing into the page, but not both at the same time, Fig. 13.5)

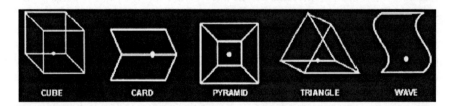

**Fig. 13.5** Reversible geometric figures, as used by Peterson [22] to investigate the neural basis of bistable percepts. Each figure can be perceived either with the dot protruding out of the page or receding into the page. The neural substrate for consciously selecting either image may also subserve other conscious choices of perspective that influence our mental life, such as what goes on in psychotherapy. Figure taken from Peterson [22] © Elsevier 2005, used with permission

[66]. Frontal–striatal circuits are active when one alternates between images, suggesting a supervisory role of these circuits in other interpretations of ambiguous stimuli, such as transference.

Westen and Gabbard [67, 68] have argued that investigation into the neural basis of transference is likely to be useful for studying psychoanalytic treatments. In particular, they point to long-standing psychoanalytic debates such as whether there is one transference or many in a given clinical moment, or whether the transference is significantly altered by real-world properties of the analyst and analytic setting (on which empirical evidence could have a useful impact). They argue that transference is predominantly a form of procedural memory. Gerber and Peterson speculate that transferential processes may have elements of multiple memory systems including procedural and associative nondeclarative systems. Neuroimaging findings using the Andersen paradigm may shed light on these questions, which may then suggest properties and constraints of the transference system that are relevant to theorizing and clinical techniques. For example, we may learn that some aspects of transference are rooted in procedural memories, by noting their association with activity in the basal ganglia. These elements of transference may be learned earlier in life, change more slowly, and are more amenable to supportive interventions than to higher level interpretations. In contrast, we may learn that other aspects of transference are rooted in implicit associative memories but associating them with activity in the frontal cortex and hippocampus. These elements may stem from later conflict and change relatively quickly in response to defense interpretations. Ultimately, neuroimaging of paradigms such as Andersen's could help us clarify different aspects of transference in the laboratory in such a way that could be directly applied to clinical technique.

Attachment theory, as originated by John Bowlby and carefully operationalized by Ainsworth, Main, and others, has been influential on psychodynamic theorizing and clinical practice [69, 70]. Empirical work in both humans and animals has suggested that the attachment system is fundamental to our social processes and is likely subserved by a distinct neural mechanism [71, 72]. Recent neuroimaging work has attempted to localize these processes using attachment-related stimuli such as pictures of one's own children [73, 74]. Progress in this area will likely be relevant to our understanding of how attachment affects and is changed within the treatment environment. Such work could help clarify the extent to which insecure or disorganized attachments are rooted in neurobiologically fixed deficits whose roots do not change in treatment (though we may develop helpful compensations) versus difficulties in higher-level processing that can be fundamentally altered by treatment. Attachment and psychodynamic theorists have argued about these very points and it is hopeful that neurobiological methods can advance the debate.

Empathy, an inherently interpersonal process, has received considerable attention in the cognitive neuroscience literature [75–77]. Researchers have shown activation in specific brain regions, in particular the insula and the anterior cingulate cortex, that relate to both an individual's experience of his/

her own distress, and his/her experience of someone else's distress. A subject's own behaviorally rated capacity for empathy is tightly correlated with the activation of these brain regions [75, 76]. In a related work, Marci has shown a link between therapist empathy and physiologic correlation between patient and therapist using a measure of skin conductance [16, 78]. Marci and Riess have shown that awareness of lack of patient–therapist concordance in physiological measures can lead to significantly improved alterations in clinical interventions, helping the therapist see previously unseen anxiety in the patient [79]. Given the highly reproduced finding that the patient–therapist alliance (a construct that overlaps with empathy) is closely related to therapeutic outcome, neurobiological investigation of empathy is relevant and important for our understanding of analytic treatments.

Conceptualization and empirical research into "theory of mind" (i.e., an individual's understanding about the content and functioning of other people's minds) began in the developmental psychology literature but has become an important part of work on psychopathology [in particular autism, borderline personality disorder (BPD), and schizophrenia] and therapeutic change (where it is often called "mentalization") [80–82]. Several neuroimaging researchers have found evidence for functional localization of theory of mind in the medial prefrontal cortex, interestingly close to, and undoubtedly related to, regions implicated in self-representations [83–86]. Further investigation into the nature of theory of mind, its properties, and its capacity for modification during treatment may be an important window into a psychodynamic mechanism of action. For example, it is widely hypothesized that in certain disorders such as autism, there is a relatively fixed deficit in theory of mind. However, some have argued that it is possible to significantly improve the ability of high functioning autistic or Asperger's individuals though therapy and it would be useful to understand whether these changes affect the same areas as the underlying disorder or are more likely to affect compensatory mechanisms. Fonagy and others have discussed impaired theory of mind in BPD; neuroimaging could help clarify whether this is more of a stable deficit or an inhibition of an underlying capacity that can be improved through treatment [80].

The term "mirror neurons" was coined in reference to premotor and parietal cells in the brain of macaque monkeys that fired *both* when the animal carried out a specific action (e.g., reaching for a banana) and when the animal observed a human experimenter performing that action [87]. The translation of this concept into humans, predominantly through functional neuroimaging experiments, has received a great deal of attention within the psychodynamic literature [88–90]. Dynamic theorists have seen in the mirror neuron literature a potential neurobiological substrate and legitimization of the psychodynamic concept of "primary identification" (i.e., a core level experience by one person of the mental state of another). However, this argument is potentially misleading in a number of ways. First, it appears to imply that the processes of empathy and identification are somehow "neurobiologically primary" and not mediated by higher level neurocognitive processes, as is well established by clinical and empirical evidence. Second, these conclusions are based on an extrapolation of a finding in nonhuman primates, where single-cell recordings are possible, to humans, where at present we can only measure activation in large groups of neurons. Finally, it is unclear how the mirror neuron literature adds to the broader theory that all concepts (including self and object representations, as well as their expected actions and affects) are stored in distributed neural representations, which are, in turn, connected to representations of behaviors being carried out both by ourselves and by others. More empirical and theoretical work is required to clarify the usefulness of the mirror neuron literature to psychodynamic therapy.

## Attention, Free Association, and Defense

The study of attentional processes is important as well for the investigation of unconscious and clinically relevant mechanisms. Although consciousness is typically thought of as a binary phenomenon – something is either accessible or inaccessible to awareness – research into attention suggests a broad continuum in which material is more or less accessible in any given context due to a variety of factors [91, 92]. A number of studies have demonstrated preferential attention for mental contents that are less objectionable according to basic psychodynamic principles [93–95]. Repression, one of the most basic of all defense mechanisms, has been studied carefully from behavioral and neurobiological perspectives [64, 96]. Evidence supports the notion that motivated forgetting relies on increased activity in the dorsolateral prefrontal cortex (which may supply the motivation) and reduced activity in the hippocampus (which fails to encode the memory) [97].

Hypnosis is an extreme example of altered consciousness often associated with Freud and psychoanalysis, yet for many years has been on unclear empirical grounds. Recently, neuroimagers have been able to investigate hypnosis in the MRI scanner and show that it has measurable consequences in terms of brain activity that closely parallel behavioral findings [98, 99]. In particular, Raz and colleagues have shown that effects of the Stroop Task, a highly reliable and well-accepted cognitive measure, can be significantly reduced using hypnosis. In the Stroop task, subjects are presented with a series of color words (e.g., "red," "blue," "green") written in either the *same* color that the word represents (i.e., a congruent trial) or a *different* color (i.e., an incongruent trial). The subject is asked to indicate for each word, the color that the word is written in, ignoring what the word itself means. Because reading is automatic, subjects take longer to respond to incongruent trials than to congruent trials, no matter how hard they try or train in the task. Giving a subject the posthypnotic suggestion that the words are "nonsense strings" effectively reduces the extent of this effect. This reduction correlated closely with decreased activity in the anterior cingulate cortex, a structure associated with managing conflict between two stimuli seeking attention [98].

Dreams have long been of interest to psychodynamic (and especially psychoanalytic) therapists, who have theorized that dream contents may reflect relational, and dynamic mental constructs that are otherwise difficult for the conscious mind to access. Recent neuroimaging findings suggest that brain regions that are highly active during rapid eye movement (REM) sleep, when most dreaming takes place, may be relevant to accessing this material [100, 101]. These regions include brain stem, limbic, and paralimbic circuitry. Deactivation of the dorsolateral prefrontal cortex, as also observed during REM, may facilitate retrieval of this material through disinhibition of limbic and other subcortical processes. Experience while awake is seen to influence subsequent dreaming activity [102]. Along these lines, it may the case that certain aspects of psychodynamic therapy engage neural circuits that are also activated (or deactivated) during dreaming, facilitating the identification and resolution of deeply held intrapsychic conflicts. Further research is needed to clarify the neurobiology common to dreaming and psychodynamic therapy process, and to understand the neural mechanics of Freud's "royal route" to the unconscious.

Early evidence is even accumulating to support one of the oldest psychodynamic notions, namely that the behavior of the mind when it is not consciously being controlled – free association – consists of more than merely background noise. Researchers have begun to describe a network of cortical regions that activate in a "default mode" when the mind otherwise appears to be at rest or wandering [103, 104]. Default mode circuits could be of crucial importance in understanding the unconscious or nonconscious mechanisms that are relevant to psychodynamic processes and treatment.

## Conclusions

Empirical data is clearly accumulating that is relevant to psychodynamic processes in a wide range of areas. Whereas at one point psychodynamic psychology was the only language and method for studying the unconscious, affect, interpersonal processes, dreams, defense mechanisms, and free association, now cognitive neuroscience offers concepts and methods for this purpose as well. A useful task of psychodynamics in this context is to integrate its own large database of clinical data and theoretical constructs with the emerging empirical findings. Several writers have begun to do so, though the explosion in research makes it difficult to identify and navigate the salient neural findings [105–110]. Advances in the years to come will reveal how these two fields fit together, hopefully with direct benefit to clinical practice.

One of the principal criticisms leveled against neuroscientific investigations of psychodynamic theory and practice has been that, neuroscience has very little to offer the clinician in terms of understanding his patients in a "dynamic" way or choosing his individual techniques [19, 111]. To date, it seems quite true that findings from the neuroscience literature have had little direct influence on the thinking of analytic clinicians and their behavior in the office. However, this promises to change in a number of ways in the not too distant future. First, dynamic clinicians have long been moving in the direction of understanding certain deficits – of cognitive functioning, affect regulation, and attachment – as related to but not the same as dynamic conflicts. This then influences their conceptualization of pathology (particularly in a developmental context) and way of speaking with their patients. This movement was driven by an entire culture of change in psychiatry, psychology, and psychoanalysis, but neuroscience has played a role in making deficits more objectifiable and real.

Second, there has been a significant movement in dynamic thinking toward an object relations approach. Though this has been stimulated by many factors, one among them is the greater emphasis in neuroscience on social functioning and the growing evidence for an attachment system. Finally, many dynamic clinicians feel that research into the process and outcome of patients with BPD has clarified the appropriateness of a supportive–expressive model of treatment versus a more purely interpretive, classical analytic approach. Kernberg and others have discussed the importance of matching the structure and depth of the treatment to the personality organization of the patient [80, 112, 113]. Neuroscientific studies of BPD and the mechanisms involved in its treatment (e.g., mentalization, theory of mind, affect regulation) are relatively recent, but are already starting to support and refine this approach to matching treatment and patient.

## Psychotherapy in the Era of Neuroimaging

Neuroimaging techniques have begun to provide us not only with a better understanding of psychotherapy components, but also of the overall effects of psychotherapy on brain function. At their fullest potential, studies of how psychotherapy affects the brain can be of tremendous value to patients, therapists, and to the field as a whole. Providing patients with information on how psychotherapy changes brain function reinforces the notion that the treatment induces meaningful changes. In the dialogue between patient and therapist, neuroimaging results can enhance the vocabulary of psychotherapy process and help concretize the goals of treatment. In some cases, it may even be possible to predict how well a given patient will do with a given therapeutic approach, based on that individual's pattern of brain activity at baseline. Finally, the notion that psychotherapy has a biological substrate places the intervention in the same category as other "medical" treatments that induce measurable changes in physiology, biochemistry, or morphology. This notion could be a powerful ally in combating the residual stigma associated with psychotherapy (and psychiatric treatment in general) that promotes hesitation in many potential patients, prevents the achievement of parity with other medical treatments, and nurtures an unfounded skepticism and mistrust within some elements of culture and society.

A healthy conglomeration of studies has now begun to deliver findings with clear implications for psychotherapy theory and practice [10, 114]. Even so, the story of how psychotherapy changes brain function is far from complete. Notably, as of the time of this writing, the effects of *psychodynamic* psychotherapy on brain activity have not yet been studied explicitly (more on what is meant by "explicitly" will follow). However, extant studies examining other psychotherapeutic modalities have clearly shed light on the same questions that will be essential to understanding how dynamic therapy changes the brain. This section will focus on how these preliminary studies have addressed three fundamental questions related to psychotherapy and brain function: (1) Does psychotherapy affect activity within brain regions known to be involved in the pathophysiology of the target disorders? (2) Does psychotherapy differ from psychopharmacology, the other mainstay of psychiatric treatment, in this regard? and (3) Do different varieties of psychotherapy that are equally effective target similar brain regions, and in similar ways?

## *Repairing Dysregulated Neural Machinery in Anxiety Disorders*

Neuroimaging studies have provided previously unimaginable insight into how and where psychiatric disorders disrupt the normal workings of the brain. While dramatic changes in the size and shape of brain structures were long ago ruled out in the study of psychiatric conditions, functional abnormalities – that is, inappropriate activation or deactivation of identified neural regions and circuits – have been clearly demonstrated in many disorders [115]. By the same token, the first test of how psychotherapy induces meaningful changes in brain function is whether these changes occur in implicated brain regions, and whether these changes restore normal levels of activity.

Perhaps the clearest example of regional brain dysfunction in psychiatric conditions is obsessive-compulsive disorder (OCD). One of the most consistently replicated findings in psychiatry neuroimaging research involves abnormal activity in cortico–striato–thalamic circuitry in OCD. Baseline activity in the orbitofrontal cortex (OFC), anterior cingulate cortex, striatum, and thalamus is increased in OCD, and this pattern is exacerbated by symptom provocation [116, 117]. Further, the degree of hyperactivity intercorrelates among these regions [118]. Within the striatum, the caudate nucleus in particular is thought to contribute to OCD symptoms by inappropriately managing cognitive and emotional impulses, leading to their dysregulated expression [119].

In the first published investigations of the neural effects of psychotherapy, Baxter, Schwartz and colleagues [118] studied the effects of behavioral therapy

(BT) on OCD. In two cohorts, the investigators found that successful BT was associated with significant reduction in caudate nucleus activity, as well as a decoupling of hyperactivation in the caudate, OFC, and thalamus. Although BT does not explicitly rely on psychodynamic formulation or technique, nonetheless, Baxter and associates were aware of at least one dynamic implication of their work:

> Another basal ganglia function, 'gating,' by which certain motor, sensory, and perhaps cognitive impulses are either allowed to proceed through to perception and behavior or are held back ('filtered') and dissipated, seems to speak to the psychodynamic concept of disordered 'repression' in OCD [118].

They also note that the emotional dysregulation seen in some individuals with Huntington's disease correlates with decreased caudate activity in these patients [120], again speaking to the role that the caudate may play in gating emotional impulses.

The neural circuitry underlying phobias has also been clearly established, involving increased activity in limbic, paralimbic, and ventral prefrontal regions. This pattern is entirely in keeping with studies associating the amygdala and adjacent structures with conditioned fear responses, and the ventral prefrontal cortex with both retention and recall of conditioned fear and in planning responses to frightening stimuli [121]. One might imagine, for example, that among individuals with specific phobias, exposure to the fear-inducing stimulus would cause increased activity in the amygdala, related to recognition and generation of the fear response, and in the prefrontal cortex, related to planning a strategy for confrontation (or retreat).

Two recent neuroimaging investigations suggest that psychotherapy for specific phobias targets these same regions. In a study of individuals with social phobia, Furmark and colleagues [122] examined the effect of cognitive-behavioral therapy (CBT) on brain activation following symptom provocation. Prior to treatment, subjects exhibited increased activity in the amygdala and other limbic structures when asked to read a speech about a personal experience in front of multiple observers. Following eight sessions of group CBT, the same individuals demonstrated significantly lower activation of these regions when performing the same task as before. Another provocation design by Paquette and associates [123] examined changes in brain activation related to group CBT for spider phobia. With successful treatment, patients exhibited a decline in parahippocampal gyrus and prefrontal cortex activation when exposed to pictures of spiders. Again, although neither of these studies was geared toward measuring effects of *psychodynamic* interactions on brain function, given the generative roles of prior (usually developmental) traumatic experiences on phobic responses and the undoing of phobias through a therapeutic relationship, it is quite likely that dynamic factors play an implicit role even in CBT for phobias [124]. It remains to be seen to what extent changes in prefrontal and limbic regions as a result of CBT actually reflect dynamic processes.

## Contrasting Effects of Psychotherapy and Psychopharmacology on Brain Function

For many psychiatric conditions, psychotherapy and psychopharmacology offer equivalent efficacy (or, in some cases, synergistic beneficial effects). However, do their similar clinical effects reflect parallel changes on brain activity? Evidence from other areas of medicine seems to challenge this notion. For example, while beta blockers, ACE inhibitors, and diuretics are all effective treatments for hypertension, each works through a unique mechanism (i.e., by affecting sympathetic or vascular tone, or circulating volume). With the complex neural pathophysiology of depression, it would not be surprising to see that different treatment modalities target different components of the disorder. Functional neuroimaging provides the ability to compare directly the neural mechanisms of action of psychotherapy and psychopharmacology. More importantly, as we shall later discuss, this information may one day be useful in predicting which type of therapy best matches up against a given individual's pattern of brain susceptibility – just as optimal selection of blood pressure medications can be guided by individual risk patterns (e.g., comorbid diabetes, heart disease, or kidney disease) [125].

The question of how psychotherapy compares to pharmacotherapy in influencing brain function has been of interest to neuroimaging investigators since Baxter and colleagues' first study of OCD. Indeed, in that investigation, BT was contrasted with fluoxetine on treatment-related changes in brain activity [118]. Both treatments, as it turned out, reduced activity in the caudate nucleus and disrupted the pattern of tandem hyperactivity in cortico–striato–thalamic circuitry. However, in a subsequent study conducted by Brody and associates [126], a strikingly different pattern emerged with respect to activity in another region implicated in OCD, the OFC. Taking a slightly different approach, Brody and colleagues examined whether baseline brain activity alone might predict response to BT versus fluoxetine. Among responders to BT, the degree of baseline activity in the left OFC cortex positively correlated with responsiveness to treatment. However, among responders to fluoxetine, the opposite pattern emerged: those with *less* baseline activity in the left OFC were more likely to respond to treatment. Offering an explanation for this pattern, the investigators proposed that "subjects with higher pretreatment metabolism in the OFC may have a greater ability to change the assignment of affective value to stimuli," a process that more explicitly relies on psychotherapy than psychopharmacology.

Comparisons of brain activity response to psychotherapy versus medication have also intrigued investigators studying depression. In an FDG (fluorodeoxyglucose)–PET study of CBT versus paroxetine, Goldapple and colleagues [127] focused on how these respective treatments changed brain function. Their report focused on prefrontal, limbic, and paralimbic structures that had previously been implicated in the pathophysiology of depression.

Once again, a provocative contrast emerged between the two treatments (despite similar efficacy). In the paroxetine group, treatment resulted in increased prefrontal activity, and diminished activity in the hippocampus and subgenual cingulate cortex. However, in those patients receiving CBT, treatment response was associated with decreased prefrontal activity, and increased hippocampal and dorsal cingulate cortex activity – almost completely opposite to the paroxetine group. This finding is also somewhat counterintuitive, given the well established role of the prefrontal cortex in stimulus appraisal, strategy planning, and direction of attentional resources – all elements that are actively re-trained during CBT. Rather, as the authors speculated:

> Hippocampal and mid and anterior cingulate increases coupled with decreases in medial frontal, dorsolateral, and ventrolateral prefrontal activity with CBT treatment might be nonetheless interpreted as correlates of CBT-conditioned increases in attention to personally relevant emotional and environmental stimuli associated with a learned ability to reduce online cortical processes at the level of encoding and retrieval of maladaptive associative memories, as well as a reduction in both ruminations and overprocessing of irrelevant information [127].

While this explanation is certainly plausible, it remains theoretical, and as we shall later consider, fails to account for other critical factors that might account for this apparent discrepancy. Impressively, though, Kennedy and colleagues have replicated their findings of decreased prefrontal deactivation in CBT responders, although in a more medial prefrontal region than previously reported. Kennedy et al. also replicated the previous finding of opposing changes in the anterior cingulate cortex in response to CBT (increased activity) versus a pharmacologic intervention, venlafaxine (decreased activity) [128].

In a second study comparing psychotherapy to paroxetine for depression, Brody and colleagues this time focused on interpersonal therapy (IPT) [129]. However, unlike the Goldapple investigation of paroxetine versus CBT, [127] in this case the two treatments similarly affected the prefrontal cortex (decreasing activity) as well as limbic and paralimbic regions (increased activity in the insula and left inferior temporal lobe). This pattern is noteworthy on two fronts: on the one hand, the same pharmacologic intervention (paroxetine) appeared to work in opposing directions relative to psychotherapy in the Goldapple and Brody studies, and on the other, differing psychotherapeutic approaches appeared to induce similar changes in both studies (Fig. 13.6).

While this pattern makes it difficult to draw conclusions about whether psychotherapy and psychopharmacology induce similar changes in brain activity, it has even more hair-raising implications for psychotherapists, who sometimes ardently prefer one therapeutic approach over another: can it be possible that, despite their dissimilarities in theory and practice, that various types of psychotherapy ultimately change the brain in similar ways?

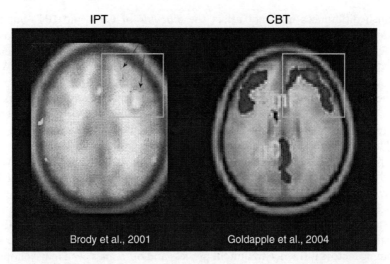

**Fig. 13.6** Decreases in prefrontal activity (white box) seen after trials IPT and CBT. © American Medical Association, used with permission

## Contrasting Effects of Varying Psychotherapeutic Approaches on Brain Function

With only few published studies available to weigh this important question – and no head-to-head investigations of the effects of different psychotherapies on brain function – it is impossible to formulate a definitive answer at present. Indeed, it is likely that the answer will require a more complex experimental design than contrasting pre- and posttreatment scans of patients in different psychotherapy groups, as well as independent replication of the results. But let us first take a step back, and carefully consider the argument for why differing effects on brain activity might be expected.

The studies mentioned thus far used either CBT or IPT to treat depression. Consistent with a wealth of clinical experience and validation, both interventions were successful in improving depression symptoms, performing comparably to antidepressant intervention. However, while IPT and CBT are similar in that they are both time-limited, manual-guided treatments, in theory, the work of therapy differs substantially in these treatments. Unlike CBT, IPT focuses primarily on improving interpersonal relationships, often drawing material directly from the patient–therapist relationship. With a greater focus on transference, certain psychodynamic elements are touched upon more explicitly in IPT. Moreover, cognitive and dynamically oriented therapies may draw on different memory systems (described in section on "Memory and Learning"), as cognitive therapy may more strongly rely on declarative memories, and dynamic therapy on implicit memories.

Such differences may not affect the *outcome* of CBT and IPT, but they certainly should affect the *process*. In this sense, it is unfortunate that most of the currently published neuroimaging studies that focus on psychotherapy failed to include process measures and measures of treatment adherence. Without such measures, it remains possible that despite the differing "brand names," elements of IPT contributed to CBT sessions, and vice versa. Along the same lines, it is possible that symptom improvement was significantly influenced by alternate therapeutic approaches.

This risk is more than theoretical: other investigators examining psychotherapy process with rigorous criteria strongly suggest that psychotherapeutic approach is often more eclectic than intended. For one manualized trial of IPT versus CBT, [130] in *both* treatment groups, process and outcome were more closely related to cognitive-behavioral techniques. Conversely, in another investigation of CBT for depression, [131] psychodynamic elements both influenced the course of treatment and the outcome [132]. Many would argue that dynamic factors influence treatment process and outcomes even in psychopharmacology [133, 134] or general medical settings, [135] even without the caregiver explicitly employing psychodynamic techniques. As such, even though psychodynamic psychotherapy has not "explicitly" been studied with neuroimaging, in all likelihood, dynamic elements influenced both outcome and brain activity even for patients receiving BT or CBT in the studies described earlier. Regardless, it is impossible to reliably disentangle the effects of varying psychotherapy techniques on brain function without measures of adherence or process.

By the same token, the oft employed "pre–post" model of comparing brain activity before and after a course of psychotherapy relates much more directly to outcome than to process. In the studies described earlier, while CBT and IPT appeared to exert very similar effects on brain function *as a result of* therapy, parallel changes may or may not occur *during* therapy. The ability to measure brain activation patterns serially over the course of psychotherapy – or, better, to measure them during psychotherapy sessions themselves – will be instrumental in addressing this question, especially when viewed alongside measures of psychotherapy process.

Thus, while the question "Does psychotherapy change brain function?" appears to be convincingly answered, the questions of "How does psychotherapy change brain function?" and, more specifically, "How do different psychotherapies change brain function?" remain largely unexplored. In the next section we will consider how these questions might best be addressed in future studies, as well as the unique implications that these studies may have on the practice of psychodynamic psychotherapy.

## Synthesis and Future Directions

Given the broad range of findings reviewed in this chapter it is a significant challenge to synthesize it into a reliable set of conclusions. However, analogous to the method of psychodynamic therapy itself, perhaps it is more useful to comment on the process of this review than on its detailed contents (though we will attempt to do some of both). We begin by suggesting several things that we feel that the literature *does* support.

First, we believe that given the sheer volume of scientifically sophisticated empirical investigations on psychotherapy, affect, social processes, and non-conscious mechanisms (including but not limited to dreams, hypnosis, free association, and defense mechanisms) it is increasingly clear that neurobiological research is relevant to psychodynamic concepts and treatment. That said, we have no doubt that controversy will continue to rage about the applicability of this work to the day-to-day thinking of psychodynamic theorists and clinicians. It is helpful and responsible to question the application of individual findings when the methods of investigation are so different. However, we believe it is irresponsible and counterproductive to the field when some generalize that criticism to a condemnation of the usefulness of all neurobiological research, particularly without a first-hand knowledge of that literature [17, 19].

To date, a number of important brain systems and associated regions have been implicated as important to psychodynamically relevant hypotheses. These include limbic and paralimbic structures (e.g., amygdala, insula, OFC), memory systems (e.g., dorsolateral prefrontal cortex and hippocampus), conflict management and affect regulatory systems (e.g., anterior cingulate cortex and medial prefrontal cortex), attentional systems (prefrontal, cingulate, and parietal cortices), and planning and procedural memory systems (basal ganglia).

It is perhaps equally, if not more important, to be open and frank about what the neurobiological literature does not do, and in some cases will never do, in reference to psychodynamic thinking. First, we believe that it is a fundamental error to look toward neurobiology to "prove" that psychodynamic thinking and therapy are fundamentally "true." The body of theory and clinical work is too vast and heterogeneous for this to be possible, nor does it seem reasonable to think that any body of concepts, particularly one that has historically isolated itself from empirical methods, is not in need of modification. This attempt is merely the flip side of the equally false argument that empirical research has "proven" psychoanalysis to have no scientific foundation [20]. Phrasing the argument in either of these ways is counterproductive as it encourages zealotry and selective interpretation of the data, as opposed to the careful scientific elaboration of complicated theories and integration of information from multiple perspectives.

It also seems increasingly clear that the neurobiological literature does not provide a consensus on the existence of the "unconscious mind" according to psychodynamic principles. On the one hand, it is now widely accepted by cognitive neuroscientists that important mental functioning takes place outside of awareness [136]. However, the properties and constraints of nonconscious systems – whether called unconscious, implicit, procedural, or by some other name – are complex and remain to be successfully elaborated. It appears likely that there are multiple brain systems involved in nonconscious processes, including implicit associative and implicit procedural memories, and that these systems may have links to alternate ways of thinking about nonconscious processes in psychodynamic theory (e.g., Oedipal vs. pre-Oedipal functioning).

Next, it is important for empirical investigators and psychodynamic theorists or clinicians to be open about the ways in which new experimental paradigms and methodologies capture some, but never *all* aspects of a clinical phenomenon. It is a central fact of all scientific investigation that one needs to reduce a complex real-world phenomenon into a set of component parts to study it usefully. This should not be taken to be equivalent to the statement that experimental models have nothing relevant to teach us about the clinical situation [22].

Finally, we must be aware of the temptation, particularly in the era of neuroimaging, to point to particular brain regions and look for localization of individual psychodynamic processes. Given the distributed nature of brain processes and the complex interdigitation of the machinery that drives cognitive, emotional, and social processes, it is difficult to imagine wholly discrete, unambiguous localization for any particular concept, whether it be the unconscious mind, repression, transference, or structural change. Suggesting otherwise may limit the success of the dialogue on these topics.

Despite these caveats, there are a number of exciting directions to which the research reviewed in this chapter seems to point. We believe that as experimental paradigms improve, accumulating data will help us identify properties and constraints of neurobiologially based systems relevant to psychodynamic theory and practice. Once these measures are well understood, it will lead to iterative testing and refinement of psychodynamic concepts and theories about normal and pathological functioning. Ultimately, these measures will also be incorporated into clinical research and lead to the iterative testing and refinement of clinical theories and techniques. Progress in clinically relevant neurobiological research will likely also depend on the further development of cutting-edge technologies that allow for measurement of brain function in the therapist's office. Psychophysiological (e.g., skin conductance, heart rate variability) and near-infrared imaging (which measures cortical activation without requiring the heavy machinery of MRI or PET) may be important in this regard, though new technologies may emerge as well [16, 137].

Though less an area of current empirical investigation, it is likely that other empirical methods now gaining currency in experimental psychiatry will become useful for psychodynamic work as well. In particular, genetics and temperament are two important (and likely related) areas of research that are undoubtedly relevant to the variability of patient outcome in psychodynamic treatment, and ultimately to our understanding of the mechanisms of psychopathology and therapeutic change. Interestingly, Freud and other psychodynamic theorists were not opposed to the importance of hereditary and temperamental factors in understanding patients, though they have had a mixed reception in the broader psychoanalytic literature [138, 139]. On the other hand, the neurobiology and genetics of temperament is a rapidly expanding area, with an abundance of recent studies establishing how certain genetic variants predispose toward affective, harm avoidance, and novelty-seeking traits through their actions on discrete neural systems [140, 141].

Though still somewhat distant, it is not difficult to imagine some of the useful consequences of a successful program of neurobiological research into psychodynamic theories and treatments. Theorists and clinicians have long wished for a better ability to predict response in patients, so as to assist in their ability to recommend which treatments for which patients. As is currently being sought with regard to other treatments in psychiatry, sophisticated research may find patterns of neurobiological activity in response to specific tasks that is predictive of psychotherapy outcome.

Two investigations of psychotherapeutic interventions have offered extremely promising preliminary results in this regard. In a study comparing BT to fluoxetine for OCD, Brody and associates [142] found that a baseline scan differentially stratified responders from nonresponders for the two treatments: patients who were to receive fluoxetine ultimately demonstrated the best response if they had low baseline activity in the left orbitofrontal cortex, while those who would receive BT exhibited better responses if they had high activity in the same brain region. After conducting baseline scans of patients with depression, Siegle and colleagues [143] found that increased activity in the amygdala, and decreased in the subgenual cingulate cortex predicted significantly better responsiveness to CBT. These results have clearly important clinical implications: they suggest that a baseline brain scan can provide objective biomarkers that, if shown to be reliable, may be used to determine the likelihood of a good treatment response for a given individual. Ongoing work by Roffman and colleagues is examining whether baseline scans likewise can predict responsiveness to psychodynamic therapy.

Equally tantalizing is the possibility that we may investigate the effectiveness of individual interventions (e.g., supportive vs. transference interpretations) using in-session neurobiological techniques. Perhaps, we will someday have more sophisticated ways to gauge when the alliance is strong enough to make deeper interpretations helpful [16, 57]. As all of medicine moves toward individualized treatments, psychodynamic psychotherapy will keep pace [14].

Even before these advances, though, clinicians can anticipate using what we learn from neurobiological research to influence their conceptualization of patients' problems and their vocabulary for discussing such concepts with their patients. Contemporary clinicians have been greatly affected in how they talk to their patients by concepts such as attachment, mentalization, and empathy, so it is not hard to imagine that new research will yield useful changes in language too.

On another practical level, psychodynamic–neurobiological research has immediate implications for the education of psychiatrists, psychologists, therapists, and other mental health professionals. Psychodynamic teaching in psychiatry residencies and psychology graduate programs has recently been under threat specifically because critics have complained that it is not tied to a scientific literature [144]; however, even in the setting of rapidly expanding neuroscience curricula, program directors for the most part remain highly committed to psychotherapy training [145]. New research will address that challenge and also improve the teaching of concepts and techniques that have often relied more on the charisma and persuasive powers of the teacher than on the merit of the ideas. Furthermore, the ideas contained in a careful discussion of psychodynamic–empirical research are likely to be useful to trainees of many kinds. Cappas and colleagues suggest seven "principles of brain-based psychotherapy" about which there is considerable (with the possible exception of Principal 5) consensus [146]:

1.  Genetics and environment interact in the brain to shape the individual
2.  Experience transforms the brain
3.  Memory systems in the brain are interactive (i.e., memory storage and retrieval depends on context and should not be treated as a perfect account of what happened).
4.  Cognitive and emotional processes work in partnership
5.  Bonding and attachment provide the foundation for change
6.  Imagery activates and stimulates the same brain systems as does real consensus
7.  The brain can process nonverbal and unconscious information

As research progresses, we will undoubtedly further refine and add to the principles that can usefully be taught to trainees along with their empirical foundations.

Without surrendering the core skepticism toward certainty that characterizes both good science and good psychodynamic thinking, we believe that the future of close collaboration between empirical researchers and psychodynamic theorists and clinicians is bright. As long as a mutually respectful dialogue is allowed to develop, the progress in this area will drive improvements in our theory and in our clinical work with patients.

# References

1.  Freud, S. *Sigmund Freud: The Origins of Psychoanalysis (1954)*. New York: Basic Books; 1895. Project for a scientific psychology.
2.  Masson JM, ed. *The Complete Letters of Sigmund Freud to Wilhelm Fleiss 1887-1904*. 3rd ed. Cambridge, MA: The Belknap Press of Harvard University Press; 1995.
3.  Kandel ER. Biology and the future of psychoanalysis: a new intellectual framework for psychiatry revisited. *Am J Psychiatry* 1999;156(4):505–24.
4.  Alexander F. *Psychosomatic Medicine: Its Principles and Applications*. New York: WW Norton; 1950.
5.  Kandel ER. A new intellectual framework for psychiatry. *Am J Psychiatry* 1998; 155(4):457–69.
6.  Price BH, Adams RD, Coyle JT. Neurology and psychiatry: closing the great divide. *Neurology* 2000;54(1):8–14.
7.  Antonuccio DO, Danton WG, DeNelsky GY. Psychotherapy versus medication for depression: challenging the conventional wisdom with data. *Professional Psychol: Res Pract* 1995;26:574–85.

8. Goldman W, McCulloch J, Cuffel B, Zarin DA, Suarez A, Burns BJ. Outpatient utilization patterns of integrated and split psychotherapy and pharmacotherapy for depression. *Psychiatr Serv* 1998;49(4):477–82.

9. U.S. Department of Health and Human Services. *Mental Health: A Report of the Surgeon General—Executive Summary*. Rockville, MD: U.S. Department of Health and Human Services, Substance Abuse and Mental Health Services Administration, Center for Mental Health Services, National Institutes of Health, National Institute of Mental Health, 1999.

10. Roffman JL, Marci CD, Glick DM, Dougherty DD, Rauch SL. Neuroimaging and the functional neuroanatomy of psychotherapy. *Psychol Med* 2005;35:1–14.

11. Roffman JL, Marci CD, Glick DM, Dougherty DD, Rauch SL. Neuroimaging and the functional neuroanatomy of psychotherapy. *Psychol Med* 2005;35(10):1385–98.

12. Westen D, Novotny CM, Thompson-Brenner H. The empirical status of empirically supported psychotherapies: assumptions, findings, and reporting in controlled clinical trials. *Psychol Bull* 2004;130(4):631–63.

13. Dougherty DD, Rauch SL, Rosenbaum JF. *Essentials of Neuroimaging for Clinical Practice*. Washington: American Psychiatric Association; 2004.

14. Jones DS, Perlis RH. Pharmacogenetics, race, and psychiatry: prospects and challenges. *Harv Rev Psychiatry* 2006;14(2):92–108.

15. Giove F, Mangia S, Bianciardi M, et al. The physiology and metabolism of neuronal activation: in vivo studies by NMR and other methods. *Magn Reson Imaging* 2003;21(10):1283–93.

16. Marci CD, Ham J, Moran E, Orr SP. Physiologic correlates of perceived therapist empathy and social-emotional process during psychotherapy. *J Nerv Ment Dis* 2007;195(2):103–11.

17. Green A. What kind of research for psychoanalysis? In: Sandler J, Sandler A-M, Davies R, eds. *Clinical and Observational Psychoanlaytic Research: Roots of a Controversy*. Madison, CT: International Universities Press; 2000:21–6.

18. Perron R. Reflections on psychoanalytic research problems – the French speaking view. In: IPA, ed. *An Open Door Review of Outcome Studies in Psychoanalysis*. London: Research Committee of the International Psychoanalytic Association; 1999:8–19.

19. Hoffman IZ. "Doublethinking" our way to scientific legitimacy: the desiccation of human experience. In: Winter Meeting of the American Psychoanalytic Association, New York, 2007.

20. Torrey EF. Does psychoanalysis have a future? No. *Can J Psychiatry* 2005;50(12):743–4.

21. Westen D. The scientific status of unconscious processes: Is Freud really dead? *J Am Psychoanal Assoc* 1999;47(4):1061–106.

22. Peterson BS. Clinical neuroscience and imaging studies of core psychoanalytic constructs. *Clin Neurosci Res* 2005;4(5):349–65.

23. Westen D. Implications of developments in cognitive neuroscience for psychoanalytic psychotherapy. *Harv Rev Psychiatry* 2002;10(6):369–73.

24. Westen D, Gabbard GO. Developments in cognitive neuroscience: I. Conflict, compromise, and connectionism. *J Am Psychoanal Assoc* 2002;50(1):53–98.

25. Lane RD, Garfield DAS. Becoming aware of feelings: integration of cognitive-developmental, neuroscientific, and psychoanalytic perspectives. *Neuro-Psychoanalysis* 2005;7(1):5–30.

26. Beutel ME, Stern E, Silbersweig DA. The emerging dialogue between psychoanalysis and neuroscience: neuroimaging perspectives. *J Am Psychoanal Assoc* 2003;51(3):773–801.

27. Ellenberger HF. *The Discovery of the Unconscious; the History and Evolution of Dynamic Psychiatry*. New York: Basic Books; 1970.

28. Sandler J, Holder A, Dare C, Dreher AU. *Freud's Models of the Mind: An Introduction*. Madison. Connecticut: International Universities Press, Inc.; 1997.

29. Kandel ER, Kupferman O, Iverson S. Learning and memory. In: Kandel ER, Schwartz JH, Jessell TM, eds. *Principles of Neural Science*. New York: McGraw-Hill; 2000:1227–46.

30. Baddeley A. Working memory: looking back and looking forward. *Nat Rev Neurosci* 2003;4(10):829–39.
31. Schacter DL, Slotnick SD. The cognitive neuroscience of memory distortion. *Neuron* 2004;44(1):149–60.
32. Smith EE, Kosslyn SM. Encoding and retrieval from long-term memory. In: *Cognitive Psychology: Mind and Brain*. Upper Saddler River, NJ: Prentice Hall; 2007:195–246.
33. Kihlstrom JF. The cognitive unconscious. *Science* 1987;237(4821):1445–52.
34. Kihlstrom JF. Availability, accessibility, and subliminal perception. *Conscious Cogn* 2004;13(1):92–100.
35. Wong PS, Bernat E, Snodgrass M, Shevrin H. Event-related brain correlates of associative learning without awareness. *Int J Psychophysiol* 2004;53(3):217–31.
36. Wong PS. Anxiety, signal anxiety, and unconscious anticipation: neuroscientific evidence for an unconscious signal function in humans. *J Am Psychoanal Assoc* 1999;47(3):817–41.
37. Ochsner KN, Chiu CY, Schacter DL. Varieties of priming. *Curr Opin Neurobiol* 1994;4(2):189–94.
38. Knowlton BJ, Squire LR, Gluck MA. Probabilistic classification learning in amnesia. *Learn Mem* 1994;1(2):106–20.
39. Knowlton BJ, Mangels JA, Squire LR. A neostriatal habit learning system in humans. *Science* 1996;273(5280):1399–402.
40. Svoboda E, McKinnon MC, Levine B. The functional neuroanatomy of autobiographical memory: a meta-analysis. *Neuropsychologia* 2006;44(12):2189–208.
41. Barrett LF, Mesquita B, Ochsner KN, Gross JJ. The experience of emotion. *Annu Rev Psychol* 2007;58:373–403.
42. LeDoux J. The emotional brain, fear, and the amygdala. *Cell Mol Neurobiol* 2003; 23(4–5):727–38.
43. Russell JA. Core affect and the psychological construction of emotion. *Psychol Rev* 2003;110(1):145–72.
44. Posner J, Russell J, Peterson BS. The circumplex model of affect: an integrative approach to affective neuroscience, cognitive development, and psychopathology. *Dev Psychopathol* 2005;17(3):715–34.
45. Gerber AJ, Posner J, Gorman D, et al. An affective circumplex model of neural systems subserving valence, arousal, and cognitive overlay during the appraisal of emotional faces. Neuropsychologia 2008;46:2129–39.
46. Paton JJ, Belova MA, Morrison SE, Salzman CD. The primate amygdala represents the positive and negative value of visual stimuli during learning. *Nature* 2006; 439(7078):865–70.
47. Ochsner KN, Bunge SA, Gross JJ, Gabrieli JD. Rethinking feelings: an FMRI study of the cognitive regulation of emotion. *J Cogn Neurosci* 2002;14(8):1215–29.
48. Etkin A, Klemenhagen KC, Dudman JT, et al. Individual differences in trait anxiety predict the response of the basolateral amygdala to unconsciously processed fearful faces. *Neuron* 2004;44(6):1043–55.
49. Insel TR. A neurobiological basis of social attachment. *Am J Psychiatry* 1997;154(6):726–35.
50. Insel TR, Young LJ. The neurobiology of attachment. *Nat Rev Neurosci* 2001;2(2):129–36.
51. Ochsner KN, Lieberman MD. The emergence of social cognitive neuroscience. *Am Psychol* 2001;56(9):717–34.
52. Mitchell JP, Heatherton TF, Macrae CN. Distinct neural systems subserve person and object knowledge. *Proc Natl Acad Sci USA* 2002;99(23):15238–43.
53. Kelley WM, Macrae CN, Wyland CL, Caglar S, Inati S, Heatherton TF. Finding the self? An event-related fMRI study. *J Cognit Neurosci* 2002;14(5):785–94.
54. Northoff G, Heinzel A, de Greck M, Bermpohl F, Dobrowolny H, Panksepp J. Self-referential processing in our brain – a meta-analysis of imaging studies on the self. *Neuroimage* 2006;31(1):440–57.

55. Lieberman MD. Social cognitive neuroscience: a review of core processes. *Annu Rev Psychol* 2007;58:259–89.
56. Cooper A. Changes in psychoanalytic ideas: transference interpretation. *J Am Psychoanal Assoc* 1987;35:77–98.
57. Hoglend P, Amlo S, Marble A, et al. Analysis of the patient-therapist relationship in dynamic psychotherapy: an experimental study of transference interpretations. *Am J Psychiatry* 2006;163(10):1739–46.
58. Luborsky L, Crits-Christoph P. *Understanding Transference: The Core Conflictual Relationship Theme Method.* 2nd ed. Washington, DC: American Psychological Association; 1998.
59. Andersen SM, Baum A. Transference in interpersonal relations: inferences and affect based on significant-other representations. *J Pers* 1994;62(4):459–97.
60. Andersen SM, Glassman NS, Chen S, Cole SW. Transference in social perception: the role of chronic accessibility in significant-other representations. *J Pers Soc Psychol* 1995;69(1):41–57.
61. Andersen SM, Reznik I, Manzella LM. Eliciting facial affect, motivation, and expectancies in transference: significant-other representations in social relations. *J Pers Soc Psychol* 1996;71(6):1108–29.
62. Berk MS, Andersen SM. The impact of past relationships on interpersonal behavior: behavioral confirmation in the social-cognitive process of transference. *J Pers Soc Psychol* 2000;79(4):546–62.
63. Glassman NS, Andersen SM. Activating transference without consciousness: using significant-other representations to go beyond what is subliminally given. *J Pers Soc Psychol* 1999;77(6):1146–62.
64. Erdelyi MH. The unified theory of repression. *Behav Brain Sci* 2006;29(5):499–511.
65. Peterson BS. Indeterminacy & compromise formation: implications for a psychoanalytic theory of mind. *Int J Psychoanal* 2002;83(Pt 5):1017–35.
66. Raz A, Lamar M, Buhle JT, Kane MJ, Peterson BS. Selective biasing of a specific bistable-figure percept involves fMRI signal changes in frontostriatal circuits: A step toward unlocking the neural correlates of top-down control and self-regulation. *Am J Clin Hypn* 2007;50:137–56.
67. Westen D, Gabbard GO. Developments in cognitive neuroscience: II. Implications for theories of transference. *J Am Psychoanal Assoc* 2002;50(1):99–134.
68. Gabbard GO. What can neuroscience teach us about transference? *Can J Psychoanal* 2000;9:1–18.
69. Cassidy J, Shaver PR, eds. *Handbook of Attachment: Theory, Research, and Clinical Applications.* New York: Guilford Press; 1999.
70. Fonagy P, Leigh T, Steele M, et al. The relation of attachment status, psychiatric classification, and response to psychotherapy. *J Consult Clin Psychol* 1996;64:22–31.
71. Leckman JF, Herman AE. Maternal behavior and developmental psychopathology. *Biol Psychiatry* 2002;51(1):27–43.
72. Insel TR. Is social attachment an addictive disorder? *Physiol Behav* 2003;79(3):351–7.
73. Bartels A, Zeki S. The neural correlates of maternal and romantic love. *Neuroimage* 2004;21(3):1155–66.
74. Buchheim A, George C, Kachele H, Erk S, Walter H. Measuring adult attachment representation in an fMRI environment: concepts and assessment. *Psychopathology* 2006;39(3):136–43.
75. Lamm C, Batson CD, Decety J. The neural substrate of human empathy: effects of perspective-taking and cognitive appraisal. *J Cogn Neurosci* 2007;19(1):42–58.
76. Singer T. The neuronal basis and ontogeny of empathy and mind reading: review of literature and implications for future research. *Neurosci Biobehav Rev* 2006;30(6):855–63.
77. Shamay-Tsoory SG, Lester H, Chisin R, et al. The neural correlates of understanding the other's distress: a positron emission tomography investigation of accurate empathy. *Neuroimage* 2005;27(2):468–72.

78. Marci CD, Orr SP. The effect of emotional distance on psychophysiologic concordance and perceived empathy between patient and interviewer. *Appl Psychophysiol Biofeedback* 2006;31(2):115–28.

79. Marci C, Reiss H. The clinical relevance of psychophysiology: support for the psychobiology of empathy and psychodynamic process. *Am J Psychother* 2005;59:213–26.

80. Fonagy P, Target M, Gergely G, Jurist EL. *Affect Regulation, Mentalization, and the Development of Self.* London: Other Press; 2002.

81. Corcoran R, Frith CD. Autobiographical memory and theory of mind: evidence of a relationship in schizophrenia. *Psychol Med* 2003;33:897–905.

82. Baron-Cohen S, Leslie AM, Frith U. Does the autistic child have a 'theory of mind'? *Cognition* 1985;21:37–46.

83. Saxe R, Moran JM, Scholz J, Gabrieli J. Overlapping and non-overlapping brain regions for theory of mind and self reflection in individual subjects. *Soc Cogn Affect Neurosci* 2006;1(3):229–34.

84. Mitchell JP, Banaji MR, Macrae CN. General and specific contributions of the medial prefrontal cortex to knowledge about mental states. *Neuroimage* 2005;28(4):757–62.

85. Happe F. Theory of mind and the self. *Ann N Y Acad Sci* 2003;1001:134–44.

86. Gallagher HL, Frith CD. Functional imaging of 'theory of mind'. *Trends Cogn Sci* 2003;7(2):77–83.

87. Iacoboni M, Dapretto M. The mirror neuron system and the consequences of its dysfunction. *Nat Rev Neurosci* 2006;7(12):942–51.

88. Olds DD. Identification: psychoanalytic and biological perspectives. *J Am Psychoanal Assoc* 2006;54(1):17–46.

89. Gallese V. Mirror neurons and intentional attunement: commentary on Olds. *J Am Psychoanal Assoc* 2006;54(1):47–57.

90. Rizzolatti G, Fadiga L, Fogassi L, Gallese V. Resonance behaviors and mirror neurons. *Arch Ital Biol* 1999;137(2-3):85–100.

91. Posner MI, Rothbart MK. Research on attention networks as a model for the integration of psychological science. *Annu Rev Psychol* 2007;58:1–23.

92. Raz A, Buhle J. Typologies of attentional networks. *Nat Rev Neurosci* 2006;7(5):367–79.

93. McGinnies E, Bowles W. Personal values as determinates of perceptual fixation. *J Pers* 1949;18(2):224–35.

94. Blum GS. An experimental reunion of psychoanalytic theory with perceptual vigilance and defense. *J Abnorm Psychol* 1954;49(1):94–8.

95. Silverman LH, Weinberger J. Mommy and I are one. Implications for psychotherapy. *Am Psychol* 1985;40(12):1296–308.

96. Shevrin H, Ghannam JH, Libet B. A neural correlate of consciousness related to repression. *Conscious Cogn* 2002;11(2):334–41; discussion 42–46.

97. Anderson MC, Ochsner KN, Kuhl B, et al. Neural systems underlying the suppression of unwanted memories. *Science* 2004;303(5655):232–5.

98. Raz A, Fan J, Posner MI. Hypnotic suggestion reduces conflict in the human brain. *Proc Natl Acad Sci USA* 2005;102(28):9978–83.

99. Raz A, Shapiro T. Hypnosis and neuroscience: a cross talk between clinical and cognitive research. *Arch Gen Psychiatry* 2002;59(1):85–90.

100. Maquet P. Functional neuroimaging of normal human sleep by positron emission tomography. *J Sleep Res* 2000;9(3):207–31.

101. Maquet P, Peters J, Aerts J, et al. Functional neuroanatomy of human rapid-eye-movement sleep and dreaming. *Nature* 1996;383(6596):163–6.

102. Maquet P, Laureys S, Peigneux P, et al. Experience-dependent changes in cerebral activation during human REM sleep. *Nat Neurosci* 2000;3(8):831–6.

103. Andreasen NC, O'Leary DS, Cizadlo T, et al. Remembering the past: two facets of episodic memory explored with positron emission tomography. *Am J Psychiatry* 1995;152(11):1576–85.

104. Mason MF, Norton MI, Van Horn JD, Wegner DM, Grafton ST, Macrae CN. Wandering minds: the default network and stimulus-independent thought. *Science* 2007;315(5810):393–5.
105. Gabbard GO, Westen D. Rethinking therapeutic action. *Int J Psychoanal* 2003;84 (Pt 4):823–41.
106. Liggan DY, Kay J. Some neurobiologiocal aspects of psychotherapy. *J Psychother Pract Res* 1999;8(2):103–14.
107. Gabbard GO. A neurobiologically informed perspective on psychotherapy. *Br J Psychiatry* 2000;177:117–22.
108. Peled A, Geva AB. Brain organization and psychodynamics. *J Psychother Pract Res* 1999;8(1):24–39.
109. Olds DD. Connectionism and psychoanalysis. *J Am Psychoanal Assoc* 1994;42:581–611.
110. Westen D. The scientific legacy of Sigmund Freud: toward a psychodynamically informed psychological science. *Psychol Bull* 1998;124(3):333–71.
111. Blass RB, Carmeli Z. The case against neuropsychoanalysis: on fallacies underlying psychoanalysis' latest scientific trend and its negative impact on psychoanalytic discourse. *Int J Psychoanal* 2007;88(1):19–40.
112. Gabbard GO, Gunderson JG, Fonagy P. The place of psychoanalytic treatments within psychiatry. *Arch Gen Psychiatry* 2002;59(6):505–10.
113. Kernberg O. Psychoanalysis, psychoanalytic psychotherapy and supportive psychotherapy: contemporary controversies. *Int J Psychoanal* 1999;80:1075–91.
114. Linden DEJ. How psychotherapy changes the brain – the contribution of functional neuroimaging. *Mol Psychiatry* 2006;11:528–38.
115. Mitterschiffthaler MT, Ettinger U, Mehta MA, Mataix-Cols D, Williams SC. Applications of functional magnetic resonance imaging in psychiatry. *J Magn Reson Imaging* 2006;23(6):851–61.
116. McGuire PK, Bench CJ, Frith CD, Marks IM, Frackowiak RS, Dolan RJ. Functional anatomy of obsessive-compulsive phenomena. *Br J Psychiatry* 1994;164(4):459–68.
117. Rauch SL, Jenike MA, Alpert NM, et al. Regional cerebral blood flow measured during symptom provocation in obsessive-compulsive disorder using oxygen 15-labeled carbon dioxide and positron emission tomography. *Arch Gen Psychiatry* 1994;51(1):62–70.
118. Baxter LR, Schwartz JM, Bergman KS, et al. Caudate glucose metabolic rate changes with both drug and behavior therapy for obsessive-compulsive disorder. *Arch Gen Psychiatry* 1992;49:681–9.
119. Baxter LR, Schwartz JM, Guze BH, Bergman K, Szuba MP. Neuroimaging in obsessive-compulsive disorder: seeking the mediating neuroanatomy. In: Jenike MA, Baer L, Minichiello WE, eds. *Obsessive-Compulsive Disorders: Theory and Management.* 2nd ed. St. Louis: Mosby-Year Book; 1990:167–88.
120. Baxter LR, Jr., Mazziotta JC, Pahl JJ, et al. Psychiatric, genetic, and positron emission tomographic evaluation of persons at risk for Huntington's disease. *Arch Gen Psychiatry* 1992;49(2):148–54.
121. Milad MR, Rauch SL, Pitman RK, Quirk GJ. Fear extinction in rats: implications for human brain imaging and anxiety disorders. *Biol Psychol* 2006;73(1):61–71.
122. Furmark T, Tillfors M, Marteinsdottir I, et al. Common changes in cerebral blood flow in patients with social phobia treated with citalopram or cognitive-behavioral therapy. *Arch Gen Psychiatry* 2002;59(5):425–33.
123. Paquette V, Levesque J, Mensour B, et al. "Change the mind and you change the brain": effects of cognitive-behavioral therapy on the neural correlates of spider phobia. *Neuroimage* 2003;18(2):401–9.
124. Menninger WW. Integrated treatment of panic disorder and social phobia. *Bull Menninger Clin* 1992;56(2 Suppl A):A61–70.

125. Chobanian AV, Bakris GL, Black HR, et al. The Seventh Report of the Joint National Committee on Prevention, Detection, Evaluation, and Treatment of High Blood Pressure: the JNC 7 report. *JAMA* 2003;289(19):2560–72.
126. Brody AL, Saxena S, Schwartz JM, et al. FDG-PET predictors of response to behavioral therapy and pharmacotherapy in obsessive compulsive disorder. *Psychiatry Res* 1998;84(1):1–6.
127. Goldapple K, Segal Z, Garson C, et al. Modulation of cortical-limbic pathways in major depression: treatment-specific effects of cognitive behavior therapy. *Arch Gen Psychiatry* 2004;61(1):34–41.
128. Kennedy SH, Konarski JZ, Segal ZV, et al. Differences in brain glucose metabolism between responders to CBT and venlafaxine in a 16-week randomized controlled trial. *Am J Psychiatry* 2007;164(5):778–88.
129. Brody AL, Saxena S, Stoessel P, et al. Regional brain metabolic changes in patients with major depression treated with either paroxetine or interpersonal therapy: preliminary findings. *Arch Gen Psychiatry* 2001;58(7):631–40.
130. Ablon JS, Jones EE. Validity of controlled clinical trials of psychotherapy: findings from the NIMH Treatment of Depression Collaborative Research Program. *Am J Psychiatry* 2002;159(5):775–83.
131. Hollon SD, DeRubeis RJ, Evans MD, et al. Cognitive therapy and pharmacotherapy for depression. Singly and in combination. *Arch Gen Psychiatry* 1992;49(10):774–81.
132. Jones EE, Pulos SM. Comparing the process in psychodynamic and cognitive-behavioral therapies. *J Consult Clin Psychol* 1993;61(2):306–16.
133. Knobel M. Psychodynamics of psychopharmacology. *J Nerv Ment Dis* 1961;133:309–15.
134. Mintz D. Psychodynamic Trojan horses: using psychopharmacology to teach psychodynamics. *J Am Acad Psychoanal Dyn Psychiatry* 2006;34(1):151–61.
135. Weyrauch KF. The personal knowledge of family physicians for their patients. *Fam Med* 1994;26(7):452–5.
136. Hassin RR, Uleman JS, Bargh JA. *The New Unconscious.* New York, NY: Oxford University Press; 2005.
137. Izzetoglu K, Bunce S, Izzetoglu M, Onaral B, Pourrezaei K. Functional near-infrared neuroimaging. *Conf Proc IEEE Eng Med Biol Soc* 2004;7:5333–6.
138. Gay P. *Freud: a Life for Our Time.* New York: Norton; 1998.
139. Hartmann H. *Ego Psychology and the Problem of Adaptation.* New York: International Universities Press; 1958.
140. Hariri AR, Drabant EM, Weinberger DR. Imaging genetics: perspectives from studies of genetically driven variation in serotonin function and corticolimbic affective processing. *Biol Psychiatry* 2006;59(10):888–97.
141. Ebstein RP. The molecular genetic architecture of human personality: beyond self-report questionnaires. *Mol Psychiatry* 2006;11(5):427–45.
142. Brody AL, Saxena S, Schwartz JM, et al. FDG-PET predictors of response to behavioral therapy and pharmacotherapy in obsessive compulsive disorder. *Psychiatry Res* 1998;84(1):1–6.
143. Siegle GJ, Carter CS, Thase ME. Use of FMRI to predict recovery from unipolar depression with cognitive behavior therapy. *Am J Psychiatry* 2006;163(4):735–8.
144. Weissman MM, Verdeli H, Gameroff MJ, et al. National survey of psychotherapy training in psychiatry, psychology, and social work. *Arch Gen Psychiatry* 2006;63(8):925–34.
145. Roffman JL, Simon AB, Prasad KM, Truman CJ, Morrison J, Ernst CL. Neuroscience in psychiatry training: how much do residents need to know? *Am J Psychiatry* 2006;163(5):919–26.
146. Cappas NM, Andres-Hyman R, Davidson L. What psychotherapists can begin to learn from neuroscience: seven principles of a brain-based psychotherapy. *Psychother Theor Res Pract Train* 2005;42(3):374–83.

# Chapter 14
# Physiologic Monitoring in Psychodynamic Psychotherapy Research

Carl D. Marci and Helen Riess

## Introduction

There is a rich history of measuring physiologic responses between patient and clinician that has infused psychodynamic psychotherapy research for over half a century. The findings complement research outside of psychotherapy that increasingly supports a significant relationship between physiological, emotional, and psychological states [1]. Indeed, investigations into how physiologic parameters change during psychotherapy offer a unique opportunity to inform clinical practice, improve training of clinicians, and illuminate change processes unique to human dyadic relationships [2]. The goal of this chapter is to review the history of physiologic monitoring during psychodynamic psychotherapy and present recent findings that complement neuroimaging results and support recent advances in interpersonal neurobiology and social neuroscience. A clinical case from a research protocol is described that demonstrates the power of insights derived from physiologic measurement and illustrates the challenges of breaking through unconscious defenses in the process of psychodynamic psychotherapy.

Through a variety of methodological approaches, the early literature on psychophysiology and psychotherapy begins to address two critical questions. First, is there a measurable, biologically based influence that emerges from the physiological responses of patient and therapist during psychotherapy? Second, what are the observable correlates of these physiologic responses and what are the implications for psychotherapy practice, training, and research? These two questions are at the core of this chapter. Prior studies on psychophysiology and psychotherapy almost exclusively use heart rate (HR) and skin conductivity (SC) as a measure of physiologic reactivity, thus the present chapter briefly reviews the origins and mechanisms of these two measures. A critical review of the rich historical literature employing psychophysiology in psychodynamic psychotherapy is presented with an update on more recent studies. Following

C.D. Marci
Department of Psychiatry, Massachusetts General Hospital, 15 Parkman Street, WAC 812, Boston, MA 02114-3117, USA
e-mail: cmarci@partners.org

R.A. Levy, J.S. Ablon (eds.), *Handbook of Evidence-Based Psychodynamic Psychotherapy*,
DOI: 10.1007/978-1-59745-444-5_14, © Humana Press 2009

the description of a clinical case, the review is placed in the context of modern neurobiology and neuroscience with a discussion of future directions.

## Psychophysiology in Psychotherapy Research

Peripheral measures of central nervous system activity have historically been used in a variety of ways in psychodynamic psychotherapy research. In the last published review in 1981, the author divides the uses of psychophysiology in psychotherapy into three categories: (1) exploration of the relationship between physiologic responses, psychopathology, and psychodynamic concepts; (2) investigation of physiologic correlates of the patient–therapist interaction; and (3) monitoring patterns within and across therapy sessions [3]. The review also expounds on the many advantages of using psychophysiology for psychotherapy research. These advantages include the relatively inexpensive, noninvasive nature of most measures, plus ease of portability resulting in the capacity to monitor in "naturalistic" or ecologically valid clinical environments outside of the laboratory. Recent emphasis on biology in the field of mental health also supports the use of psychophysiology in psychotherapy research [4]. These measures are biologically based and free of the self-report and observer bias found in most self-report research tools [5]. Few other technologies offer an objective measure that reflects conscious and unconscious responses to intrapersonal and interpersonal stimuli in real-time during real therapy. The multiple advantages afford the opportunity to place psychotherapy research on a firm biological foundation in parallel with pharmacological interventions and neuroimaging techniques [6].

The two most common parameters used in psychotherapy research, HR and SC, have been studied extensively during different emotional states and cognitive tasks outside of psychotherapy [1]. Different patterns of skin conductance and HR response have been observed in normal versus psychopathological populations [7]. While still in the early stages, multiple studies have integrated physiologic responses into neuroimaging studies leading to increased understanding of the relationship between central and peripheral nervous system activity [8, 9]. This understanding offers intriguing opportunities to advance knowledge in studies of social interaction in general and models of interpersonal neurobiology relevant to psychotherapy in particular. Over time, biologically based models of social interaction have the potential to inform and improve clinical practice and training in psychotherapy as clinicians understand the powerful yet subtle influence of their physiologic responses on their patients.

### *Measures of Heart Rate*

For several hundred years, physicians using a stethoscope for listening to the internal sounds of the heart have noted shifting heartbeat rhythms associated with illness and psychological states [10]. Initially beginning as a central component of traditional Chinese medical practice, scientific investigation into cardiac monitoring increased with advancing technology from the relatively primitive kymograph, through ink-writing polygraphs to modern digital signal processing systems [11]. Development of the electrocardiogram (ECG) methodology around the turn of the century allowed heart rhythms to be monitored with three noninvasive electrodes typically placed on the arms and leg of the individual. The ECG now typically utilizes a 12-lead configuration for a more detailed and critical evaluation of cardiac pathology, while advances in portable single-lead devices allow for more continuous monitoring [12].

Recent neuroanatomical and neurophysiological evidence indicates that central HR regulation involves structures within the brain stem, subcortex, and cortex [8, 13, 14]. While the brain stem circuits function mostly in homeostatic regulation, the cortical and subcortical networks, including the areas involved in emotion regulation, influence the nonhomeostatic activity of the heart. The structures of the subcortex and limbic system primarily responsible for emotion generation, particularly the amygdala and insula, are involved in pairing emotional responses to stimuli and also influence brain stem activity [8]. The outputs of these structures provide direct control of cardiac activity via the sympathetic and parasympathetic divisions of the autonomic nervous system. A more detailed account of the central mechanisms of HR regulation can be found elsewhere [10]. The majority of psychophysiological investigations examines the reactivity of HR to stressful stimuli and focus on the impact of heart disease and hypertension. However, more recently, brief changes in HR and derived measures of HR variability have also been used to index behavioral, emotional, and cognitive functions [15, 16].

## Measures of Skin Conductivity

First employed over 100 years ago, measures of electrical changes in the human skin remain a widely used indicator of general physiological arousal and reactivity. Furthering investigations by Charcot and Vigouroux a decade earlier, Féré in 1888 found that by passing an electrical current across two electrodes placed on the fingers he could detect momentary changes in SC in response to various stimuli [17]. Some of the important features of the SC signal identified in this early work, the tonic and phasic components, continue to be used today. The tonic aspect of SC refers to an individual's absolute SC level at a given time without a phasic response. The phasic response is a momentary change in SC level and is sometimes further described by its peak amplitude, rise time, slope, and one-half recovery time. SC is best measured from the palmar surface of the hands where there is a high concentration of eccrine sweat glands generally resulting in good signal quality and sensitivity [18]. While the majority of monitoring devices still utilize two leads attached to the nondominant hand, modern portable devices are available for continuous monitoring of everyday activities [19].

The activity of human eccrine sweat glands as measured by SC is predominately controlled by the sympathetic nervous system [20]. Central mechanisms of both excitatory and inhibitory influence on SC activity are divided into three primary pathways involving the brain stem, subcortex, and cortex [9, 21–24]. Specifically, these pathways involve the reticular formation in the brain stem, the premotor cortex, and subcortical basal ganglia, and the prefrontal cortex and subcortical limbic system. The diversity of the structures involved reflects the various influences on SC activity that include thermoregulation, muscle tone, gross and fine motor control, emotion processing, attention, and other higher-processing functions [25]. Measures of SC activity have been utilized in a diverse range of applications including the study of attention, learning, and emotion as well as a marker for response to treatment and correlates of psychopathology [15].

## History of Psychophysiology in Psychotherapy Research

Beginning in the mid-1950 s, several studies began to investigate the emotional states and physiologic responses of patients and therapists during psychotherapy. The introduction of psychophysiology to psychotherapy research began with the analysis of HR in a series of patient and therapist dyads [26]. In their methods, the authors introduced the Bales Interaction Coding System (BICS), an observer measure of social–emotional process in the patient and the therapist that categorizes responses into three main groups [27]. These groups include social–emotional positive (solidarity, tension release, or agreement), neutral (giving or asking for suggestions, opinions, or orientation), and negative (disagreement, tension, or antagonism). The authors attempted to relate the BICS social–emotional states with physiologic responses in the patients and therapists but differences were small and no significance levels were reported. However, in companion data that compared a single interview of each of three patients with three different therapists, all three patients consistently exhibited a lower HR, independent of BICS coding, with one of the three therapists. This finding was the first to imply that unique therapist characteristics may have a strong influence on the physiologic states of patients – a view recently put forward in a theoretical paper on the influence of "sociophysiology" on all patient–doctor relationships [28].

The authors also discuss data from a series of 38 interviews between a single patient and therapist. In this unusual early longitudinal single case study, the authors claim that therapy sessions containing a higher frequency of positive BICS categories for the patient tended to be associated with higher mean HR, while those sessions containing a higher frequency of negative Bales categories tended to be associated with lower mean HR. Interestingly, in analyzing patient and therapist HR data from the case study, the authors note some moments of "concordance," when patient and therapist HR appeared to increase and decrease in unison. The authors speculate that concordance might provide a valuable tool as a measure of "therapeutic rapport." It is difficult to evaluate the significance of these findings as no data or statistical analysis are shown or further described. However, despite the lack of statistical analyses, these early findings laid the groundwork for defining a relationship between affective states and physiologic responses in the psychotherapeutic relationship.

In a follow-up case report, evidence for a physiologic relationship between patient and therapist was presented as an in-depth investigation of 44 therapy sessions [29]. The researchers examined the therapist–patient HR and patient affect ratings using an adaptation of the BICS in which affective ratings for anxiety, hostility, and depression were analyzed independently. The authors report that patient HR was significantly higher during periods when the patient showed anxiety, intermediate during those periods when the patient showed hostility, and lowest during those periods when the patient showed depression. Interestingly, analysis of therapist HR during these same interactions resulted in a less robust but statistically significant parallel pattern with the highest therapist HR observed with patient anxiety, intermediate therapist HR with patient hostility, and lowest therapist HR with patient depression.

The authors also attempt to define "physiological" empathy. To do this, rankings of each session were made based on patient and therapist physiology and therapist notes following each session. In the case of the physiology, the ranking was based on two factors: (1) the extent to which therapist HR increased with patient hostility and decreased with patient depression, and (2) the similarity of therapist and patient HR response to these categories. In the case of the therapist notes, the ranking was based on the number of disturbance words found in therapist postsession notes (e.g., statements in the notes reflecting the therapist "unresolved conflicts"). The surprising finding was that the degree of physiologic relationship between patient and therapist within a session was inversely proportionate to the number of disturbance words found in the therapist's notes made after that session. Thus, at times when the therapist did not feel connected to the patient due to a disturbance or distraction in his or her psychological state, the similarity in physiology between patient and therapist was lowest. The authors speculate that the physiological relationship between therapist and patient might be a reflection of the psychological relationship and, by extension, that physiologic "concordance" might be a predictor of psychological empathy [29]. Interestingly, evidence for a "physiologic" basis to empathy during psychotherapy has been reproduced in recent studies while convergent evidence comes from modern neuroimaging techniques investigating the role of "mirror" mechanisms during empathy (see below).

In 1957, another report by the same authors used a new adaptation of the BICS to explore the relationship between affective content and patient and therapist HR [30]. This study measured the mean HR per session of a single patient–therapist pair over the course of 12 therapy sessions. Consistent with the prior studies, the authors showed that higher mean patient and therapist HR per session were significantly correlated with sessions in which the patient showed more negatively rated affect as measured by a higher frequency of "tension units" on the modified BICS. During sessions in which the patient showed more positively rated affect as measured by a higher frequency of "tension release units," significant decreases in patient mean HR per session, and small but nonsignificant decreases in therapist mean HR per session were noted. In contrast, during sessions when the patient showed antagonism toward the therapist, the patient mean HR per session showed a small, nonsignificant decrease, while the therapist's mean HR per session increased significantly. Thus, patient manifestations of "antagonism" toward the therapist, tended to affect patient and therapist HR in opposite directions. The authors give little explanation as to why this may have been so, although one might hypothesize that antagonistic statements from the patient might serve as a tension release for the patient but serve as a source of tension for the therapist, resulting in opposing effects on HR.

Also in 1957, another study was published that used stories based on the thematic appreciation test (TAT) cards created by 19 female neurotic patients [31]. Patients were randomized into two groups according to whether they received "praise" or "criticism" from the study interviewer using a scripted dialogue after the presentation of each story. Each period of praise or criticism was followed by a period of questioning and reassurance by a second interviewer. It is important to note that this study consisted of scripted rather than a psychotherapeutic interaction as seen in other studies. Nonetheless, this study provides interesting insights into the relationship between interpersonal affective and physiological phenomenon relevant to psychotherapy. In agreement with previous studies, the results showed that patient HR responses were significantly higher during and immediately after periods when they experienced criticism (negative affect) relative to periods during and immediately after which they experienced praise (positive affect).

The authors also found a significant effect of the baseline emotional state of the interviewer on the HR of the patient. As part of their experimental design, the first interviewer was asked to rate their own affective state (i.e., whether they were having a "good" or a "bad" day) immediately prior to each interview. The results indicated that interviewer "bad" days were associated with significant elevation of patient HR relative to interviewer "good" days. Interestingly, these changes in patient HR were noted during an initial instruction period, and independent of any other experimental variables (including examiner's HR). The authors suggest that subtle differences in quality and pitch of voice might account for this effect. Regardless, the results are extremely interesting in that they suggest that the therapist's emotional state prior to the start of a therapy session may have a significant mediating influence on a patient's physiologic and psychological state. Taken together, these early data demonstrate the bidirectional influence of the patient–therapist relationship and reinforce the idea that whereas criticism, tension, or negative affect tend to increase patient HR, praise, tension release or positive affect tends to decrease patient HR.

The first study to examine SC in both the patient and therapist was published in 1971 and examined 12 individual patient and therapist dyads in the first session of psychodynamic psychotherapy [32]. Notably, six of the therapists were experienced psychiatrists and six were inexperienced medical students. The authors rated all therapist verbalizations according to increasing levels of confrontational content as follows: (1) reflection, (2) interrogation, (3) interpretation, and (4) confrontation. The results suggest that both patient and therapist arousal, as measured by the amplitude of SC response, varied as a function of the degree of verbal confrontation of the therapist.

It is also interesting to note that this group found significant differences between the experienced psychiatrists compared with the inexperienced medical students as therapists. The authors found that patients interviewed by inexperienced student therapists tended to have significantly higher mean SC response amplitudes than patients interviewed by experienced psychiatrists. Similar to the finding reviewed above of an individual study therapist having a consistent "calming" effect on each study patient [26], this finding further suggests a specific physiologic influence of the therapist on the patient. Furthermore, the authors found that inexperienced therapists showed less arousal with their own confrontational remarks compared to experienced therapists under similar conditions. The authors speculate that inexperienced therapists may not be as sensitive to or aware of the potential effects of their confrontational remarks, and therefore display less autonomic reactivity in these conditions. These data indicate a strong link between affective content of a therapeutic interaction and autonomic activity of both patient and therapist.

The next study examined the relationship between ratings of affect intensity and four physiologic measures of sympathetic activation including HR, SC, respiration, and plethysmography (a measure of pulse wave intensity) in a single patient [33]. While the therapist was not monitored in this study, the first and last 10 min of multiple psychotherapy sessions were rated for affect intensity by experienced therapists. Affect intensity scores were then correlated with the mean value for each physiologic parameter. The authors found significant correlations between intensity of affect and several of the physiologic variables for all interviews. These data further indicate that affect intensity has an influence on autonomic activity in the psychotherapeutic relationship.

Until the 1980s, analyses and methodological considerations of psychophysiology in psychotherapy research relied on observer and therapist ratings of emotional or affective responses of patients and therapists. In 1982, an attempt was made to move away from the relationship between affective states and physiological variables and focus again on patterns of concordance of physiological phenomenon within dyads and their relationship with subjective ratings of empathy [34]. Specifically, the authors examined SC in student volunteers playing the role of "clients" and graduate level therapists in 21 independent sessions. Therapist empathy was measured with the Barrett-Lennard Relationship

Inventory of Empathic Understanding Subscale (EUS) from the interviewee perspective [35]. Analyses of the physiologic data attempted to determine whether, and to what degree, concordance in SC correlated with perceptions of therapist empathy. The results showed a high and statistically significant relationship between concordant, rapid (i.e., within 7 s), large amplitude SC responses, and subjective empathy scores. No significant correlation was found between slower (i.e., within 40 s) or lower amplitude SC responses and perceived empathy scores. Thus, the authors found that subjective empathy scores correlated only with rapid and large amplitude responses occurring within a short time frame. Although not in a clinical population, these findings not only support previous notions of physiologic concordance but also the need to relate findings to the subjective experience of the patient. In addition, the results highlight the importance of using a time-series approach to capture the dynamic, moment-to-moment fluctuations in physiologic responses during the entire psychotherapy session.

## Recent Developments in Psychophysiology and Psychotherapy Research

One of the major weaknesses of the studies reviewed above is a relative lack of sophistication in the signal processing and statistical analysis of the physiologic and nonphysiologic variables. With the development of modern computing power and more sophisticated statistical theory, however, more precise methods of statistical approaches have become available [36]. Several recent articles expand on the earlier historical work and add additional signal processing methods and modern statistical analyses. Three recent studies using simultaneous recordings of SC in patient–therapist dyads during psychodynamic psychotherapy illustrate the application of new methods and new approaches that build on the prior research.

The first study reported in 2004 demonstrated the interpersonal role of laughter during psychotherapy [37]. The study built on research on laughter outside of psychotherapy over the last decade that has revealed that the majority of laughter is not primarily related to humor, joking, or ridicule, rather it serves to moderate social relationships and communication [38]. Ten unique patient–therapist dyads in established psychotherapies were analyzed. Observers coded videotapes for precisely defined "laugh episodes" while changes in arousal as measured by the difference between SC 5 s immediately before and 5 s immediately after were calculated. The data were analyzed using a two-factor analysis of variance. While there was no significant difference between arousal patterns between patients and their therapists, there was a significant difference in the overall level of arousal when both patient and therapist laughed suggesting a physiologic contagion of laughter during psychotherapy. Interestingly, therapist SC increased significantly when the patients laughed *regardless* of whether the therapist laughed or not suggesting an internal generation of an implicit or empathic physiologic response to the patient by the therapist. This response is largely unconscious and is consistent with modern views of empathy as an automatic emotional response [39].

The next study examined physiologic concordance suggested by prior studies reviewed above [26, 29, 34] using a novel scoring algorithm, a behavioral manipulation, and patient perception of empathy. In the study, patients from a mental health clinic with mood and anxiety disorders were interviewed briefly by a single psychiatrist on a scripted neutral topic (i.e., their thoughts on the weather) with simultaneous measures of SC from both patient and the interviewer [40]. The study introduces a unique time-series approach to measure physiologic concordance that calculates the running correlation in the rate of change in SC in two simultaneous signals. Emotional distance was manipulated by creating two interview conditions that varied by amount of gaze toward the patient by the interviewer. The results found significant differences between the emotionally neutral condition (normal eye-gaze) and the emotionally distant condition (low eye-gaze) in both patients' self-report of interviewer empathy and the amount of physiologic concordance between patient and interviewer. While the results are unique in that they employed a time-series approach to the entire arousal curve for both patient and interviewer, they are also consistent with prior studies on physiologic concordance.

The third and most recent study extended these findings further in a clinical population of 20 patient–therapist dyads in established psychodynamic psychotherapy [41]. Modeled in part after Robinson et al. [34], the study used the same time-series approach and the same empathy scale as in the gaze study but applied it to patients and their therapists during a live clinical encounter. The results were consistent in that patient reports of their therapist empathy during the monitored session were significantly correlated with the amount of physiologic concordance for that session. Additional analyses used videotaped segments of the highest and lowest moments of physiologic concordance for each patient–therapist dyad. Observers blinded to the goals of the study and trained in the BICS, rated each second for both patient and therapist for the highest and lowest 1-min moments. The results showed significantly greater solidarity and positive regard from both patients and therapists during the highest compared with the lowest moments of physiologic concordance.

## Clinical Relevance of Psychophysiology

The following case report involves a patient and therapist who participated in a psychotherapy research protocol using simultaneous measures of SC [41]. Described in the context of the research protocol exploring the relationship between patient and clinician physiology and perceived empathy, the present case uses psychophysiology as a clinical and diagnostic aide that moves the therapist toward a richer, deeper understanding and appreciation of the patient's symptoms. In contrast to the studies described above, physiologic data from the research protocol were reported to the patient clinically and had a significant impact on the process and outcome of the case. The results illustrate the clinical relevance of psychophysiologic measures in understanding aspects of psychodynamic psychotherapy process and broaden the discussion of potential uses of this technology.

As mentioned above, a large number of research studies use psychophysiology in the study of psychopathology [7]. Two consistent findings in the literature involve depression and anxiety disorders. Depressed patients tend to show changes in SC including decreased overall SC levels, decreased frequency of response, and decreased amplitude of response when compared with nondepressed patients [42, 43, 44]. In contrast, it is well documented that anxious patients have increased autonomic arousal, manifested by higher SC levels, more frequent spontaneous fluctuations, and higher response amplitudes [45].

The following case which has been published in its entirety elsewhere [2], illustrates the subtle complexity and psychobiology of social interaction during clinical psychotherapy practice. Data normally not available to clinicians enhanced the therapeutic process and outcome. Specifically, the therapist's knowledge of the patient's physiologic reactions during the therapy session facilitated an empathic recognition and deeper understanding of a profound disconnection between the patient's history of depression and externally stolid, well-controlled demeanor and the more intense, chaotic internal milieu of high-sympathetic arousal more reflective of anxiety. The empathic validation of the patient's hidden inner-anxious state, in the context of a psychodynamic formulation involving the role of the patient's mother in her behavior, had significant therapeutic and clinical benefits.

## Clinical Case Report

Jane is a 40-year-old married, white, professional female who was referred for psychotherapy after a consultation with a nutritional counselor for weight loss. Jane was 70 lb over her ideal body weight, a fact that caused her a great deal of self-consciousness and embarrassment. At the time of her consultation she was unable to complete a record of her food intake because of the intense feelings that surfaced about her mother's attempt to control her eating for most of her life. The nutritionist felt she could not help until Jane worked through the anger and depression related to her mother's control. Jane began psychodynamic psychotherapy and focused the first 2.5 years on distancing herself from her mother's constant verbal abuse and obsession about Jane's weight. This was very difficult because Jane and her mother had had daily phone contact. Despite the difficulties communicating about food, she was her mother's closest confidant and care taker, a role she had known all her life.

Jane had always felt the need to be "perfect" for her mother so she would not add to her burdens, and she learned to soothe herself with unhealthy eating habits and a sedentary lifestyle. An important variable for Jane's mother was the fact that she had been so overwhelmed by her other four children, all of whom had special needs and one who had died. After much progress was made in therapy toward changing the relationship with her mother from one of dependency and verbal abuse to a mutually respectful one, Jane initiated conversations in therapy about becoming physically fit and eventually wanting to lose weight. These subjects had been remarkably avoided during her therapy. She started a personal training program in which she exercised with a trainer for 6 months, resulting in a 5 lb weight *gain*. Jane expressed frustration and hopelessness, and considered changing trainers when her trainer blamed her entirely for the lack of progress. This dynamic activated a powerful reaction in Jane.

At about this time, Jane was asked if she would participate in a psychotherapy and psychophysiology research study assessing therapist empathy by using simultaneous recording of patient and therapist skin conductance. The findings revealed that there was a high degree of physiologic concordance between patient and therapist. This correlated with the patient's perception of a high level of therapist empathy on the questionnaire for the monitored session [41]. There was, however a very surprising finding in the analysis of Jane's SC. Although the overall tracing of Jane's skin conduction matched almost identically in shape to that of her therapist's, the amplitude and reactivity of her SC revealed unusually high tonic arousal, high frequency of nonspecific fluctuations, and high-amplitude responses in her SC. This was especially significant because her arousal level was nearly two to three times higher than that of her therapist, despite the relatively high overall concordance. The finding was also surprising because the patient appeared very calm, even tempered, and tended toward a depressed presentation with almost no outward indications or expressions of anxiety.

After reviewing the psychophysiology data with the researcher, the therapist asked Jane if she were interested in the findings. Interestingly, Jane was not surprised by the revelation of her high-anxiety state. She said, "No one has ever seen my pain. I live with this every day. . . . I am so used to feeling like this. . . it has always been my job to take care of other peoples' anxiety and not to focus on my own." In subsequent sessions, Jane stated she felt extremely validated by what her therapist learned form the research. As a result, the therapist became increasingly attuned to very subtle signs of anxiety that Jane demonstrated. The therapist became aware that she had subtly been enlisted to miss the full range of her patient's inner needs, just as Jane's mother had. With the increased empathy the therapist had for Jane's internal anxiety state by virtue of the data from the physiologic "X-ray" of her patient's psyche, Jane came to realize she had been using unhealthy eating and exercise habits to manage her own anxiety all her life.

After her anxiety was validated by her therapist, Jane considered new ways of managing it that were less self-defeating. Jane had had a lifelong history of subjugating her own emotional needs in the service of meeting the needs of the people on whom she depended. She had worked very hard, both consciously and unconsciously to appear self-sufficient, thus winning the approval, and ironically, the dependency, of those on whom she yearned to depend. Her anxiety was suffused with fear and anger about the lack of responsiveness that her caregivers were giving her as well as feelings of guilt and shame that she would be a burden to others if she allowed others to be aware of her needs. A part of her believed that she should be responsible and responsive to her caregivers at the expense of having her own needs met to ensure attachment and engagement.

Armed with compassion for herself and greater empathy from her therapist, Jane used the therapy to analyze her relationship to her current trainer, discover its psychodynamic roots, and ultimately to find the courage to fire her personal trainer who was taking no responsibility for Jane's lack of improvement. Through active research Jane was able to find and hire a new trainer who was much more empathic and responsive to Jane's needs. The act of firing her first trainer was the subject of many agonizing psychotherapy sessions, where Jane had to confront her own fears of inciting anger in her trainer as well as asserting her own needs above this authority figure, who was interested in collecting Jane's money but less interested in the results she and Jane were able to achieve in their collaboration. With great difficulty Jane was able to identify her own needs for greater self-acceptance and self-love and place these above the needs of her trainer. Jane became empowered to place her own desire to become more physically fit, healthy, and attractive above the apparent needs of her trainer to keep Jane as a client, however dissatisfied Jane was with the results. Jane ultimately fired her trainer and engaged a new exercise coach. Interestingly, Jane had no trouble completing a food diary for the new coach – a task that she could not complete for the dietician prior to therapy.

In the year following the psychophysiology research, with continuous work in psychotherapy emphasizing Jane's personal needs, Jane had a startling result: *She lost 40 lb!* This represented the first weight loss in her life. She had transformed herself from a sedentary lifestyle to a pattern of exercising three times a week. By focusing on her own needs rather than the needs of those caring for her, Jane replaced a self-defeating dependency on others to an empowered advocacy for herself. In addition to achieving her personal goals, Jane has also emerged as a leader in her community (after purposely avoiding groups all her life) and in addition, she has a much healthier and more enjoyable relationship with her mother.

Jane has continued to lose weight, continues to exercise, and her overall sense of contentment and agency in her life have dramatically improved. By having her inner emotional state seen and objectively validated by the physiologic monitoring in the context of a psychodynamically oriented psychotherapy, Jane has become empowered to verbally ask for her needs to be met and no longer uses self-defeating behaviors such as overeating to manage her feelings. Jane has traversed the landscape of using food to manage her feelings to the richer world of genuine engagement with the people in her life who can appropriately respond to her needs. She reports being much less anxious and more confident in her ability to identify and ask for her needs to be met, and she has been delightfully surprised by the responses she has received.

Jane's case illustrates the complex nature of the therapeutic process as well as the limits of empathic understanding, even with an experienced therapist, in the context of a good therapeutic alliance. Prior to involvement in the research protocol, the psychodynamic formulation of the case by the therapist emphasized the patient's awareness of her mother's overwhelming experience of having a child with special needs. The patient feared that if she expressed her own physical and emotional needs, she would be rejected, thus protecting her mother from the burden of additional "defects" in her children. In response, the patient learned to mask her own age-appropriate needs for mirroring and nurturance from her caregivers and to present an illusion of a self-sufficient false self. After arriving at this psychological compromise, this patient, aided by psychodynamic psychotherapy, has moved form a state of chronic frustration of unconscious wishes for nurturance and depression stemming from feeling slighted and unimportant from the failure of her primary caregivers, to a state of responsiveness to her wishes for affection and engagement. She was able to engage her therapist in becoming more attuned to the nuances of her emotional state, and in turn, she has become more able to attune and to attend to her own relational needs through awareness and comfortable expression of her needs and longings with others. The responsiveness of her therapist has now been echoed by the responsiveness to this patient from her inner circle of friends and family.

This case demonstrates the vital importance of full empathic attunement on the part of the psychotherapist in supporting psychodynamic interventions aided by psychophysiological monitoring in helping to bridge the gap between basic science research and clinical practice, providing unique information in a way that informs the therapist's understanding of the patient during psychotherapy in a clinically relevant and meaningful way.

## Modern Perspectives, Future Directions, and Conclusions

One of the questions proposed in the introduction to this chapter relates to whether there is a role for psychophysiology in psychotherapy research. The studies reviewed above, despite limitations of size or statistical sophistication of the early work, all suggest a role for the use of psychophysiology as an objective, biologically based bridge between the intrapersonal and interpersonal psychology of emotions of patients and their therapists during psychodynamic psychotherapy. This deeper understanding of the two-person psychology in psychotherapy helps shift explanatory models away from the traditional focus on patient or therapist variables alone to a more appropriate focus on interaction variables that uniquely emerge out of the patient and therapist communication [46].

Taken together, the results of the past and present studies suggest a biological model of patient–therapist interpersonal process during psychotherapy. The interpersonal response is suggested by evidence that therapist physiologic reactivity is specific to the emotional responses of patients [30, 32]. There is also evidence that patients respond differentially to therapists of comparable training [26] and therapists with different levels of training and experience [32]. In addition, patients are physiologically sensitive to positive versus negative feedback from therapists as well as the therapists' state of mind [31]. Finally, there are multiple studies suggesting moments of physiologic concordance related to emotional responses between patients and therapists during psychotherapy and that these moments may underlie important prosocial constructs including empathy and establishing rapport [26, 29, 34, 40, 41, 47].

The studies reviewed above complement recent neuroimaging studies (see below) and offer potential insights into a clinically relevant, biologically based model of interpersonal interaction between patients and therapists during psychotherapy. This model is predicated on the overlap between neurobiological control of physiologic responses and structures implicated in neuroimaging studies of socially relevant phenomenon. In regard to the neurobiology of physiologic responses, several studies implicate the prefrontal cortex and anterior cingulate cortex in the control of SC and HR responses [8, 9, 23, 24, 48]. Moreover, neuroimaging studies on the neurobiology of emotional responses [49–51], empathy and empathy-related tasks [52–54], and social interaction [55–58] consistently implicate similar regions. Given that emotional and attitudinal states have physiologic and neurobiologic bases [49, 59, 60], it is not surprising that shared emotional and attitudinal states would also have shared physiologic and neurobiologic bases. For example, a recent study demonstrated that females watching their significant other receive a shock activated the affective component of a well-defined "pain matrix" in the observer even when the observer was not receiving a shock [54]. The authors also reported a direct correlation between activity in the observers' anterior cingulate cortex and self-reported level of empathic sensitivity. Other studies used responses to pictures of emotional faces to demonstrate similar but attenuated activation in a brain network (including the inferior frontal, insular, and premotor cortices) while participants were merely observing compared with imitating the emotion in the picture [53].

These results suggest a distinct neural network for emotional responsiveness informed by recent increases in our understanding of "mirror" mechanisms in humans that are implicated in the ability to take another's emotional perspective [61–63]. These mechanisms reflect the ability of neurons to react in a similar, albeit attenuated manner, when an individual observes versus performs an action. Thus, there is accumulating evidence for a definition of emotional responsiveness that involves a "shared representational network," which creates common representations of mental states of "self" and "other" [64]. This ability is dependent on the insula and prefrontal cortex that plays an integral role in coordinating and contrasting these cognitive representations [65]. Thus, in the present context, it is perhaps also not surprising that a measure of SC concordance between patient–therapist dyads during psychotherapy resulted in associations with patient perceptions of therapist empathic relatedness and shared positive social–emotional states. If similar brain networks are in some way involved in empathic and autonomic responses, then emotional responsiveness and empathic experiences may be regulated via a shared or concordant neuropsychobiology of representational networks.

In addition to the neuroimaging results describing a neurobiology to empathy, recent dyadic models informed by neurobiology suggest that human interpersonal experience emerges from patterns in the flow of verbal and nonverbal information within and between brains mediated by the interaction of internal physiologic processes [66]. This physiology is multidetermined, with factors including early interpersonal experiences combined with genetically determined programmed maturation of the nervous system. This view is increasingly supported by longitudinal animal and human studies of development [67, 68]. In his influential paper entitled "Biology and the Future of Psychoanalysis," Kandel argues that neurobiology is important for the future of psychotherapy research and should focus on social and biological determinants of behavior [4]. At the same time, developmentally informed models of the process of change in psychotherapy have evolved to include a more interpersonal perspective [69, 70]. As evidenced by this review, physiologic monitoring during psychotherapy has a long history with convergent results that support a biological basis to interpersonal models of patient–therapist interactions and answers the calls for a basic science approach to psychotherapy research [71, 72].

Two questions were posed in the beginning of this chapter. The research reviewed supports the existence of a measurable, biologically based influence that emerges from the physiologic responses between patient and therapist during psychotherapy. The observable correlates are most frequently related to strong negative emotion (e.g., antagonism) and strong positive emotions (e.g., positive reassurance). However, several important questions remain. Future research should include additional types of psychotherapy (e.g., cognitive-behavioral therapy), additional physiologic measures (e.g., respiratory rate, facial coding), consideration of the role of different types of psychopathology, and use of prospective study designs with gender controls utilizing other important psychotherapy constructs such as the therapeutic alliance. Importantly, a shift in research focus toward a determination of whether physiologic infuences between patient and therapist vary over time, and what, if any, is the relationship between these physiologic influences and outcomes in psychotherapy. Future research should also include models on whether trainees can learn complex social skills such as empathic listening and improve communication with patients. While several studies support the possibility of improved empathic awareness following targeted training [73, 74], a systematic application or study of empathy training has not been developed. Thus, it is possible that biologically based models presented in a neuroscience perspective with examples including physiologic measures could be used in conjunction with didactic sessions to enhance clinician training in interpersonal skills to optimize physiologic influences for the benefit of their patients.

Research that allows for the translation of the explosion of clinically relevant neuroscience into everyday practice is needed to further advance the therapeutic impact of psychosocial interventions. Psychophysiology as a measure of the subtle but powerful mutual influence of patients and therapists has the potential to aid in both generating empirically testable hypotheses and in bridging the gap between research and clinical practice. Moreover, physiologic monitoring during psychotherapy offers an opportunity for translational research and complements other process measures used in psychotherapy research. The technology used to collect psychophysiology is relatively inexpensive compared with neuroimaging modalities and new sensor technologies that are minimally intrusive are increasingly available allowing for continuous measurement of social interaction in a variety of clinical settings [12]. Given the growing understanding of the neurobiological mechanisms that control physiologic responses and the need for better understanding of human social interaction, physiologic monitoring during psychotherapy, as argued in the present chapter, offers exciting opportunities to build clinically relevant and applicable models of emotional influence and psychotherapy process well into the future.

**Acknowledgments** The authors wish to thank the patient for giving permission to present her case material in this chapter. Some of the details of the case have been disguised to protect anonymity.

# References

1. Cacioppo, J. T., & Tassinary, L. G. (2000). *Handbook of psychophysiology* (2nd ed.). New York, NY: Cambridge University Press.
2. Marci, C. D., & Riess, H. (2005). The clinical relevance of psychophysiology: Support for the psychobiology of empathy and psychodynamic process. *American Journal of Psychotherapy, 59*, 213–226.
3. Glucksman, M. L. (1981). Physiological measures and feedback during psychotherapy. *Psychotherapy and Psychosomatics, 36*, 185–199.
4. Kandel, E. R. (1999). Biology and the future of psychoanalysis: A new intellectual framework for psychiatry revisited. *American Journal of Psychiatry, 156*(4), 505–524.
5. Benbassat, J., & Baumal, R. (2004). What is empathy and how can it be promoted during clinical clerkships? *Academic Medicine, 79*(9), 832–839.
6. Roffman, J. L., Marci, C. D., Glick, D. M., Dougherty, D. D., & Rauch, S. L. (2005). Neuroimaging and the functional neuroanatomy of psychotherapy. *Psychological Medicine, 35*, 1–14.
7. Keller, J., Hicks, B., & Miller, G. (2000). Psychophysiology in the study of psychopathology. In J. T. Cacioppo, L. G. Tassinary & G. G. Berntson (Eds.), *Handbook of psychophysiology* (2nd ed.). Cambridge, UK: Cambridge University Press.

8. Critchley, H. D., Corfield, D. R., Chandler, M. P., Mathias, C. J., & Dolan, R. J. (2000). Cerebral correlates of autonomic cardiovascular arousal: A functional neuroimaging investigation in humans. *Journal of Physiology, 523*(1), 259–270.
9. Critchley, H. D., Elliott, R., Mathias, C. J., & Dolan, R. J. (2000). Neural activity relating to generation and representation of galvanic skin conductance responses: A functional magnetic resonance imaging study. *Journal of Neuroscience, 20*(8), 3033–3040.
10. Berntson, G. G., Bigger, T., Eckberg, D. L., Grossman, P., Kaufmann, P. G., Malik, M., Nagaraja, H. N., Porges, S. W., Saul, J. P., Stone, P. H., & Van Der Molen, M. W. (1997). Heart rate variability: Origins, methods, and interpretive caveats. *Psychphysiology, 34*, 623–648.
11. Cooper, J. (1986). Electrocardiography 100 years ago: Origins, pioneers, and contributors. *New England Journal of Medicine, 315*(7), 461–464.
12. Sung, M., Marci, C. D., & Pentland, A. (2005). Wearable feedback systems for rehabilitation. *Journal of NeuroEngineering and Rehabilitation, 2*(2), 2–17.
13. Buchanan, S. L., Valentine, J., & Powell, D. A. (1985). Autonomic responses are elicited by electrical stimulation of the medial but not lateral frontal cortex in rabbits. *Behavioural Brain Research, 18* (1), 51–62.
14. Oppenheimer, S. M., Gelb, A., Girvin, J. P., & Hachinski, V. C. (1992). Cardiovascular effects of human insular cortex stimulation. *Neurology, 42*, 1727–1732.
15. Fraguas, R., Marci, C. D., Fava, M., Iosifesco, D. V., Bankier, D., Loh, R., & Dougherty, D. D. (2007). Autonomic reactivity to induced emotion as a potential predictor of response to antidepressant treatment. *Psychiatry Research, 151*, 169–172.
16. Marci, C. D., Glick, D. M., Loh, R., & Dougherty, D. D. (2007). Autonomic and prefrontal cortex responses to autobiographical recall of emotions. *Cognitive, Affective, & Behavioral Neuroscience, 7*(3), 243–250.
17. Boucsein, W. (1992). *Electrodermal response*. New York: Plenum.
18. Hugdahl, K. (1995). Electrodermal activity. In: K. Hugdahl (Ed.), *Psychophysiology: The mind-body perspective* (pp. 101–130). Cambridge, MA: Harvard University Press.
19. Bell, G., & Gemmell, J. (2007). A digital life. *Scientific American, 296*(3), 58–65.
20. Lidberg, L., & Wallin, B. G. (1981). Sympathetic nerve discharges in relation to amplitude of skin resistance responses. *Psychophysiology, 18*, 268–270.
21. Tranel, D., & Damasio, A. R. (1994). Neuroanatomical correlates of electrodermal skin conductance responses. *Psychophysiology, 31*, 427–438.
22. Mangina, C. A., & Beuzeron-Mangina, J. H. (1996). Direct electrical stimulation of specific human brain structures and bilateral electrodermal activity. *International Journal of Psychophysiology, 22*, 1–8.
23. Fredrickson, M., Furmark, T., Olsson, M. T., Fischer, H., Andersson, J., & Langstrom, B. (1998). Functional neuranatomical correlates of electrodermal activity: A positron emission tomographic study. *Psychophysiology, 35*(2), 179–185.
24. Patterson, J. C., Ungerleider, L. G., & Bandettini, P. A. (2002). Task-independent functional brain activity correlation with skin conductance changes: An fMRI study. *Neuroimage, 17*(4), 1797–1806.
25. Venables, P. H. (1991). Autonomic activity. *Annals of the New York Academy of Sciences, 620*, 191–207.
26. Di Mascio, A., Boyd, R. W., Greenblatt, M., & Solomon, H. C. (1955). The psychiatric interview: A sociophysiologic study. *Diseases of the Nervous System, 16*, 4–9.
27. Bales, R. F. (1951). *Interaction process analysis: A method for the study of small groups.* Cambridge, MA: Addison-Wesley Press, Inc.
28. Adler, H. M. (2002). The sociophysiology of caring in the doctor-patient relationship. *Journal of General Internal Medicine, 17*, 883–890.
29. Coleman, R., Greenblatt, M., & Solomon, H. C. (1956). Physiological evidence of rapport during psychotherapeutic interviews. *Diseases of the Nervous System, 17*, 71–77.

30. Di Mascio, A., Boyd, R. W., & Greenblatt, M. (1957). Physiological correlates of tension and antagonism during psychotherapy: A study of "interpersonal change". *Psychosomatic Medicine, 19*(2), 99–104.
31. Malmo, R. B., Boag, T. J., & Smith, A. A. (1957). Physiological study of personal interaction. *Psychosomatic Medicine, 19*(2), 105–119.
32. McCarron, L. T., & Appel, V. H. (1971). Categories of therapist verbalizations and patient-therapist autonomic response. *Journal of Consulting and Clinical Psychology, 37*(1), 123–134.
33. Roessler, R., Bruch, H., Thum, L., & Collins, F. (1975). Physiologic correlates of affect during psychotherapy. *American Journal of Psychotherapy, 29*, 26–36.
34. Robinson, J. W., Herman, A., & Kaplan, B. J. (1982). Autonomic responses correlate with counselor-client empathy. *Journal of Counseling Psychology, 29*(2), 195–198.
35. Barrett-Lennard, G. T. (1962). Dimensions of therapist response as causal factors in therapeutic change. *Psychological Monographs: General and Applied, 76*(43), 1–36.
36. Gottman, J. M. (1981). *Time-series analysis: A comprehensive introduction for social scientists* (Vol. 1). Cambridge: Cambridge University Press.
37. Marci, C. D., Moran, E. K., & Orr, S. P. (2004). Physiologic evidence for the interpersonal role of laughter during psychotherapy. *Journal of Nervous and Mental Disease, 192*, 689–695.
38. Provine, R. B. (2000). Natural history of laughter. In *Laughter: A scientific investigation* (pp. 23–53). New York, NY: Viking.
39. Preston, S. D., & De Waal, F. B. M. (2002). Empathy: Its ultimate and proximate bases. *Behavior and Brain Sciences, 25*, 1–72.
40. Marci, C. D., & Orr, S. P. (2006). The effects of emotional distance on psychophysiologic concordance and perceived empathy between patient and interviewer. *Applied Psychophysiology and Biofeedback, 31*, 115–128.
41. Marci, C. D., Ham, J., Moran, E. K., & Orr, S. P. (2007). Physiologic correlates of empathy and social-emotional process during psychotherapy. *Journal of Nervous and Mental Disease, 195*(2), 103–111.
42. Iacono, W. G., Lykken, D. T., Peloquin, L. J., Lumry, A. E., Valentine, R. H., & Tuason, V. B. (1983). Electrodermal activity in euthymic unipolar and bipolar affective disorders. *Archives of General Psychiatry, 40*, 557–565.
43. Ward, N. G., Doerr, H. O., & Storrie, M. C. (1983). Skin conductance: A potentially sensitive test for depression. *Psychiatry Research, 10*(4), 295–302.
44. Thorell, L. H., Kjellman, B., & D'Elia, G. (1987). Electrodermal activity in relation to diagnostic subgroups and symptoms of depressive patients. *Acta Psychiatrica Scandinavica, 76*(6), 693–701.
45. Ashcroft, K. R., Guimaraes, F. S., Wang, M., & Deakin, J. F. (1991). Evaluation of a psychophysiological model of classical fear conditioning in anxious patients. *Psychopharmacology, 104*, 215–219.
46. Ablon, J. S., & Marci, C. D. (2004). Psychotherapy process: The missing link: Comment on Westen, Novotny, and Thompson-Brenner (2004). *Psychological Bulletin, 130*(4), 664–668.
47. Stanek, B., Hahn, P., & Mayer, H. (1973). Biometric findings on cardiac neurosis: Changes in ECG and heart rate in cardiopathic patients and their doctor during psychoanalytical initial interviews. *Psychotherapy and Psychosomatics, 22*, 289–299.
48. Critchley, H. D., Mathias, C. J., Josephs, O., O'Doherty, J., Zanini, S., Dewar, B., Cipolotti, L., Shallice, T., & Dolan, R. J. (2003). Human cingulate cortex and autonomic control: Converging neuroimaging and clinical evidence. *Brain, 126*, 2139–2152.
49. Cacioppo, J. T., & Gardner, W. L. (1999). Emotion. *Annual Review of Psychology, 50*, 191–214.
50. Phan, K. L., Wager, T., Taylor, S. F., & Liberzon, I. (2002). Functional neuroanatomy of emotion: A meta-analysis of emotion activation studies in PET and fMRI. *Neuroimage, 16*(2), 331–348.

51. Murphy, F. C., Nimmo-Smith, I., & Lawrence, A. D. (2003). Functional neuroanatomy of emotion: A meta-analysis. *Cognitive, Affective, & Behavioral Neuroscience, 3*(3), 207–233.
52. Farrow, T., Zheng, Y., Wilkinson, I., Spence, S., Deakin, J., Tarrier, N., Griffiths, P., & Woodruff, P. (2001). Investigating the functional anatomy of empathy and forgiveness. *Neuroreport, 12,* 2433–2438.
53. Carr, L., Iacoboni, M., Dubeau, M., Mazziotta, J. C., & Lenzi, G. L. (2003). Neural mechanisms of empathy in humans: A relay from neural systems for imitation to limbic areas. *Proceedings of the National Academy of Science, 100*(9), 5497–5502.
54. Singer, T., Seymour, B., O'Doherty, J., Kaube, H., Dolan, R. J., & Frith, C. D. (2004). Empathy for pain involves the affective but not the sensory components of pain. *Science, 303,* 1157–1161.
55. Berthoz, S., Armony, J. L., Blair, R. J., & Dolan, R. J. (2002). An fMRI study of intentional and unintentional (embarrassing) violations of social norms. *Brain, 125,* 1696–1708.
56. Eisenberger, N. I., Lieberman, M. D., & Williams, K. D. (2003). Does rejection hurt? An fMRI study of social exclusion. *Science, 302,* 290–292.
57. Iacoboni, M., Lierberman, M. D., Knowlton, B. J., Molnar-Szakacs, I., Moritz, M., Throop, C. J., & Fiske, A. P. (2004). Watching social interactions produces dorsomedial prefrontal and medial parietal bold fMRI signal increases compared to a resting baseline. *NeuroImage, 21,* 1167–1173.
58. Ruby, P., & Decety, J. (2004). How would you feel versus how do you think she would feel? A neuroimaging study of perspective-taking with social emotions. *Journal of Cognitive Neuroscience, 16,* 988–999.
59. Cacioppo, J. T., & Petty, R. E. (1981). Attitudes and cognitive response: An electrophysiologic approach. *Journal of Personality and Social Psychology, 37,* 2181–2199.
60. Ochsner, K. N., & Feldman Barrett, L. (2001). A multiprocess perspective on the neuroscience of emotion. In G. A. Bonanno (Ed.), *Emotions: Current issues and future directions* (pp. 38–81). New York, NY: Guilford Press.
61. Kohler, E. (2002). Hearing sounds, understanding actions: Action representation in mirror neurons. *Science, 297,* 846–848.
62. Iacoboni, M., Molnar-Szakacs, I., Gallese, V., Buccino, G., Mazziotta, J. C., & Rizzolatti, G. (2005). Grasping the intentions of others with one's own mirror neuron system. *PLoS Biology, 3,* 529–535.
63. Miller, G. (2005). Reflecting on another's mind: Mirror mechanisms built into the brain may help us understand each other. *Science, 308,* 945–947.
64. Decety, J., & Sommerville, J. A. (2003). Shared representations between self and other: A social cognitive neuroscience view. *Trends in Cognitive Sciences, 7*(12), 527–533.
65. Lamm, C., Batson, C. D., & Decety, J. (2007). The neural substrate of human empathy: Effects of perspective-taking and cognitive appraisal. *Journal of Cognitive Neuroscience, 19*(1), 42–58.
66. Siegel, D. J. (1999). *The developing mind.* New York: Guilford Press.
67. Schore, A. N. (1994). Orbitofrontal influences on the autonomic nervous system. In *Affect regulation and the origin of the self* (pp. 320–336). Hillsdale, NJ: Lawrence Erlbaum Associates, Inc.
68. Lyons Ruth, K. (2003). Dissociation and the parent-infant dialogue: A longitudinal perspective from attachment research. *Journal of the American Psychoanalytic Association, 51*(3), 883–991.
69. Fonagy, P. (1998). Moments of change in psychoanalytic theory: Discussion of a new theory of psychic change. *Infant Mental Health Journal, 19*(3), 346–353.
70. Tronick, E. Z., Bruschweiler-Stern, N., Harrison, A. M., Lyons-Ruth, K., Morgan, A. C., Nahum, J. P., Sander, L., & Stern, D. N. (1998). Dyadically expanded states of consciousness and the process of therapeutic change. *Infant Mental Health Journal, 19*(3), 290–299.

71, Borkovec, T. D. (1997). On the need for a basic science approach to psychotherapy research. *Psychological Science, 8*(3), 145–147.
72. Mayes, L. C. (2003). Partnering with the neurosciences. *Journal of the American Psychoanalytic Association, 51*(3), 745–753.
73. Nerdrum, P. (1997). Maintenance of the effect of training in communication skills: A controlled follow-up study of level of communicated empathy. *British Journal of Social Work, 27*(5), 705–722.
74. Hammond, D. C., Hepworth, D. H., & Smith, V. G. (2002). *Improving therapeutic communication: A guide for developing effective techniques.* San Francisco: Jossey-Bass.

# Part V
# Letters on Research in Psychodynamic Psychotherapy

# Chapter 15
# A Letter to My Friend and Researcher Colleague, Professor Sy Entist

Rolf Sandell

In this letter—somewhat edited in the interest of confidentiality—I argue that divergence or dispersion is much more typical of psychotherapy outcomes in a sample of cases than convergence and communality. The typical outcome picture is that few patients show very considerable improvement, while some deteriorate and the majority are widely scattered in-between. This fact, that people are different, has wide implications for the way outcome research data should be represented and presented. As the patient and the therapist factors are partially confounded, a remaining interesting theoretical issue is how the responsibility for this variation should be divided between the patient and the therapist. There are indications that researchers—and therapists—so far have tended to underestimate the accountability of therapist factor.

Dear Sy,

Heartfelt congratulations to your paper in the October issue of the *Journal of Psychotherapeutic Science*! The issue landed yesterday, and I couldn't wait to read it. I admire your productivity—and feel a bit envious about your success, I must admit. But it's absolutely well deserved, no doubt about that. Not only have you developed your Relaxed Cognition Systems Affect-Based Psychotherapy (RCSABP) on your own for the suffering post-partum depressions (PPDs); you've also personally provided them the treatment and, not least, evaluated it, and with quite good results, at that! Effects sizes between the 0.60's and the 0.80's are respectable, indeed. Maybe I could do a replication study in support? You know I have my own ideas about treating PPD with my Affect-Liberating Mindfulness Cognitive Dynamic Therapy (ALMCDT) that I wrote about in the *Journal* a few years ago, but as an objective scientist I'm sure I can control any bias as well as I'm sure you have in your study. One thing I really would like to do is to prolong the follow-up after the 3 months you had (and I had, too, in my study) and see what's happening in, say, a 1- or 2-year perspective. That would

R. Sandell
Fredrikshovsgatan 3A, SE-11523 Stockholm, Sweden
e-mail: rolf.sandell@liu.se

R.A. Levy, J.S. Ablon (eds.), *Handbook of Evidence-Based Psychodynamic Psychotherapy*,
DOI: 10.1007/978-1-59745-444-5_15, © Humana Press 2009

be kind of a nice innovation in psychotherapy research, relatively speaking, wouldn't you say?

However, there's one thing that I found intriguing in your report, tying in with a concern which has been with me for some time now. In your Table 2, I find on the AFSQ scale a within-groups effect size of 0.86 and on the OHGS scale a somewhat smaller one, 0.63. Then I took some other figures in the same table and used my hand calculator to compute the variation across your cases. As I did not have all the figures I needed, I had to make some assumption about the correlation between the pre-treatment and post-treatment scores, which usually is between 0.50 and 0.70, so I took 0.60 as my best guess.

Then I found out that the standard deviation of the change scores across all patients were about twice as large as their mean change on the OHGS and almost one-and-a-half times larger than the mean change on the AFSQ. Inter-estingly enough, this almost exactly replicates what I myself have found in our own data on the ALMCDT, and just to emphasize the implications of this, I enclose a graph of what it looks like when I plotted our patients from start to finish on the two scales. My concern is that I find it quite difficult, absurd really, with such images in view, to speak of any effect of ALMCDT in general terms, like averages. You know, "This is a very effective treatment," "This is a better treatment than this other one," etcetera, etcetera, the way we usually do. Even if we report the standard deviations around these averages, I'm sure neither our readers, nor ourselves, will really realize the extent of the variation and the futility to predict what will be happening with any individual patient (Fig. 15.1).

To begin with, I think we have to find a way of summarizing our data so that at least something of this huge variation is preserved. In my opinion the average becomes a bizarre misrepresentation. You have probably seen this poster, you know, in the subway these days, "The average human," it says, "has 1.7 children." And then, "Have you seen anyone with 1.7 children." This is to promote greater tolerance for disadvantaged and handicapped people, but I think it has much wider implications. You know, in our obsession with group statistics I think we tend to forget one of the really important insights we had in our differential psychology course, if you remember: *People are different.* Not only in a random fashion, but systematically.

In our research group we have tried a kind of clustering procedure which makes our accounts of treatment effects at least a bit closer to reality. I will not tire you with the technicalities but it's a nice software (DATAMINE or D-MINE) by a German guy which sorts patients into more or less homogeneous subgroups on the basis of their patterns of change.

The fact that people are systematically different is of course why we might improve our prediction to the extent that we may find these systematic patient factors that correlate with change scores. I don't know about your patients, but we have found some such relations in our data, though not very strong. But when we divide the patients in D-MINE clusters, the patient samples split sharply in subtypes which perform differently in therapy, at least in ALCMDT. And at least our subtypes were significantly different in terms of personality

**Fig. 15.1** Change trajectories on the AFSQ (upper panel) and the OGHS (lower panel) across a 1-year treatment plus 3-month follow-up, sorted by patients

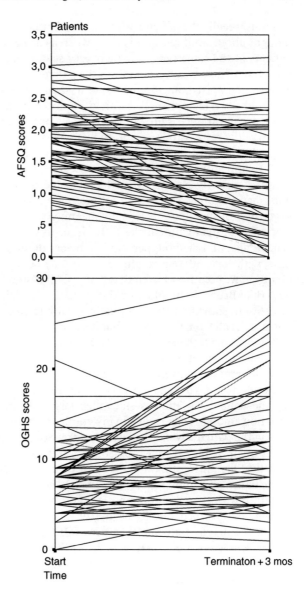

disorders, primarily (borderline, schizoid, phobic, narcissistic, and obsessive) in our ALCMDT sample. Also, SASB-defined personality variables as being vindictive and self-occupied uniquely predicted cluster membership in that particular context. And when we have tried grouping patients in other samples on the basis of outcome on health-care and sickness-related variables, diagnostic factors (Axis-I diagnoses, Global Assessment of Functioning, Vocational Impairment, problem history) have been found predictive.

But is it really the patients who perform better or worse? One thing I haven't thought about until recently is that, whereas a therapist generally has several patients at the same time, a patient very seldom has several therapists at the same time. Thus, we cannot know if the patient would fare better or worse with another therapist than the one (s)he has. In treatment studies, as well as in reality, the two factors are therefore partially confounded in what we call cases, and the case variance is no doubt very large, but we don't know the two parties' shares of the responsibility for it. In fact, when I have sorted the cases I showed before by therapists, instead of by patients, and plotted each therapist's average (sic!) treatment results, the resulting picture is almost as chaotic. Look at this graph! Especially chaotic when I plot some data from this other study we published the other year with a lot more therapists, 219 to be exact, as in the lower part of the figure. Is it really meaningful to speak of "the treatment" or "the effect of the treatment" here, Sy? It seems to me we are dealing here with a general idea of a method, personified in very different ways by different therapists, with very different results. But this may be so just with my ALMCDT? I don't know, because I haven't seen any similar summaries before. True, some guys (like Bruce Wampold, and dolls, like Irene Elkin) have juggled with their statistics to show that the therapist variation is quite large (say some guys) or not large at all (some dolls say), but it's really too sophisticated for me to grasp, although I like to believe I'm fairly good at statistics. (And how do you think our clinician friends could grasp it?) And how on earth can they come to such very different conclusions? (Fig. 15.2).

But even though some guys claim that the therapist variation is large, they say the patient variation is still much larger. I doubt that. In my eyes, the variation among the therapists in my graph seems much as large as the variation among the patients which I showed before. So, as you didn't report any data I could use in your article, I took some of my own data again and did my own statistical juggling, estimating the error component and the "true" component in the patient variation (within therapists) and then comparing the true patient variation with the variation among therapists' "average patient." And lo and behold, they turned out to be pretty much the same! It varied somewhat between different outcome measures (OFGS and AFSQ and MBDI) but, apart from an extreme value with AFSQ at one point of follow-up, the patient-to-therapist variance ratio was astoundingly close to 1.

Thus, however much, as therapists, we dislike the idea, as researchers we have to reckon with the idea that our treatment results may have as much to do with us as therapists as with our patients. My good patients might be difficult (or bad, as we sometimes say!) and my difficult patients might be good, with my colleague next door at the clinic! And with some therapists it seems like good patients really are the exception! That must be a truly unpleasant thought for any therapist, to suspect that he or she is more or less chronically suboptimal, to put it nicely, for his or her patients! We have also followed-up these findings by looking for factors that seem to account for some of these quality differences among therapists. For instance, therapeutic attitudes seem to matter, that is,

**Fig. 15.2** Change
trajectories on the AFSQ
across a 1-year treatment
plus 3-month follow-up
(upper panel) and a 3-year
treatment plus 3-year
follow-up (lower panel),
sorted by therapists

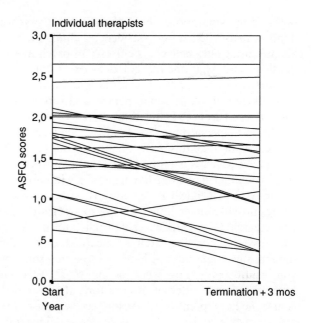

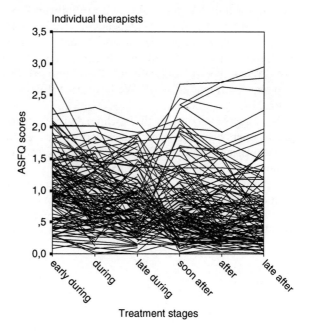

one's basic assumptions about the nature of psychotherapy and the human mind, such as whether one considers psychotherapy as a form or art or rather a science; what ones believes is curative in psychotherapy, such as warmth and kindness; and what one recognizes as one's style as a therapist, such as being supportive or not. We also found that the chronically suboptimal therapists are more likely to have personal therapy and supervision longer and more often. But it doesn't seem to help—that's how we interpreted it, anyway.

I know this is becoming too long, Sy, and I ask you to bear with me that I get so excited about all this. After all, it was your paper that set me going! Before I stop I have to tell you a funny thing that happened to me—or was it embarrassing? The other day I was having coffee with, you know Clee Nician, the guy whom we had Clinical Psychology II with. Now and then we meet, and he always provokes me a little by being so arrogantly uninterested in psychotherapy research. He says the ratio of insight gained to reading time is much below 1 when psychotherapy research is concerned. Can you imagine? Now, anyway, I thought this might interest him, so I told him some pieces of what I have told you. And do you know what the guy says? "Welcome to reality! Didn't you know people are different; it goes for patients and therapists, too?" And, of course, he has a point there. As long as we continue to treat the patients as an average, while clinicians know each one is unique, our work will lack credibility—and validity. What could we do to improve? Well, one thing might be to analyze our studies from the dependent variable point of view instead of from the point of view of the independent variable. Thus, instead of asking, "Is there a difference in average outcome between these treatment groups?" we might ask, "What types of outcome are there, and are those types associated with different treatment groups?" We have tried it on several data sets now, and it works!

Sy, we have to consider this a while. As researchers, maybe we are alienating practitioners by not minding this very obvious fact, that we should focus on the variations, not the averages? Now we don't seem to be of much help to the clinicians. We might improve this deplorable state of affairs by describing the variations and teasing out what underlies them. And then, let's not put all the light on the patient, let's not ignore the therapist factor.

Well, I won't go on, as I might, indefinitely. I'd love to hear your reactions, Sy. I hope Sue and the kids are sound and well and hope to see you some time in the near future.

Best wishes,
Rolf

# Chapter 16
# The Perils of *p*-Values: Why Tests of Statistical Significance Impede the Progress of Research

## An Open Letter to Psychotherapy Researchers

John M. Kelley

Imagine that you conduct an experiment to determine whether a new form of psychotherapy is more effective than treatment as usual. You analyze the data and find them to be statistically significant with a *p*-value that is less than 5%. How accurately does the following paragraph describe your understanding of the meaning of these results?

Because the data are statistically significant, I know that they are reliable. In other words, if I were to repeat the experiment in the same manner, I would most likely get statistically significant results again. More specifically, the *p*-value indicates that there is less than a 5% chance that a replication would not be statistically significant. In other words, at least 95% of the time a replication would again produce a statistically significant result. In addition, a *p*-value below 5% means that it is at least 95% certain that the new therapy is better than treatment as usual. The *p*-value also indicates that the difference in patient improvement between the new therapy and treatment as usual is important. The lower the *p*-value, the greater the clinical significance of the findings. In other words, a *p*-value of 1% indicates a greater clinical effect than a *p*-value of 5%. And finally, if the results had not been statistically significant, then I would know that any difference between the new therapy and treatment as usual probably just occurred by chance, and that the true difference between the new therapy and treatment as usual is probably zero.

Surprisingly, every sentence of the preceding paragraph is false. In particular, statistical significance on its own tells you nothing about: (1) the probability of replication; (2) the effect size; or (3) the clinical significance of the findings. Most surprising of all, statistical significance does not even tell you what you most want to know: the probability that the effect you found is genuine! My assumption is that you could pick out several sentences in the previous paragraph as being false, but that at least one of the interpretations of *p*-values seemed correct to you. My purpose in this paper is to point out some common errors in thinking about statistical tests and to correct them. Before beginning,

J.M. Kelley
376 Hale Street, Beverly, MA 01915, USA
e-mail: JKelley@Endicottt.Edu

R.A. Levy, J.S. Ablon (eds.), *Handbook of Evidence-Based Psychodynamic Psychotherapy*,     367
DOI: 10.1007/978-1-59745-444-5_16, © Humana Press 2009

I should note two things. First, I am by no means the first person to identify these common errors (e.g., [1–6]). Sadly, however, these misinterpretations of statistical significance are remarkably resistant to eradication, hence the need for periodic reminders. Second, even though I am keenly aware of these common errors in thinking about statistical significance, I must confess that I fall prey to them myself at times. Indeed, the meaning of statistical significance is so strongly counter-intuitive that nearly everyone is lead astray at some point.

Anyone who has ever read a published research article is familiar with $p$-values. When the $p$-value is less than 5%, the researcher rejoices – the study is statistically significant and has a good chance of being published. In contrast, when the $p$-value is greater than 5%, the researcher despairs. No matter how interesting the theory or how suggestive the data; if the $p$-value is greater than 5%, it is difficult to get the work published in a peer-reviewed journal. Thus, one meaning of $p$-values that is certainly true is that our journals seem to consider them the single most important aspect of any empirical study. This is, I am afraid, a grave mistake, and it has had a pernicious effect on progress in the behavioral sciences.

I believe that the confusion regarding statistical significance arises from the convoluted logic that underlies hypothesis testing in the behavioral sciences. In the natural sciences, researchers often test specific hypotheses that can be captured by precise mathematical equations. For example, one of the laws of physics is expressed by the equation: force = mass × acceleration. This law can be tested directly by collecting many pieces of data and then seeing how closely the data match the predicted equation.

In contrast, in the behavioral sciences, our hypotheses almost never achieve such precision. In comparing a new form of psychotherapy against treatment as usual, we merely predict that patients receiving the new therapy will be better off than those receiving treatment as usual. We are never able to precisely quantify the difference between the groups. Thus, our hypotheses are directional rather than exact – we specify the direction of the effect, but not its magnitude.

Because our hypotheses are imprecise, we cannot test them in a straightforward manner. Instead, we use null hypothesis testing. The logic of null hypothesis testing is as follows. First, we set up two hypotheses that cover all possible experimental outcomes. The null hypothesis is that there is *no* effect – there is no difference in efficacy between the new therapy and treatment as usual. The alternative hypothesis (or research hypothesis) is that there *is* an effect – there is a difference in efficacy between the new therapy and treatment as usual. If we can show that one of the two hypotheses is false, then we know that the other hypothesis must be true.

We *assume* that the null hypothesis is true. That is, we assume that the efficacy of the new therapy is exactly the same as treatment as usual. We then gather data to test the null. Remember, we are testing the null because it specifies an exact value for the strength of the effect (i.e., the difference in efficacy between the two treatment groups will be zero). Most of the time however, even if the null is true, there will be *some* difference between the two groups due to various sources of error.

If we conduct a study and find a difference between two treatment groups, how can we decide whether the observed difference is due to error or to a genuine treatment effect? This is where the *p*-value comes in. *The p-value is the probability of the data given the assumption that the null hypothesis is true.* More specifically, when the *p*-value is less than 5%, this means that, *if the null is true*, there is less than a 5% chance of obtaining a difference between the two treatment groups that was as large as (or larger than) the observed difference.

Let's assume that we obtain a *p*-value below 5%. Since the probability of getting such a large difference between the two groups is less than 5%, we decide to reject the null hypothesis, to say that we believe it to be false. And therefore, if the null is false, then the alternative must be true. We conclude that the new therapy is more effective than treatment as usual. The researcher can then report that the results were statistically significant at the $p < 0.05$ level, publish the study in a peer-reviewed journal, and eventually achieve tenure if she can repeat this feat many times.

Here, however, is where the trouble begins. Most people who read research articles do not completely understand the logic underlying null hypothesis statistical testing. And perhaps even more disturbing, there are several empirical studies that suggest that many active researchers in the behavioral sciences have similar difficulties in properly interpreting what statistical significance really means [7–9].

So how *should* you interpret *p*-values? The *p*-value has a very narrow and restricted meaning. When the *p*-value is below 5% then, *if the null is true*, there is only a 5% probability the data could have occurred by chance. Unfortunately, that is *all* that you can properly conclude. *P*-Values by themselves provide no information whatsoever about how large an effect is, or how clinically meaningful an effect is, or how likely it is that an effect would be replicated. Most unfortunate of all, a statistically significant result doesn't even tell us what we most want to know – how probable is it that the effect that I have found is genuine? This last phrase captures the meaning of statistical significance that is most difficult to give up. After all, aren't we conducting the statistical test to determine whether the research hypothesis is true? I myself have found it very difficult to accept the fact that the *p*-value by itself offers no information on the likelihood that the research hypothesis is true. A straightforward numerical example may help clarify this point.

Figure 16.1 illustrates the fate of 1000 research studies. Let's assume that 10% of the time the research hypothesis is true (this is often referred to as the *prior probability* because it represents the probability that a research hypothesis is true *prior* to a study being conducted). Ten percent prior probability will seem a bit low for your own hypotheses (and, I must admit, for my own as well), but perhaps not unreasonable for the hypotheses of others! This means that the null is true for 900 of the studies. If we use a *p*-value of 5% as the standard for statistical significance, 45 of these studies will incorrectly claim that the research

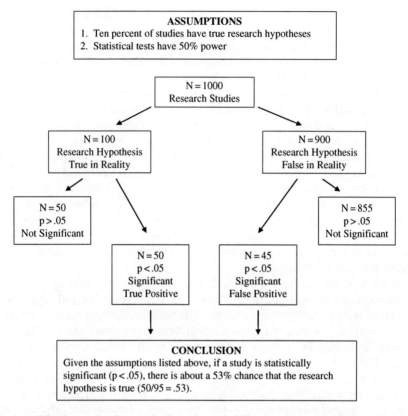

**Fig. 16.1** Why the *p*-value does not indicate the probability that the research hypothesis is true

hypothesis is correct. Let's also assume that statistical power is about 50%. Empirical evidence suggests that this may be a generous estimate of statistical power in the social sciences [7, 8]. This means that of the 100 studies in which the research hypothesis is correct, only 50 will be statistically significant. Now, considering the entire body of 1000 research studies, what is the probability that the research hypothesis is correct given that the study was statistically significant? The answer is 53% (50/95 = 0.53). Under different assumptions, of course, this probability can vary widely.

Table 16.1 summarizes the probability that the research hypothesis is true given a statistically significant test ($p < 0.05$) under various conditions. In the table, this probability varies from a low of 18% to a high of 99% in spite of the fact that in all cases the test is statistically significant ($p < 0.05$). The two factors that affect this probability are statistical power and the prior probability that the research hypothesis is true. As these factors increase, the probability that the research hypothesis is true increases. The first line of the table shows that when the prior probability is low (10%), a statistically significant study that has very high power (90%) will have only a two-thirds chance of correctly identifying a

**Table 16.1** Probability that the research hypothesis is true under different assumptions (all probabilities are expressed as percentages)

| Actual percentage of research hypotheses that are true | Statistical power | Probability that the research hypothesis is true given a significant test ($p < 0.05$) |
|---|---|---|
| 10 | 10 | 18 |
|    | 30 | 40 |
|    | 50 | 53 |
|    | 70 | 61 |
|    | 90 | 67 |
| 30 | 10 | 46 |
|    | 30 | 72 |
|    | 50 | 81 |
|    | 70 | 86 |
|    | 90 | 88 |
| 50 | 10 | 67 |
|    | 30 | 86 |
|    | 50 | 91 |
|    | 70 | 93 |
|    | 90 | 95 |
| 70 | 10 | 82 |
|    | 30 | 93 |
|    | 50 | 96 |
|    | 70 | 97 |
|    | 90 | 98 |
| 90 | 10 | 95 |
|    | 30 | 98 |
|    | 50 | 99 |
|    | 70 | 99 |
|    | 90 | 99 |

true research hypothesis. This fact is captured by the familiar phrase: extraordinary claims require extraordinary proof. In other words, when the research hypothesis is implausible, a $p$-value below 5% should not necessarily be considered as strong evidence that the hypothesis is true. Conversely, as can be seen in the bottom section of Table 16.1, when the prior probability is high (90%), then a statistically significant study provides strong evidence that the research hypothesis is true even under conditions of low power (10%). The bottom line is this: the $p$-value on its own cannot tell us the probability that the research hypothesis is true.

   $P$-Values and statistical significance provide no information about a number of important scientific issues, and yet many researchers and consumers of research act as if they do. Misinterpreting the meaning of statistical significance has had a negative impact on the progress of behavioral science in a number of ways. First, a finding of statistical significance is often interpreted as essentially proof that one's research hypothesis is correct. As we saw in Table 16.1, although a statistically significant result should increase one's confidence in the research hypothesis, it does not provide an estimate of the probability that your hypothesis is correct (i.e., that probability could vary from a low of 18% to a high of 99%). Second, as a result of the first problem, replication studies have been inappropriately devalued. If statistical significance is misinterpreted as meaning that there is a high probability that research hypotheses are correct, then it makes little sense to conduct replications. Third, because statistical significance is often confused with clinical significance, small effects with limited clinical impact are sometimes touted as being more important than they really are simply because they are statistically significant (this situation occurs when sample sizes are very large yielding high statistical power). Fourth, large effects that have important implications for clinical practice can easily be missed if sample sizes are small and statistical significance is not achieved (this is the problem of low statistical power). Fifth, if there are a number of studies on a particular topic of interest, the studies with significant effects are much more likely to be published, whereas the other studies are likely to be relegated to the "file drawer." As a result, meta-analysis of the published data will yield an inflated effect size (i.e., the "file drawer effect," [10]). Sixth, excessive focus on $p$-values encourages dichotomous thinking (i.e., if $p < 0.05$, then my theory is true; and if $p > 0.05$ then my theory is false). As Rosnow and Rosenthal [5] put it, "Surely God loves the .06 nearly as much as the .05."

An example of the problems that can flow from misinterpretation of statistical significance is the Food and Drug Administration's (FDA) use of the $p$-value as the standard by which new medications are approved. The FDA requires two statistically significant randomized controlled trials, but it does not put any limit on the total number of trials that a drug company could perform to achieve this standard. Given a sufficient number of attempts with reasonably large sample sizes, it is highly probable that two significant effects will be found even if the medication has only marginal efficacy or potentially no efficacy at all. A recent meta-analysis of randomized controlled trials of the selective serotonin reuptake inhibitors (SSRIs) dramatically illustrated this problem [11]. It would make a great deal more sense for the FDA to consider effect sizes and clinical significance, and use meta-analysis to consider all of the relevant clinical trials rather than focusing solely on the presence or absence of two statistically significant trials.

Regrettably, the American Psychological Association (APA) has followed the FDA's lead in requiring two statistically significant randomized controlled trials by independent research teams as the gold standard by which it will determine that a specific mode of psychotherapy is "empirically supported." Let me make clear that I support the use of randomized controlled trials as a way to evaluate the effectiveness of psychotherapy. Moreover, I agree that evidence of statistical significance from a randomized controlled trial should certainly increase one's confidence in the effectiveness of the therapy examined. In other words, there is nothing inherently wrong with the empirically supported designation. Rather, the problem is one of interpretation – it is too easy to make sweeping judgments about the relative value of different forms of psychotherapy. The dichotomous thinking encouraged by statistical hypothesis testing can lead one to conclude that forms of psychotherapy that have achieved statistical significance in a randomized controlled trial have been definitively proven effective, and forms of therapy that have not achieved statistical significance have been definitively proven ineffective. One might even be tempted to conclude that the only forms of psychotherapy that can be ethically practiced are those that the APA has designated as empirically supported [12]. This strikes me as severe over-reaching. If a statistical test cannot even tell us the probability that the research hypothesis is true, how can it possibly serve as a guide to ethical practice? Let me re-iterate that I am not against randomized controlled trials of psychotherapy. Rather, I simply want us to acknowledge their limitations so as to avoid dichotomous thinking and the illusion of certainty that their misuse can foster. For additional detailed discussion of the limitations of the empirically supported therapy movement, see Watson et al. [13].

An especially cautionary note was struck by an analysis of 29 head-to-head trials pitting various treatments for psychological disorders against one another. Luborsky et al. [14] showed that the allegiance of the first author was an extraordinarily good predictor of which treatment fared better ($r = 0.85$, $p < 0.001$). One final note: although I have lumped the FDA and APA together by criticizing both for their excessive reliance on statistical significance, the problems that arise from that reliance are quite different for the two institutions. The drug companies who seek approval for their medications have enormous financial resources at their command. They can (and do) conduct large numbers of randomized controlled trials of their medications in the search for two statistically significant findings (e.g., for the six most popular SSRIs approved between 1987 and 1999, the drug companies conducted 42 trials – an average of seven trials per drug, [11]). As I have argued, such a process has the potential to result in approval for medications of minimal efficacy. The situation in psychotherapy research is precisely the opposite. Because most psychotherapy researchers have limited funding, they may have difficulty financing a randomized controlled trial, and any trials that they do conduct are likely to have limited sample sizes (hence reduced power). The result is that many forms of psychotherapy may never receive an adequate trial. Concluding that such therapies are ineffective on the basis of a single (possibly underpowered) study is not scientifically justified.

A better understanding of the logic underlying null hypothesis statistical testing is crucial if we want to avoid the misinterpretations discussed in this paper. Instead of focusing so intently on statistical significance, we should pay greater attention to estimates of effect size and clinical significance. These two ideas are closely related in that they both assess the magnitude of the effect that has been observed in the research. Clinical significance is difficult to define – nevertheless, I suspect that many clinicians would agree with the sentiments of Supreme Court Justice, Stewart Potter, who in 1964 wrote about obscenity, "I know it when I see it."

Several quantitative methods have been proposed for defining clinical significance (see [15] for a comparison of these methods). The most popular method is the one proposed by Jacobson and Traux [16]. These authors recommend using three categories: (1) recovered; (2) improved but not recovered; and (3) unchanged or deteriorated. The recovered category is defined in three different ways depending on the available data: (1) improvement that places the patient more than two standard deviations above the dysfunctional mean; (2) improvement that places the patient within two standard deviations of the normal mean; and (3) improvement that places the patient above the midpoint dividing the normal mean from the dysfunctional mean. Each of these criteria is an attempt to define recovery as change that moves the patient out of the dysfunctional range and into the normative range, which seems to be a reasonable definition of recovery. The second category, improved but not recovered, is comprised of those patients who have shown statistically significant change (i.e., they have improved by more than twice the standard error of the difference between the pre- and post-treatment means), but who have not crossed the cutoff point for recovery. All other patients are labeled as unchanged or deteriorated.

Although I like the quantitative rigor of this method for assessing clinical significance, I worry that the subtleties associated with the method will be glossed over. For example, consider two patients: the first whose outcome is just one point above the recovery cutoff, and the second whose outcome is just one point below the cutoff. Does it really make sense to put these two patients in different categories? Furthermore, imagine that the first patient at baseline had a relatively mild illness, while the second patient had a severe illness. In this case, the second patient has improved vastly more than the first, and yet the simple categories suggest the reverse (i.e., the first patient is categorized as recovered, and the second as improved but not recovered). Although it is often easier to think in terms of categories, taking a continuous measure and making it categorical inevitably results in a loss of information. Therefore, we should be cautious in interpreting categorical measures of clinical significance.

In spite of the fuzziness of the concept, psychotherapy researchers should always address clinical significance in their research reports by describing in the clearest terms possible what effects they found. For example, in addition to indicating the proportion of patients who achieved a clinically significant improvement, it would also be helpful to report something like the following: "On average, patients in the new psychotherapy group improved 5 points more on the Beck Depression Inventory as compared to patients in the treatment as usual group." Simplicity and clarity of presentation will allow the reader to assess how for him or herself how clinically meaningful the results might be.

In contrast to clinical significance, there is considerable consensus on standardized effect size measures. Standardized effect sizes are particularly important to include in any research report because they help facilitate the process of meta-analysis. Meta-analysis is a statistical technique for quantitatively combining data from similar research studies to produce an average effect size for the phenomenon of interest. For the difference between two treatment groups, the most common measure of effect size is Cohen's *d*, which is defined as follows: $d = (\text{mean } 1 - \text{mean } 2)/\text{pooled standard deviation}$. Cohen's *d* tells you how many standard deviations apart the means for two groups fall. If $d = 0$, the two group averages are identical. If $d = 1$, the two group averages differ by one standard deviation. An effect size of $d = 1$ means that the average person in one group scores at the 68th percentile as compared to the other group. Table 16.2 presents a variety of effect sizes and their associated percentiles, as well as Cohen's [17] suggested definitions for small, medium, and large effect sizes in the social sciences. Although it is tempting to rely exclusively on Cohen's conventional definitions, I again urge researchers to report their findings in a manner that is as clear as possible to clinicians, and to consider also reporting quantitative measures of clinical significance.

In addition to standardized effect size estimates and quantitative measures of clinical significance, researchers should also provide 95% confidence intervals around these estimates. Confidence intervals are a range of numbers within which the true population parameter is likely to lie. In particular, if a study were to be repeated 100 times in precisely the same manner, 95% of the time the confidence interval would correctly contain the true population parameter. In addition to indicating a range of plausible values within which the true population parameter is likely to lie, confidence intervals also make clear the level of precision of the point estimate.

In conclusion, both researchers and consumers of research should be careful to assign to statistical significance only its proper meaning and not any of the tempting misinterpretations that I have discussed. In addition, much more attention should be paid to estimating how large an effect is, regardless of its statistical significance. We should be routinely reporting a standardized

**Table 16.2** Percentile equivalents for effect sizes

| Effect size | Description | Percentile |
|---|---|---|
| 0 | No effect | 50 |
| 0.1 | Trivial | 54 |
| 0.2 | | 58 |
| 0.3 | Small | 62 |
| 0.4 | | 66 |
| 0.5 | | 69 |
| 0.6 | Medium | 73 |
| 0.7 | | 76 |
| 0.8 | | 79 |
| 1.0 | | 84 |
| 1.2 | | 88 |
| 1.4 | Large | 92 |
| 1.6 | | 95 |
| 1.8 | | 96 |
| 2.0 | | 98 |

measure of effect size such as Cohen's *d* with its associated confidence interval, as well as a clear description of the clinical significance of the findings. Journal editors, grant-funding agencies, and tenure evaluation committees continue to place enormous importance on tests of statistical significance, and consequently, we researchers must also be concerned with statistical significance. However, the most important question is one that is often not sufficiently addressed. We should always be asking: How clinically meaningful are our findings and what does our study have to say about clinical practice?

## Summary

A number of common misconceptions regarding the meaning of statistical significance are discussed. These include (1) that statistical significance indicates the probability of a successful replication; (2) that statistical significance is a measure of effect size; (3) that a lack of statistical significance means that there is no effect; and (4) that statistical significance gives information about the probability that the alternative hypothesis is true. The logic underlying null hypothesis statistical testing is clarified so that the true meaning of statistical significance can be better understood. Statistical significance has a narrow and restricted meaning, and consequently, has only limited implications. By convention, an experiment is statistically significant if the *p*-value is less than 5%. *The p-value is the probability of the data given the assumption that the null hypothesis is true.* Any other meanings attached to the *p*-value or to statistical significance are mistaken. I argue that progress in the behavioral sciences has been impeded by a lack of understanding of the meaning of statistical significance. Finally, regardless of statistical significance, I suggest that much more attention should be paid to estimating standardized effect sizes with confidence intervals, and to describing clinical significance as clearly as possible. The most important question is one that is often not addressed. We should always be asking: How clinically meaningful is this effect?

**Acknowledgment** This publication was made possible by Grant Number 1 R21 AT002564 from the National Center for Complementary and Alternative Medicine (NCCAM). Its contents are solely the responsibility of the author and do not necessarily represent the official views of the NCCAM, or the National Institutes of Health.

## References

1. Bakan, D. (1966). The test of significance in psychological research. *Psychological Bulletin, 66*, 1–29.
2. Cohen, J. (1990). Things I have learned (so far). *American Psychologist, 45*, 1304–1312.
3. Cohen, J. (1994). The earth is round (*p*<.05). *American Psychologist, 49*, 997–1003.
4. Lykken, D. E. (1968). Statistical significance in psychological research. *Psychological Bulletin, 70*, 151–159.

5. Rosnow, R. L. & Rosenthal, R. (1989). Statistical procedures and the justification of knowledge in psychological science. *American Psychologist, 44*, 1276–84.
6. Rozeboom, W. W. (1960). The fallacy of the null hypothesis significance test. *Psychological Bulletin, 57*, 416–428.
7. Cohen, J. (1962). The statistical power of abnormal-social psychological research: A review. *Journal of Abnormal and Social Psychology, 69*, 145–153.
8. Sedlmeier, P. & Gigerenzer, G. (1989). Do studies of statistical power have an effect on the power of studies. *Psychological Bulletin, 105*, 309–316.
9. Zuckerman, M., Hodgkins, H. S., Zuckerman, A., & Rosenthal, R. (1993). Contemporary issues in the analysis of data: A survey of 551 psychologists. *Psychological Science, 4*, 49–53.
10. Rosenthal, R. (1979). The "file drawer problem" and tolerance for null results. *Psychological Bulletin, 86*, 638–641.
11. Kirsch, I., Moore, T. J., Scoboria, A., & Nicholls, S. S. (2002). The emperor's new drugs: An analysis of antidepressant medication data submitted to the U.S. Food and Drug Administration. Prevention and Treatment, 5, Article 23, available at http://content.apa.org/journals/pre/5/1/23.
12. McFall, R. M. (1991). Manifesto for a science of clinical psychology. *American Psychologist, 44*, 75–88.
13. Weston, D., Novotny, C. M., & Thompson-Brenner, H. (2004). The empirical status of empirically supported psychotherapies: Assumptions, findings, and reporting in controlled clinical trials. *Psychological Bulletin, 130*, 631–663.
14. Luborsky, L., Diguer, L., Seligman, D. A., Rosenthal, R., Krause, E. D., Johnson, S., et al. (1999). The researcher's own therapy allegiances: A "wild card" in comparisons of treatment efficacy. *Clinical Psychology. Science and Practice, 6*, 95–106.
15. Atkins, D. C., Bedics, J. D., McGlinchey, J. B., & Beauchaine, T. P. (2005). Assessing clinical significance: Does it matter which method we use. *Journal of Consulting and Clinical Psychology, 73*, 982–989.
16. Jacobson, N. S. & Truax, P. (1991). Clinical significance: A statistical approach to defining meaningful change in psychotherapy research. *Journal of Consulting and Clinical Psychology, 59*, 12–19.
17. Cohen, J. (1988). *Statistical power analysis for the behavioral science, 2nd edn.* Hillsdale, NJ: Erlbaum.

# Chapter 17
# From Psychoanalyst to Psychoanalyst/Researcher

## A Personal Journey

Ira Lable

This letter is to all the readers of this book and especially to psychoanalysts. I was asked to share my recent journey as an evidence-based researcher and practicing psychoanalyst. I have had a hidden demon on my unconscious for a very long time, inaccessible to me over the last 25 years. Having worked hard for many years at my institute and at the American Psychoanalytic Association as a teacher, administrator, and supervisor of candidates while serving as a training analyst, there remained a part of me that envied the empirical researcher. The world of research grants, statistical analysis, and evidenced-based treatment was essentially off limits to most psychoanalysts due to the culture of relative isolation from typical scientific methods thought not to apply to our field. There was a feeling, I believe, that only someone analytically trained could understand psychoanalysis, thus we really couldn't trust others to explore aspects of our realm. These issues were addressed by thoughtful and creative thinkers in the area of psychotherapy and psychoanalytic research, but I didn't have the tools to understand their efforts nor the encouragement to learn them. Then I joined the Psychotherapy Research Program at the Massachusetts General Hospital.

When I began, I never thought I would become more than an "analyst consultant," probably expecting to tell the group that what they did was inherently misleading and misguided. I asked, "Why do analysts need to prove their ideas? " Instead I have opened up a new way of thinking about being an analyst and being true to my patients by adding another form of inquiry besides inductive reasoning to explore the dynamic unconscious and psychoanalytic process. I have become aware of a dedicated group (larger that I expected) of psychotherapists and psychoanalysts who hope to answer questions through innovative evidence-based research. One of my wishes in this regard is that psychoanalytic institutes, both faculty and candidates have access to this kind of creative exploration of our work. I have learned how essential it is

I. Lable
Department of Psychiatry, Massachusetts General Hospital, WACC 805, 15 Parkman St., Boston, MA 02114, USA
e-mail: ira_lable@hms.harvard.edu

R.A. Levy, J.S. Ablon (eds.), *Handbook of Evidence-Based Psychodynamic Psychotherapy*,
DOI: 10.1007/978-1-59745-444-5_17, © Humana Press 2009

for the beginning researcher to have a knowledgeable group of collaborators to guide one through the maze of research administration and development.

I had a wonderful mentor and friend at the beginning of my psychoanalytic career. Jerry Sashin was a psychoanalyst, teacher, and psychoanalytic researcher. He studied and published papers on his empirical studies of analyzability. We had a mutual interest in neuroscience and with his guidance, we began a Discussion Group called "Mind, Brain, and Psychoanalysis" at the American Psychoanalytic Association meetings twice a year. Our first discussion was about the book by Changeux entitled "Neuronal Man." I remember bringing a plastic model of a brain into the meeting under my coat feeling somewhat mischievous. We consulted with a neurologist colleague of mine, Brian Woods, who was recently appointed to develop a MRI service at McLean Hospital in Belmont, Massachusetts. We asked whether this "new" technology could tell us anything about the changes that take place during or after an analysis. Even at that time, we may have been responding to a larger public education issue that included the scientific community, that psychoanalysis "works." Somehow if we could visualize that change on an X-ray of the brain, we could join that community and be accepted. The change that was beginning to be documented by MRI was volume measurements of certain brain structures. As we began discussing where to put our energy, Jerry died suddenly. This was a terrible loss for all of us. I continued the Discussion Group at the American Psychoanalytic Association for the next 20 years though I no longer had a research collaborator and partner.

The excitement that I have experienced with empirical research at the Psychotherapy Research Program and continue to enjoy is the sense of discovery of a different kind than the individual therapeutic adventure of clinical psychoanalytic discovery and immersion. Some similarities exist, like the sense of the unknown, the struggle to understand the "data" and the immersion in a process of discovery. One of the most rewarding aspects of the researcher is the camaraderie and group development, which is "organic" in its growth. People are always interested in exploring new ideas and how they can be studied. This delight with the opening up of new ideas to study with ever changing methods is a joy to behold.

Psychoanalysts are missing a wonderful piece of the larger intellectual community, which includes empirical researchers. Psychoanalysis can be studied empirically and not destroyed in its essence which is what I suspect is the fear. We may even get closer to defining what psychoanalysis is through these studies. I emphasize that I see empirical research being an addition to the larger psychoanalytic debate not a replacement. I also do not feel this is necessary for psychoanalysis to survive, but rather to thrive. There is a fear among some analysts that the truth of the unique and irreplaceable psychoanalytic treatment experience, which is the shared experience of being known by another and that one is knowable, can't be studied empirically. The shared experience of being open to one's unconscious liberates and educates one's core self and the chance that the many routes to that experience would be lost is almost unthinkable.

Thus, it is guarded sometimes, by the fiercest attitudes, including a kind of solipsistic involutional isolation. I don't feel that the inclusion of forms of empirical research with its enormous creative thrust will injure psychoanalysis but rather enlighten all of us to the unique clinical and theoretical urgency of psychoanalysis.

Analysts are the master of change and the owners of a burgeoning literature of how people change. It is another essence of psychoanalysis that there is meaningful change for those stuck in the mire of symptomatic repetition. Yet we are in the position to be alienated from the kind of change that might emerge from research of all kinds.

The use of the couch and the frequency of sessions are obvious researchable questions though there are also less obvious questions to study. The whole debate about self disclosure versus neutrality or the "blank screen" could be studied. Instead of listing the myriad possibilities for study, I wonder more how to develop a climate in our institutes and professional meetings where this kind of endeavor is valued and rewarded. We must be open to a new way of developing psychoanalytic ideas and techniques. I especially feel research would create a wonderful way of delineating psychoanalytic theories (a gold mine of thinking) and technique. We must get over the idea that to study psychoanalysis will necessitate "observation" and we will need to change the experience so profoundly that it won't even approximate analysis any more.

As part of my transformation to a clinical researcher, I received a grant from the International Psychoanalytic Association to study the effects of the use of the couch in psychoanalysis. We will be using the Psychotherapy Process Q-Sort to evaluate analyses that highlight the change from sitting up to lying down. It is a requirement of graduation from an institute of the American Psychoanalytic Association that the patient lie down the entire treatment. Currently, if this does not occur, it is not "analysis." Perhaps the results of my study will provide interesting input into the rationale for this requirement. It may reinforce the requirement or question it. I don't know the answer, but I am eager for empirical inquiry to guide our thinking. There are other treatment issues, that is, time, both frequency and length of treatment, as well as who gets an analysis, about which empirical research may provide insight.

As a Principal Investigator, I am part of the general MGH research email list. To be included is to enter an unfamiliar world that analysts in general would not be privy to. I receive e-mails directed to me personally and also to the general research community. I have had to upgrade my Institutional Review Board eligibility yearly. I also received an offer to buy cloned cell lines and I wondered what it would be like to need them and participate in a laboratory environment. I have been become immersed in a world of buying and studying books on statistical analysis and now have some beginning ideas about how the Statistical Program for the Social Sciences (SPSS) is an incredible tool to explore the meaning of the data we collected. I discuss with colleagues about the importance of the "power" of a project design. I wonder how to balance and combine any data analysis with the clinical assessments and biases of my work. I wonder how decades of clinical work and study of a particular way of understanding how people change through psychoanalysis can be reconciled with the use of video- and audiotaped clinical hours and the standardized rating of the therapeutic process subjected to statistical analysis. From my clinical perch, this process can be daunting, alien and a little subversive.

To cope with my status as a researcher-in-progress I can become a little self-deprecating over my relatively small grant. I had visions of advertising for subjects on the radio and on the commuter trains. What would I say to interest a listener or traveler to participate in a "research" psychoanalysis? I think of the "true" researchers who get millions of dollars and how we lament our lack of recognition. Though, I do wonder (as an analyst to the core) whether there is some pleasure in being the underdog and having this "unappreciated" status. We are David fighting the crude and uncouth Goliaths of the world. There are other myths involved in this struggle I'm sure. We have a kind of purity of method for we include and try to capture the "human" qualities of others and ourselves. I have the clear experience of being thrilled to be part of the Psychotherapy Research group fighting to bring answers to long-asked questions where answers were based only on personal belief, unique clinical experience, and the theories of brilliant men and women. I am also now linked to a larger group of researchers of all kinds all through the ages.

I also feel the ambivalence of the psychoanalytic community toward empirical research. There are strong voices encouraging the development of a research focus in all aspects of organized psychoanalysis especially institutes, that is, from Edward Glover to Otto Kernberg. Candidates should be exposed to evidence based projects to give voice to their creative and imaginative selves encouraged by faculty. Psychoanalysis, like any discipline, has a history of shunning those who oppose the status quo – Horney and Bowlby to mention two. Yet psychoanalysts are imbedded in a culture of asking the most hidden and difficult questions facing all of us. We open up dialogue and question meanings as a routine part of our daily clinical work. There is a strong and growing movement in psychoanalysis to appropriate those aspects of the general research and scientific community to study all aspects including the analytic situation and setting. Questions remain about what can be studied without changing the basic nature of the object studied, especially the inviolability of the unique psychoanalytic encounter. Can data collected indirectly (child development, attachment research, psychotherapy) be applied to psychoanalysis?

I feel personally the fear of losing the special nature of psychoanalysis and psychodynamic psychotherapy and the access to the nature of the dynamic unconscious that is their unique contribution. I believe that psychoanalysis and psychodynamic psychotherapy overlap in their ability to access unconscious meanings and develop insight through affective understanding. And yet, I remain in conflict, a part of me continuing to believe that 4–5 times a week on the couch remains the gold standard for thorough treatment aimed at modification of multiple transferences and accessing the unconscious. I also feel psychoanalysis needs to be preserved and protected against the forces of repression and resistance, a struggle that is as old as psychoanalysis itself. However, there is a stronger "drive" that is a basic part of the psychoanalytic community, to explore the functions of the mind, and especially to ask questions and devise ways of answering them. I feel being an evidence based psychoanalytic researcher/psychoanalyst is part of the long psychoanalytic tradition.

# Chapter 18
# Clinicians' Love/Hate Relationship with Clinical Research

Anne Alonso

It's a rare pleasure to be invited to put forth my thoughts about clinical research. It is usually assumed that a practitioner has neither familiarity nor interest in the area. While this is not the case, it is also fair to say that I have not actively sought to join in this conversation. The divide serves us all ill, so I welcome the chance to explore resistances on both sides.

For the purposes of this letter, I want to distinguish between clinicians conducting research and clinicians reading the research in the field and incorporating the new findings into clinical practice and training. It is a given in my mind that responsible practitioners, just as a matter of intellectual integrity and the spirit of lifelong learning, will stay abreast of the newest thinking in our field.

The divide between clinician/analysts and research/analysts in regard to conducting research originates from several sources.

1. Clinical training
2. Practice constraints
3. The definition of research
4. Language
5. Political attitudes

*Training* for psychodynamic clinicians places great emphasis on the frame of the clinical hour and views intrusions on that frame as at best, enactments, and at worst, destructive to the alliance and the outcome of analytic work.

The theory privileges the symbolic over the concrete, and emphasizes that introducing concrete matters flies in the face of the fundamental rule, that is, the need to allow the patients' associations to emerge in a relationship with the clinician who listens, invites, and abstains from a focus on external reality in favor of internal forces. Some of this attitude probably still emanates from the early Freudian model of clinical neutrality and abstinence, some

A. Alonso
Center for Psychoanalytic Studies and Department of Psychiatry, Massachusetts General Hospital, Boston, MA, USA

R.A. Levy, J.S. Ablon (eds.), *Handbook of Evidence-Based Psychodynamic Psychotherapy*,
DOI: 10.1007/978-1-59745-444-5_18, © Humana Press 2009

from tried-and-true experience about the value of listening in greater depth and over time to the patient's own agendas, and learning to "lead from behind."

Thus, the idea of introducing the clinician's agenda feels antithetical, or at least confusing.

Clinicians and researchers often employ different epistemologies. The loosely hovering attention of the analyst/practitioner values free association, hunches, and attention to subtleties of mood and affect. These non-specific factors are difficult to examine in a quantitative way, so it is encouraging to see quantitative research efforts that are also clinically sophisticated. Many of the contributing authors to this volume stand as stellar examples of the best of this kind of research, and it is important that clinicians see their work.

Analyst/practitioners need to make a much more vigorous effort to include psychotherapy process research into our curricula and into our supervisory conversations. And perhaps these practitioners turned practitioner/researchers can learn how to minimize intrusion in order to be able to gather data for the purpose of studying treatments to improve the impact of psychotherapy.

To that end, research that does not intrude into the hour with the patient will be a far more acceptable model for many of us who are still very committed to maintaining the frame of the clinical hour. Hopefully, the emphasis of some of the authors in this book to link clinical examples to the research findings will make that translation easier for all of us.

## Definitions of Research

It is misleading to think of research in only one model, that is, quantitive research based in a logical-positivist model. Longitudinal studies are a far more attractive model for long-term psychoanalytic clinicians who are by definition committed to thinking of developmental changes over an extended treatment. For example, Jonathan Shedler and Drew Westen have developed the Shedler–Westen Assessment Procedure (SWAP) which is a clinician-rated measure that describes 200 personality characteristics and serves to measure developmental changes of interest to dynamic thinkers.

Other forms of research are more apt to attract many clinicians: single case research, narrative research, and other qualitative models sit between the two extremes of clinician versus empirical researcher. It is true that they bring to mind a different set of assumptions about how we know and construct knowledge. If the lens though which we define research is wide enough, I expect that many more of us will be eager to be both clinicians and researchers. This book aims to achieve this balance.

*The constraints of the practice milieu* play a large part in the reluctance of practitioners to engage in research. It is one thing to work with a team of colleagues in an academic setting where there is both moral and practical support for conducting research. Cameras and other equipment are rarely available in most private offices, and research assistants are a distant fantasy. Worries about HIPAA, the need to fill precious clinical hours, and a deep resistance to additional burdensome paperwork all combine to add to clinicians' disinclination to be involved in research.

The patient population in private practice is another factor constraining clinicians' efforts to engage in research. The cost of individual psychodynamic treatment and the unwillingness of most insurance companies to support it means that many of the patients in long-term open-ended psychodynamic treatment tend to be wealthy and prominent. They may be very concerned about maintaining therapist confidentiality and protecting their reputations in the community. Introducing them to a research protocol can feel intimidating and risky while leaving the clinician open to potential legal/ethical problems. If the clinician fears rupturing the alliance and losing the patient and/or alienating the referral source, then the barrier is even greater. Here again, researchers represented in this book are attending to matters such as the alliance, all of which will encourage clinicians to pursue this kind of exploration and research.

Perhaps one effective way to promote an alliance is to place more research focus on the clinician's countertransference, on their own changes in the work along the life cycle, both positive and negative, and their questions about how their own development affects the work with their patients.

## Language

Analysts have been properly chastised for resorting to arcane jargon in their publications, rendering them unintelligible to all but the inner circle, and inviting ridicule in New Yorker cartoons. On the contrary, researchers similarly have been bound to write in the language of statistics and design methodologies that are off-putting to the less linear clinical mind. Neither side has spent enough time translating their ideas into plain English. It takes a very devoted and busy researcher, unfamiliar with the concepts, to dig deeply into the meanings of words such as "transmuting internalizations" or, for that matter, for a non-researcher clinician to pore through page after page of dense statistical tables. It is in the middle ground between those extremes that a common space that we can all inhabit can be developed.

One suggestion for improving this situation is to read and edit one another's work, contribute to each others' curricula, and ask the "dumb" questions when the language gets murky. Writing together will make us feel more familial and familiar.

## Politics

Psychoanalysis and psychotherapy began as a small "ma and pa" shop in Vienna, and like all pioneer groups the members were bound together in a spirit of creativity and intimacy .They fought among themselves, analyzed one another and each others' children, and felt themselves to be an elite group. The pioneering zest resulted in deeply solidifying the ideas of Freud and his followers in the public domain. They flourished until the last three decades, when other modalities and ideas began to challenge their shibboleths. The next generation came along, and like in most organizations, sought to define the founders as old fogies who were holding back progress. To some extent, this is true, yet the wealth of theory and practice that had brought forth the movement was not held in high esteem, giving way to some scorn and unfortunate schisms between the traditionalist and the researchers, pharmacologists, and briefer and more applied modalities. Researchers tended to ally with the briefer therapeutic modalities and with psychopharmacology, and were thus able to find funding for their growth.

Departments rely on research funding to advance their programs, so they have valued the researchers as the "favorites" in most training departments, often leaving the old loyalist clinicians feeling like they have been marginalized and at risk of losing their place in the academy. A quick look at leaders of training programs would indicate that their fears were justified. Still, Hegel had a point, and we have begun to see the pendulum swing toward the middle once again.

Armed camps of body versus mind are finally giving way to a more mature and less polarized understanding that synergy serves our patients' best interests. Mercifully, psychodynamic researchers have underscored the place of the therapeutic relationship as central to all our work with patients. To the extent that we can move from competition to collaboration, recognize the limits of any single viewpoint, and be of help to each other in a challenging time for mental health service and research, our own working alliance will flourish.

This invitation to write this letter is a great step in that direction, and I appreciate the chance to be included in the dialogue.

# Chapter 19
# Measuring and Enhancing the Impact of Psychodynamic Psychotherapy Research

## An Open Letter to Scientists and Clinicians

Anthony P. Weiss

It is a great pleasure to be able to contribute to this groundbreaking collection of papers regarding the evidence base for psychodynamic psychotherapy. My involvement in this text is as something of an outside observer of the field. Although I received training and supervision in dynamic therapy, I am not a psychotherapist. I am a clinical scientist with an interest in the process by which research findings get applied in clinical practice. My comments here are therefore not on the *content* of psychodynamic psychotherapy research (of which I have only cursory knowledge), but rather on the *process* of incorporating this research into the actual care of patients.

Evidence-based medicine (EBM) is an approach to patient care that requires (1) a body of evidence regarding effective treatments and (2) the application of those treatments that work (and abandonment of those that do not). Over the past decade and a half, EBM has become the predominant paradigm across all medical disciplines, now even within the laggardly field of psychiatry. In this context, those treatments for which evidence is lacking are in jeopardy of banishment from the medical/psychiatric mainstream. As one of the last outposts of resistance to the EBM perspective, dynamic therapy risks this fate, making this text (and other recent publications) of utmost import for those in the field.

## What is the Path from Research to Clinical Practice?

The goal of medical research is ultimately to improve the health and well-being of patients. Yet the path leading from research to this desired benefit is a tortuous one, filled with twists and dead ends.[1] When straightened and simplified, the path looks something like this:

---

[1] For more discussion on the path from research to clinical practice, see Weiss AP (2007): Measuring the impact of medical research: moving from outputs to outcomes. *American Journal of Psychiatry* 164:206–214.

A.P. Weiss
Department of Psychiatry, Massachusetts General Hospital, One Bowdoin square, Room 734, Boston, MA 02114, USA
e-mail: aweiss@partners.org

R.A. Levy, J.S. Ablon (eds.), *Handbook of Evidence-Based Psychodynamic Psychotherapy*,
DOI: 10.1007/978-1-59745-444-5_19, © Humana Press 2009

RESEARCH → AWARENESS → IMPLEMENTATION → PATIENT BENEFIT

Thus, the conduct of research leads to some evidence, which then needs to be disseminated to promote awareness. Once clinicians are aware of the evidence, they will apply the therapy in clinical practice, ultimately leading to an improvement in the patient's condition. Of course, these downstream effects (implementation and patient benefit) are not certainties; there is a big difference between knowing and doing, for example. But it all starts with awareness.

## How is Awareness Measured?

Research findings are published in academic journals, and it is the degree to which these journals are read that would probably serve as the best measure of awareness. Although the number of journals circulated can be determined, the number of these journals that are actually read cannot be known with certainty. Some journals sit on tables unread, while some journals circulated to libraries are read by dozens of patrons. Determining the readership level of a specific article within a journal is even more difficult. In addition, clinicians may obtain their information regarding a particular research result not by reading the article itself, but through secondary and tertiary distributors (review articles, colleagues, newspapers, etc.).

Because of these limitations, the degree of awareness is often based on the number of times this journal (or a specific article within the journal) is cited by other papers. This value is sometimes known as a citation index or an impact factor. These values are part of a growing branch of library science called bibliometrics (or scientometrics) and can be found in storehouses of information, such as the ISI Web of Knowledge.[2] Although these metrics have their own limitations (e.g., they reflect the dissemination of information to other scientists who are writing articles, not necessarily dissemination to clinicians) they can provide some valuable information regarding the spread of scientific ideas over time.

## The Island of Psychodynamic Literature

For this letter I conducted a bibliometric analysis of the psychodynamic literature using the ISI Web of Science.[3] Here are the key findings:

---

[2] ISI Web of Knowledge is a suite of products from the Thomson Corporation (Stamford, CT)

[3] Accessed on July 29, 2007. Search was limited to the years 1997–2006, constrained to full-length articles in the English-language literature, and used the terms "psychodynamic" and "dynamic psychotherapy" connected by a Boolean OR.

1. Over the past 10 years there have been 1160 full-length English-language articles published on this topic. Note that limiting the search to "psychodynamic *research*" reduces the total to 226. The publication rate over this period is essentially flat, with a compound annual growth rate of 1%. This is in contrast to the well-documented exponential growth rate of the overall medical/scientific body of publications, often cited as being in the 5–15% range annually.[4]
2. The publications are highly concentrated amongst a few prominent centers located in two cities (New York and Boston). Of the 1160 papers, fully 180 (15.5%) come from authors based in New York or Boston.
3. Although these papers were published in 301 distinct journals, the distribution amongst these journals is highly skewed. That is, the top three journals (in terms of number of psychodynamic psychotherapy publications), *Psychotherapy Research*, *Psychotherapy*, and the *American Journal of Psychotherapy*, account for nearly 15% of all psychodynamic publications during this period.
4. The impact factors of the journals publishing these articles are extremely low, with the majority at or below a value of 1.[5] This means that at best, an average article in one of these journals will be cited once over a 2-year period.
5. As shown schematically in Fig. 19.1, the citation flow amongst the top journals for psychotherapy research is quite meager, particularly when compared to the network of citation flow associated with the leading journals within general psychiatry. A paper published in the top journals of general psychiatry (e.g., *Archives of General Psychiatry*, *American Journal of Psychiatry*) gains access to a robust awareness network.[6] This is not true for even the top publication venues for psychodynamic psychotherapy research (e.g., *Psychotherapy Research*, *Psychotherapy*). Importantly, there is almost no connection between these two networks.

The picture that emerges is that of a psychodynamic island, with a steady buzz of communication between members on the island, but little communication with the outside world.

## Message in a Bottle?

The present situation is not necessarily bad. To the degree that these publications are meant for an audience already practicing psychodynamic therapy, this type of internal communication is exactly what is necessary. For example,

---

[4] See, for example, DJD Price. Little Science, Big Science...and Beyond. Columbia University Press, New York, 1986.

[5] Journal citation data obtained from Journal Citation Reports (Thomson Corp., Stamford CT) and are based on calendar year 2006.

[6] Take, for example, the paper by Perry et al. (*American Journal of Psychiatry* 156:1312–1321, 1999) on psychotherapy effectiveness, which has been cited 89 times.

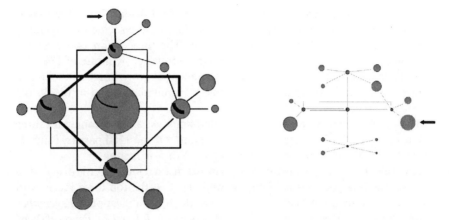

**Fig. 19.1** Schematic illustrating the flow of science in general psychiatry research (left) and psychodynamic psychotherapy research (right). Each circle represents a journal, with the diameter of the circle scaled to match that journal's 2006 impact factor. The central circle on the right represents *Psychotherapy Research* (impact factor = 0.93) while the central circle on the left represents the *Archives of General Psychiatry* (impact factor = 13.94). Lines extending from the circles represent the citation flow for papers published in a particular journal, with thickness of the line scaled to represent the total number of citations over a 10-year period (1997–2006). Curved lines represent same-journal citations (e.g., a particular article in *Psychotherapy Research* cited by other articles published in *Psychotherapy Research*). Here displayed are the five leading avenues (including same-journal citation) for publications appearing in the center journal followed by the five leading avenues of citation flow for each of these "first-generation" journals. Note that papers published in the *Archives of General Psychiatry* are cited in mass amounts by journals that are, in turn, cited in mass amounts – like a major highway system connecting large metropolitan regions. Papers published in *Psychotherapy Research* have low rates of citation by journals that themselves are minimally (if at all) cited – like a footpath connecting small hamlets. Note also that there is almost no overlap in these networks – the arrows indicate the single journal (*Schizophrenia Bulletin*) found in both

papers providing data on a nuanced modification to psychodyamic practice belongs in these journals, to be read by the very therapists engaged in this type of work.

To the degree that these publications are meant for an outside audience, however, the current publication pattern will be ineffective. Papers meant to convince general psychiatrists or psychologists on the merits of a psychodynamic approach will not find this audience through publication in dynamically oriented journals. This is not at all meant as a criticism of the quality or content of these journals; it simply reflects the niche status of these journals in a sea of publications. To raise awareness, there must be at least a few messages sent in bottles to the greater body of mental health providers, through mainstream publication channels.

Of course this has been something of a Catch-22, as many of these mainstream publications have been cool toward psychodynamic therapy. There are signs of change, however. Within the past few months there have been four psychodynamically focused articles published within the *American Journal of Psychiatry*, a manuscript with a broad and diverse readership.[7] This may portend a greater awareness of the body of literature described in this book and ultimately, greater incorporation of evidence-based psychodynamic practices within mainstream psychiatry.

---

[7] The four articles are: Horowitz MJ 164:24–27; Rusch et al., 164:500–508; Clarkin et al., 164:922–928, and Diener et al., 164:936–941.

# Subject Index

Lightning Source UK Ltd.
Milton Keynes UK
19 September 2010

160021UK00008B/46/P

616-8914   LOV